HEALTH AND HUMAN DEVELOPMENT

SOCIAL AND HEALTH ISSUES AMONG OLDER ADULTS IN INDIA

HEALTH AND HUMAN DEVELOPMENT

JOAV MERRICK - SERIES EDITOR

NATIONAL INSTITUTE OF CHILD HEALTH
AND HUMAN DEVELOPMENT,
MINISTRY OF SOCIAL AFFAIRS, JERUSALEM

Social and Health Issues among Older Adults in India
Supa Pengpid, Karl Peltzer and Joav Merrick (Editors)
2021. ISBN: 978-1-53619-937-6 (Hardcover)
2021. ISBN: NA (eBook)

Mexico: Health and Aging
Supa Pengpid, Karl Peltzer and Joav Merrick (Editors)
2020. ISBN: 978-1-53617-950-7 (Hardcover)
2020. ISBN: 978-1-53617-951-4 (eBook)

Clinical Oncology: An Encompassing Overview
Joav Merrick, Ariel Tenenbaum, Victoria Rico and Carlo DeAngelis (Editors)
2020. ISBN: 978-1-53617-933-0 (Hardcover)
2020. ISBN. 978-1-53617-934-7 (eBook)

Animal-Assisted Interventions for Health and Human Service Professionals
Carlie J. Driscoll
2020. ISBN: 978-1-53617-433-5 (Hardcover)
2020. ISBN: 978-1-53617-434-2 (eBook)

Cancer Management in Latin America II: Melanoma to Cost-Effectiveness
Maurício F Silva, Gustavo Nader Marta, Luis CM Antunes, Fiona Lim, Bo Angela Wan, Beatriz Amendola, Joav Merrick (Editors)
2020. ISBN: 978-1-53616-735-1 (Hardcover)
2020. ISBN: 978-1-53616-736-8 (eBook)

Pain: Perspectives on Acute and Chronic Pain
Patricia Schofield, Ariel Tenenbaum, Joav Merrick (Editors)
2020: ISBN: 978-1-53617-748-0 (Hardcover)
2020: ISBN: 978-1-53617-749-7 (eBook)

Cancer Management in Latin America I: Nasopharyngeal to Renal Cancer
Maurício F Silva, Gustavo Nader Marta, Luis CM Antunes, Fiona Lim, Bo Angela Wan, Beatriz Amendola, Joav Merrick (Editors)
2020. ISBN: 978-1-53616-733-7 (Hardcover)
2020. ISBN: 978-1-53616-734-4 (eBook)

Clinical Art Psychotherapy with War Veterans
Alexander Kopytin and Alexey Lebedev
2018. ISBN: 978-1-53612-975-5 (Softcover)
2017. ISBN: 978-1-53612-976-2 (eBook)

Cancer and Exercise
Leila Malek, Fiona Lim, Bo Angela Wan, Patrick L Diaz, Edward Chow, Joav Merrick (Editors)
2018. ISBN: 978-1-53612-747-8 (Hardcover)
2018. ISBN: 978-1-53612-748-5 (eBook)

Brennan Healing Science: An Integrative Approach to Therapeutic Intervention
Nina Koren, Muriel Moreno and Joav Merrick (Editors)
2018. ISBN: 978-1-53612-825-3 (Hardcover)
2018. ISBN: 978-1-53612-826-0 (eBook)

Alternative Medicine Research Yearbook 2017
Joav Merrick (Editor)
2018. ISBN: 978-1-53613-726-2 (Hardcover)
2018. ISBN: 978-1-53613-727-9 (eBook)

Psychosocial Needs: Success in Life and Career Planning
Daniel TL Shek, Janet TY Leung, Tak Y Lee and Joav Merrick (Editors)
2017. ISBN: 978-1-53611-951-0 (Hardcover)
2017. ISBN: 978-1-53611-971-8 (eBook)

Cannabis: Medical Aspects
Blair Henry, Arnav Agarwal, Edward Chow, Hatim A Omar, and Joav Merrick (Editors)
2017. ISBN: 978-1-53610-510-0 (Hardcover)
2017. ISBN: 978-1-53610-522-3 (eBook)

Palliative Care: Oncology Experience from Hong Kong
Louisa Cheuk-Yu Lui, Kam-Hung Wong, Rebecca Yeung, Joav Merrick (Editors)
2017. ISBN: 978-1-53612-397-5 (Softcover)
2017. ISBN: 978-1-53612-430-9 (eBook)

Palliative Care: Psychosocial and Ethical Considerations
Blair Henry, Arnav Agarwal, Edward Chow, and Joav Merrick (Editors)
2017. ISBN: 978-1-53610-607-7 (Hardcover)
2017. ISBN: 978-1-53610-611-4 (eBook)

Oncology: The Promising Future of Biomarkers
Anthony Furfari, George S Charames, Rachel McDonald, Leigha Rowbottom, Azar Azad, Stephanie Chan, Bo Angela Wan, Ronald Chow, Carlo DeAngelis, Pearl Zaki, Edward Chow and Joav Merrick (Editors)
2017. ISBN: 978-1-53610-608-4 (Hardcover)
2017. ISBN: 978-1-53610-610-7 (eBook)

Public Health Yearbook 2016
Joav Merrick (Editor)
2017. ISBN: 978-1-53610-947-4 (Hardcover)
2017. ISBN: 978-1-53610-956-6 (eBook)

Alternative Medicine Research Yearbook 2016
Joav Merrick (Editor)
2017. ISBN: 978-1-53610-972-6 (Hardcover)
2017. ISBN: 978-1-53611-000-5 (eBook)

Pain Management Yearbook 2016
Joav Merrick (Editor)
2017. ISBN: 978-1-53610-949-8 (Hardcover)
2017. ISBN: 978-1-53610-959-7 (eBook)

Medical Cannabis: Clinical Practice
Shannon O'Hearn, Alexia Blake, Bo Angela Wan, Stephanie Chan, Edward Chow and Joav Merrick (Editors)
2017. ISBN: 978-1-53611-907-7 (Softcover)
2017. ISBN: 978-1-53611-927-5 (eBook)

Cancer: Treatment, Decision Making and Quality of Life
Breanne Lechner, Ronald Chow, Natalie Pulenzas, Marko Popovic, Na Zhang, Xiaojing Zhang, Edward Chow, and Joav Merrick (Editors)
2016. ISBN: 978-1-63483-863-4 (Hardcover)
2015. ISBN: 978-1-63483-882-5 (eBook)

Cancer: Bone Metastases, CNS Metastases and Pathological Fractures
Breanne Lechner, Ronald Chow, Natalie Pulenzas, Marko Popovic, Na Zhang, Xiaojing Zhang, Edward Chow, and Joav Merrick (Editors)
2016. ISBN: 978-1-63483-949-5 (Hardcover)
2015. ISBN: 978-1-63483-960-0 (eBook)

Cancer: Spinal Cord, Lung, Breast, Cervical, Prostate, Head and Neck Cancer
Breanne Lechner, Ronald Chow, Natalie Pulenzas, Marko Popovic, Na Zhang, Xiaojing Zhang, Edward Chow and Joav Merrick (Editors)
2016. ISBN: 978-1-63483-904-4 (Hardcover)
2015. ISBN: 978-1-63483-911-2 (eBook)

Cancer: Survival, Quality of Life and Ethical Implications
Breanne Lechner, Ronald Chow, Natalie Pulenzas, Marko Popovic, Na Zhang, Xiaojing Zhang, Edward Chow and Joav Merrick (Editors)
2016. ISBN: 978-1-63483-905-1 (Hardcover)
2015. ISBN: 978-1-63483-912-9 (eBook)

Cancer: Pain and Symptom Management
Breanne Lechner, Ronald Chow, Natalie Pulenzas, Marko Popovic, Na Zhang, Xiaojing Zhang, Edward Chow, and Joav Merrick (Editors)
2016. ISBN: 978-1-63483-905-1 (Hardcover)
2015. ISBN: 978-1-63483-881-8 (eBook)

Alternative Medicine Research Yearbook 2015
Joav Merrick (Editor)
2016. ISBN: 978-1-63484-511-3 (Hardcover)
2016. ISBN: 978-1-63484-542-7 (eBook)

Quality, Mobility and Globalization in the Higher Education System: A Comparative Look at the Challenges of Academic Teaching
Nitza Davidovitch, Zehavit Gross, Yuri Ribakov, and Anna Slobodianiuk (Editors)
2016. ISBN: 978-1-63484-986-9 (Hardcover)
2016. ISBN: 978-1-63485-012-4 (eBook)

Public Health Yearbook 2015
Joav Merrick (Editor)
2016. ISBN: 978-1-63484-511-3 (Hardcover)
2016. ISBN: 978-1-63484-546-5 (eBook)

Alternative Medicine Research Yearbook 2014
Joav Merrick (Editor)
2015. ISBN: 978-1-63482-161-2 (Hardcover)
2015. ISBN: 978-1-63482-205-3 (eBook)

Pain Management Yearbook 2014
Joav Merrick (Editor)
2015. ISBN: 978-1-63482-164-3 (Hardcover)
2015. ISBN: 978-1-63482-208-4 (eBook)

Public Health Yearbook 2014
Joav Merrick (Editor)
2015. ISBN: 978-1-63482-165-0 (Hardcover)
2015. ISBN: 978-1-63482-209-1 (eBook)

Forensic Psychiatry: A Public Health Perspective
Leo Sher and Joav Merrick (Editors)
2015. ISBN: 978-1-63483-339-4 (Hardcover)
2015. ISBN: 978-1-63483-346-2 (eBook)

Leadership and Service Learning Education: Holistic Development for Chinese University Students
Daniel TL Shek, Florence KY Wu and Joav Merrick (Editors)
2015. ISBN: 978-1-63483-340-0 (Hardcover)
2015. ISBN: 978-1-63483-347-9 (eBook)

Mental and Holistic Health: Some International Perspectives
Joseph L Calles Jr, Donald E Greydanus, and Joav Merrick (Editors)
2015. ISBN: 978-1-63483-589-3 (Hardcover)
2015. ISBN: 978-1-63483-608-1 (eBook)

India: Health and Human Development Aspects
Joav Merrick (Editor)
2014. ISBN: 978-1-62948-784-7 (Hardcover)
2014. ISBN: 978-1-62948-794-6 (eBook)

Alternative Medicine Research Yearbook 2013
Joav Merrick (Editor)
2014. ISBN: 978-1-63321-094-3 (Hardcover)
2014. ISBN: 978-1-63321-144-5 (eBook)

Health Consequences of Human Central Obesity
Kaushik Bose and Raja Chakraborty (Editors)
2014. ISBN: 978-1-63321-152-0 (Hardcover)
2014. ISBN: 978-1-63321-181-0 (eBook)

Public Health: Improving Health via Inter-Professional Collaborations
Rosemary M Caron and Joav Merrick (Editors)
2014. ISBN: 978-1-63321-569-6 (Hardcover)
2014. ISBN: 978-1-63321-594-8 (eBook)

Public Health Yearbook 2013
Joav Merrick (Editor)
2014. ISBN: 978-1-63321-095-0 (Hardcover)
2014. ISBN: 978-1-63321-097-4 (eBook)

Textbook on Evidence-Based Holistic Mind-Body Medicine: Holistic Practice of Traditional Hippocratic Medicine
Søren Ventegodt and Joav Merrick
2013. ISBN: 978-1-62257-105-5 (Hardcover)
2012. ISBN: 978-1-62257-174-1 (eBook)

Textbook on Evidence-Based Holistic Mind-Body Medicine: Sexology and Traditional Hippocratic Medicine
Søren Ventegodt and Joav Merrick
2013. ISBN: 978-1-62257-130-7 (Hardcover)
2012. ISBN: 978-1-62257-176-5 (eBook)

Health and Happiness from Meaningful Work: Research in Quality of Working Life
Søren Ventegodt and Joav Merrick (Editors)
2013. ISBN: 978-1-60692-820-2 (Hardcover)
2009. ISBN: 978-1-61324-981-9 (eBook)

Textbook on Evidence-Based Holistic Mind-Body Medicine: Healing the Mind in Traditional Hippocratic Medicine
Søren Ventegodt and Joav Merrick
2013. ISBN: 978-1-62257-112-3 (Hardcover)
2012. ISBN: 978-1-62257-175-8 (eBook)

Conceptualizing Behavior in Health and Social Research: A Practical Guide to Data Analysis
Said Shahtahmasebi and Damon Berridge
2013. ISBN: 978-1-60876-383-2 (Hardcover)
2013. ISBN: 978-1-53611-212-2 (eBook)

Adolescence and Sports
Dilip R Patel, Donald E Greydanus, Hatim Omar and Joav Merrick (Editors)
2013. ISBN: 978-1-60876-702-1 (Hardcover)
2010. ISBN: 978-1-61761-483-5 (eBook)

Pediatric and Adolescent Sexuality and Gynecology: Principles for the Primary Care Clinician
Hatim A Omar, Donald E Greydanus, Artemis K. Tsitsika, Dilip R. Patel and Joav Merrick (Editors)
2013. ISBN: 978-1-60876-735-9 (Softcover)

Human Development: Biology from a Holistic Point of View
Søren Ventegodt, Tyge Dahl Hermansen and Joav Merrick
2013. ISBN: 978-1-61470-441-6 (Hardcover)
2011. ISBN: 978-1-61470-541-3 (eBook)

Building Community Capacity: Case Examples from Around the World
Rosemary M Caron and Joav Merrick (Editors)
2013. ISBN: 978-1-62417-175-8 (Hardcover)
2013. ISBN: 978-1-62417-176-5 (eBook)

Managed Care in a Public Setting
Richard Evan Steele
2013. ISBN: 978-1-62417-970-9 (Softcover)
2013. ISBN: 978-1-62417-863-4 (eBook)

Bullying: A Public Health Concern
Jorge C Srabstein and Joav Merrick (Editors)
2013. ISBN: 978-1-62618-564-7 (Hardcover)
2013. ISBN: 978-1-62618-588-3 (eBook)

Bedouin Health: Perspectives from Israel
Joav Merrick, Alean Al-Krenami and Salman Elbedour (Editors)
2013. ISBN: 978-1-62948-271-2 (Hardcover)
2013: ISBN: 978-1-62948-274-3 (eBook)

Health Promotion: Community Singing as a Vehicle to Promote Health
Jing Sun, Nicholas Buys and Joav Merrick (Editors)
2013. ISBN: 978-1-62618-908-9 (Hardcover)
2013: ISBN: 978-1-62808-006-3 (eBook)

Public Health Yearbook 2012
Joav Merrick (Editor)
2013. ISBN: 978-1-62808-078-0 (Hardcover)
2013: ISBN: 978-1-62808-079-7 (eBook)

Alternative Medicine Research Yearbook 2012
Joav Merrick (Editor)
2013. ISBN: 978-1-62808-080-3 (Hardcover)
2013: ISBN: 978-1-62808-079-7 (eBook)

Advanced Cancer: Managing Symptoms and Quality of Life
Natalie Pulenzas, Breanne Lechner, Nemica Thavarajah, Edward Chow, and Joav Merrick (Editors)
2013. ISBN: 978-1-62808-239-5 (Hardcover)
2013: ISBN: 978-1-62808-267-8 (eBook)

Treatment and Recovery of Eating Disorders
Daniel Stein and Yael Latzer (Editors)
2013. ISBN: 978-1-62808-248-7 (Softcover)

Health Promotion: Strengthening Positive Health and Preventing Disease
Jing Sun, Nicholas Buys and Joav Merrick (Editors)
2013. ISBN: 978-1-62257-870-2 (Hardcover)
2013: ISBN: 978-1-62808-621-8 (eBook)

Pain Management Yearbook 2011
Joav Merrick (Editor)
2013. ISBN: 978-1-62808-970-7 (Hardcover)
2013: ISBN: 978-1-62808-971-4 (eBook)

Pain Management Yearbook 2012
Joav Merrick (Editor)
2013. ISBN: 978-1-62808-973-8 (Hardcover)
2013: ISBN: 978-1-62808-974-5 (eBook)

Suicide from a Public Health Perspective
Said Shahtahmasebi and Joav Merrick
2013. ISBN: 978-1-62948-536-2 (Hardcover)
2014: ISBN: 978-1-62948-537-9 (eBook)

Food, Nutrition and Eating Behavior
Joav Merrick and Sigal Israeli (Editors)
2013. ISBN: 978-1-62948-233-0 (Hardcover)
2013: ISBN: 978-1-62948-234-7 (eBook)

Public Health Concern: Smoking, Alcohol and Substance Use
Joav Merrick and Ariel Tenenbaum (Editors)
2013. ISBN: 978-1-62948-424-2 (Hardcover)
2013. ISBN: 978-1-62948-430-3 (eBook)

Mental Health from an International Perspective
Joav Merrick, Shoshana Aspler and Mohammed Morad (Editors)
2013. ISBN: 978-1-62948-519-5 (Hardcover)
2013. ISBN: 978-1-62948-520-1 (eBook)

Adolescence and Chronic Illness. A Public Health Concern
Hatim Omar, Donald E Greydanus, Dilip R Patel and Joav Merrick (Editors)
2012. ISBN: 978-1-60876-628-4 (Hardcover)
2010. ISBN: 978-1-61761-482-8 (eBook)

Child and Adolescent Health Yearbook 2009
Joav Merrick (Editor)
2012. ISBN: 978-1-61668-913-1 (Hardcover)
2012. ISBN: 978-1-62257-095-9 (eBook)

Child and Adolescent Health Yearbook 2010
Joav Merrick (Editor)
2012. ISBN: 978-1-61209-788-6 (Hardcover)
2012. ISBN: 978-1-62417-046-1 (eBook)

Child Health and Human Development Yearbook 2010
Joav Merrick (Editor)
2012. ISBN: 978-1-61209-789-3 (Hardcover)
2012. ISBN: 978-1-62081-721-6 (eBook)

Public Health Yearbook 2010
Joav Merrick (Editor)
2012. ISBN: 978-1-61209-971-2 (Hardcover)
2012. ISBN: 978-1-62417-863-4 (eBook)

Health Risk Communication
Marijke Lemal and Joav Merrick (Editors)
2012. ISBN: 978-1-62257-544-2 (Hardcover)
2012. ISBN: 978-1-62257-552-7 (eBook)

Alternative Medicine Yearbook 2010
Joav Merrick (Editor)
2012. ISBN: 978-1-62100-132-4 (Hardcover)
2011. ISBN: 978-1-62100-210-9 (eBook)

The Astonishing Brain and Holistic Consciousness: Neuroscience and Vedanta Perspectives
Vinod D Deshmukh
2012. ISBN: 978-1-61324-295-7 (Hardcover)
2012. ISBN: 978-1-62808-677-5 (eBook)

Translational Research for Primary Healthcare
Erica Bell, Gert P Westert and Joav Merrick (Editors)
2012. ISBN: 978-1-61324-647-4 (Hardcover)
2012. ISBN: 978-1-62417-409-4 (eBook)

Building Community Capacity: Minority and Immigrant Populations
Rosemary M Caron and Joav Merrick (Editors)
2012. ISBN: 978-1-62081-022-4 (Hardcover)
2012. ISBN: 978-1-62081-032-3 (eBook)

Applied Public Health: Examining Multifaceted Social or Ecological Problems and Child Maltreatment
John R Lutzker and Joav Merrick (Editors)
2012. ISBN: 978-1-62081-356-0 (Hardcover)
2012. ISBN: 978-1-62081-388-1 (eBook)

Our Search for Meaning in Life: Quality of Life Philosophy
Søren Ventegodt and Joav Merrick
2012. ISBN: 978-1-61470-494-2 (Hardcover)
2011. ISBN: 978-1-61470-519-2 (eBook)

Randomized Clinical Trials and Placebo: Can You Trust the Drugs are Working and Safe?
Søren Ventegodt and Joav Merrick
2012. ISBN: 978-1-61470-067-8 (Hardcover)
2011. ISBN: 978-1-61470-151-4 (eBook)

Treatment and Recovery of Eating Disorders
Daniel Stein and Yael Latzer (Editors)
2012. ISBN: 978-1-61470-259-7 (Hardcover)
2012. ISBN: 978-1-61470-418-8 (eBook)

Human Immunodeficiency Virus (HIV) Research: Social Science Aspects
Hugh Klein and Joav Merrick (Editors)
2012. ISBN: 978-1-62081-293-8 (Hardcover)
2012. ISBN: 978-1-62081-346-1 (eBook)

AIDS and Tuberculosis: Public Health Aspects
Daniel Chemtob and Joav Merrick (Editors)
2012. ISBN: 978-1-62081-382-9 (Softcover)
2012. ISBN: 978-1-62081-406-2 (eBook)

Public Health Yearbook 2011
Joav Merrick (Editor)
2012. ISBN: 978-1-62081-433-8 (Hardcover)
2012. ISBN: 978-1-62081-434-5 (eBook)

Alternative Medicine Research Yearbook 2011
Joav Merrick (Editor)
2012. ISBN: 978-1-62081-476-5 (Hardcover)
2012. ISBN: 978-1-62081-477-2 (eBook)

Building Community Capacity: Skills and Principles
Rosemary M Caron and Joav Merrick (Editors)
2012. ISBN: 978-1-61209-331-4 (Hardcover)
2012. ISBN: 978-1-62257-238-0 (eBook)

Textbook on Evidence-Based Holistic Mind-Body Medicine: Basic Principles of Healing in Traditional Hippocratic Medicine
Søren Ventegodt and Joav Merrick
2012. ISBN: 978-1-62257-094-2 (Hardcover)
2012. ISBN: 978-1-62257-172-7 (eBook)

Textbook on Evidence-Based Holistic Mind-Body Medicine: Basic Philosophy and Ethics of Traditional Hippocratic Medicine
Søren Ventegodt and Joav Merrick
2012. ISBN: 978-1-62257-052-2 (Hardcover)
2013. ISBN: 978-1-62257-707-1 (eBook)

Textbook on Evidence-Based Holistic Mind-Body Medicine: Research, Philosophy, Economy and Politics of Traditional Hippocratic Medicine
Søren Ventegodt and Joav Merrick
2012. ISBN: 978-1-62257-140-6 (Hardcover)
2012. ISBN: 978-1-62257-171-0 (eBook)

Behavioral Pediatrics, 3rd Edition
Donald E Greydanus, Dilip R Patel, Helen D Pratt and Joseph L Calles, Jr (Editors)
2011. ISBN: 978-1-60692-702-1 (Hardcover)
2009. ISBN: 978-1-60876-630-7 (eBook)

Rural Child Health: International Aspects
Erica Bell and Joav Merrick (Editors)
2011. ISBN: 978-1-60876-357-3 (Hardcover)
2011. ISBN: 978-1-61324-005-2 (eBook)

International Aspects of Child Abuse and Neglect
Howard Dubowitz and Joav Merrick (Editors)
2011. ISBN: 978-1-60876-703-8 (Hardcover)
2010. ISBN: 978-1-61122-049-0 (Softcover)
2010. ISBN: 978-1-61122-403-0 (eBook)

Environment, Mood Disorders and Suicide
Teodor T Postolache and Joav Merrick (Editors)
2011. ISBN: 978-1-61668-505-8 (Hardcover)
2011. ISBN: 978-1-62618-340-7 (eBook)

Positive Youth Development: Evaluation and Future Directions in a Chinese Context
Daniel TL Shek, Hing Keung Ma and Joav Merrick (Editors)
2011. ISBN: 978-1-60876-830-1 (Hardcover)
2011. ISBN: 978-1-62100-175-1 (Softcover)
2010. ISBN: 978-1-61209-091-7 (eBook)

Understanding Eating Disorders: Integrating Culture, Psychology and Biology
Yael Latzer, Joav Merrick and Daniel Stein (Editors)
2011. ISBN: 978-1-61728-298-0 (Hardcover)
2011. ISBN: 978-1-61470-976-3 (Softcover)
2011. ISBN: 978-1-61942-054-0 (eBook)

Advanced Cancer Pain and Quality of Life
Edward Chow and Joav Merrick (Editors)
2011. ISBN: 978-1-61668-207-1 (Hardcover)
2010. ISBN: 978-1-61668-400-6 (eBook)

Positive Youth Development: Implementation of a Youth Program in a Chinese Context
Daniel TL Shek, Hing Keung Ma and Joav Merrick (Editors)
2011. ISBN: 978-1-61668-230-9

Social and Cultural Psychiatry Experience from the Caribbean Region
Hari D Maharajh and Joav Merrick (Editors)
2011. ISBN: 978-1-61668-506-5 (Hardcover)
2010. ISBN: 978-1-61728-088-7 (eBook)

Narratives and Meanings of Migration
Julia Mirsky
2011. ISBN: 978-1-61761-103-2 (Hardcover)
2010. ISBN: 978-1-61761-519-1 (eBook)

Self-Management and the Health Care Consumer
Peter William Harvey
2011. ISBN: 978-1-61761-796-6 (Hardcover)
2011. ISBN: 978-1-61122-214-2 (eBook)

Sexology from a Holistic Point of View
Soren Ventegodt and Joav Merrick
2011. ISBN: 978-1-61761-859-8 (Hardcover)
2011. ISBN: 978-1-61122-262-3 (eBook)

Principles of Holistic Psychiatry: A Textbook on Holistic Medicine for Mental Disorders
Soren Ventegodt and Joav Merrick
2011. ISBN: 978-1-61761-940-3 (Hardcover)
2011. ISBN: 978-1-61122-263-0 (eBook)

Clinical Aspects of Psychopharmacology in Childhood and Adolescence
Donald E Greydanus, Joseph L Calles, Jr, Dilip P Patel, Ahsan Nazeer and Joav Merrick (Editors)
2011. ISBN: 978-1-61122-135-0 (Hardcover)
2011. ISBN: 978-1-61122-715-4 (eBook)

Climate Change and Rural Child Health
Erica Bell, Bastian M Seidel and Joav Merrick (Editors)
2011. ISBN: 978-1-61122-640-9 (Hardcover)
2011. ISBN: 978-1-61209-014-6 (eBook)

Rural Medical Education: Practical Strategies
Erica Bell, Craig Zimitat and Joav Merrick (Editors)
2011. ISBN: 978-1-61122-649-2 (Hardcover)
2011. ISBN: 978-1-61209-476-2 (eBook)

Advances in Environmental Health Effects of Toxigenic Mold and Mycotoxins
Ebere Cyril Anyanwu
2011. ISBN: 978-1-60741-953-2
2011. ISBN: 978-1-53611-209-2

Public Health Yearbook 2009
Joav Merrick (Editor)
2011. ISBN: 978-1-61668-911-7
(Hardcover)
2011. ISBN: 978-1-62417-365-3
(eBook)

Child Health and Human Development Yearbook 2009
Joav Merrick (Editor)
2011. ISBN: 978-1-61668-912-4

Alternative Medicine Yearbook 2009
Joav Merrick (Editor)
2011. ISBN: 978-1-61668-910-0
(Hardcover)
2011. ISBN: 978-1-62081-710-0
(eBook)

The Dance of Sleeping and Eating among Adolescents: Normal and Pathological Perspectives
Yael Latzer and Orna Tzischinsky (Editors)
2011. ISBN: 978-1-61209-710-7
(Hardcover)
2011. ISBN: 978-1-62417-366-0
(eBook)

Drug Abuse in Hong Kong: Development and Evaluation of a Prevention Program
Daniel TL Shek, Rachel CF Sun and Joav Merrick (Editors)
2011. ISBN: 978-1-61324-491-3
(Hardcover)
2011. ISBN: 978-1-62257-232-8
(eBook)

Chance Action and Therapy: The Playful Way of Changing
Uri Wernik
2010. ISBN: 978-1-60876-393-1
(Hardcover)
2011. ISBN: 978-1-61122-987-5
(Softcover)
2011. ISBN: 978-1-61209-874-6
(eBook)

Bone and Brain Metastases: Advances in Research and Treatment
Arjun Sahgal, Edward Chow and Joav Merrick (Editors)
2010. ISBN: 978-1-61668-365-8
(Hardcover)
2010. ISBN: 978-1-61728-085-6
(eBook)

Children and Pain
Patricia Schofield and Joav Merrick (Editors)
2009. ISBN: 978-1-60876-020-6
(Hardcover)
2009. ISBN: 978-1-61728-183-9
(eBook)

Challenges in Adolescent Health: An Australian Perspective
David Bennett, Susan Towns, Elizabeth Elliott and Joav Merrick (Editors)
2009. ISBN: 978-1-60741-616-6 (Hardcover)
2009. ISBN: 978-1-61668-240-8 (eBook)

Obesity and Adolescence: A Public Health Concern
Hatim A Omar, Donald E Greydanus, Dilip R Patel and Joav Merrick (Editors)
2009. ISBN: 978-1-60692-821-9 (Hardcover)
2009. ISBN: 978-1-61470-465-2 (eBook)

Poverty and Children: A Public Health Concern
Alexis Lieberman and Joav Merrick (Editors)
2009. ISBN: 978-1-60741-140-6 (Hardcover)
2009. ISBN: 978-1-61470-601-4 (eBook)

Living on the Edge: The Mythical, Spiritual, and Philosophical Roots of Social Marginality
Joseph Goodbread
2009. ISBN: 978-1-60741-162-8 (Hardcover)
2013. ISBN: 978-1-61122-986-8 (Softcover)
2011. ISBN: 978-1-61470-192-7 (eBook)

Alcohol-Related Cognitive Disorders: Research and Clinical Perspectives
Leo Sher, Isack Kandel and Joav Merrick (Editors)
2009. ISBN: 978-1-60741-730-9 (Hardcover)
2009. ISBN: 978-1-60876-623-9 (eBook)

Complementary Medicine Systems: Comparison and Integration
Karl W Kratky
2008. ISBN: 978-1-60456-475-4 (Hardcover)
2008. ISBN: 978-1-61122-433-7 (eBook)

Pain in Children and Youth
Patricia Schofield and Joav Merrick (Editors)
2008. ISBN: 978-1-60456-951-3 (Hardcover)
2008. ISBN: 978-1-61470-496-6 (eBook)

Adolescent Behavior Research: International Perspectives
Joav Merrick and Hatim A Omar (Editors)
2007. ISBN: 978-1-60021-649-

HEALTH AND HUMAN DEVELOPMENT

SOCIAL AND HEALTH ISSUES AMONG OLDER ADULTS IN INDIA

SUPA PENGPID
KARL PELTZER
AND
JOAV MERRICK
EDITORS

nova
Medicine & Health
New York

Library of Congress Cataloging-in-Publication Data

ISBN: 978-1-53619-937-6

Published by Nova Science Publishers, Inc. † New York

CONTENTS

INTRODUCTION

In: Social and Health Issues … ISBN: 978-1-53619-937-6
Editors: S Pengpid, K Peltzer et al.

Chapter 1

SOCIAL AND HEALTH ISSUES AMONG OLDER ADULTS IN INDIA

Supa Pengpid[1], MPH, DrPH, MBA, Karl Peltzer[2,*], MA Clin Psych, PhD, Dr Habil and Joav Merrick[3-6], MD, MMedSci, DMSc

[1]ASEAN Institute for Health Development, Mahidol University, Salaya, Phutthamonthon, Nakhon Pathom, Thailand

[2]Department of Research Administration and Development, University of Limpopo, Turfloop, South Africa

[3]National Institute of Child Health and Human Development, Jerusalem, Israel

[4]Department of Pediatrics, Mt Scopus Campus, Hadassah Hebrew University Medical Center, Jerusalem, Israel

[5]Kentucky Children's Hospital, University of Kentucky, Lexington, Kentucky, United States

[6]Center for Healthy Development, School of Public Health, Georgia State University, Atlanta, United States

---

* *Correspondence*: Professor Karl Peltzer, Department of Research Administration and Development, University of Limpopo, Turfloop Campus, Private Bag X1106, Sovenga 0727, South Africa. Email: kfpeltzer@gmail.com.

ABSTRACT

With longevity and declining fertility rates, the population of older persons (60 years and above) is globally growing faster than the general population. The percentage of the elderly in India for example has been growing at an increasing rate in recent years and the trend is likely to continue in the coming decades. The share of population over the age of 60 years is projected to increase from 8 percent in 2015 to 19 percent in 2050. By the end of the century, the elderly will constitute nearly 34 percent of the total population in the country. In this book we aimed to identify trajectories of health and their associations with lifestyle factors in a nationally representative cohort study of middle-aged and older Indians. We discuss self-rated health status, age discrimination, major injuries, recurrent falls, perceived everyday discrimination, elder abuse, hypertension, diabetes, angina pectoris, stroke, arthritis, back pain or problems, oral health problems, cataract, edentulism, hearing loss, tobacco use, alcohol use, loneliness, health care discrimination, weight discrimination, religiosity and well-being. We hope that the findings may aid public policy and programmes for middle-aged and older adults in India.

INTRODUCTION

"India is projected to become the world's most populous nation by 2028, with a population of some 1.45 billion" [1]. "With longevity and declining fertility rates, the population of older persons (60 years and above) is globally growing faster than the general population. The percentage of the elderly in India has been increasing at an increasing rate in recent years and the trend is likely to continue in the coming decades. The share of population over the age of 60 years is projected to increase from 8 percent in 2015 to 19 percent in 2050. By the end of the century, the elderly will constitute nearly 34 percent of the total population in the country" [2].

"Poor health and morbidity diminish the quality of life and wellbeing of the elderly while increasing psychological distress and perception of vulnerability. Chronic diseases are a leading cause of death among elderly in India, increasingly so over the past 25 years. Mental health status also worsened with advancing age indicating higher mental health vulnerabilities among the oldest old. Overall, health related vulnerabilities are high in old age. With the increase in age, disability becomes a major concern, seriously limiting functioning in daily life and hence increasing the care-giving burden. The National Policy on Older Persons (NPOP) in India has been formulated as a forward-looking vision of the government for improving quality of life of older people in India through increased income security, health and nutrition, shelter, education, empowerment and welfare" [2].

In this book we aimed to identify trajectories of health and their associations with lifestyle factors in a nationally representative cohort study of middle-aged and older Indians. We used secondary data from the Longitudinal Aging Study in India (LASI) Wave 1, 2017-2018 [3]. The LASI is the world's largest survey providing data on the older population in broad domains of social, health and economic well-being. LASI is a joint undertaking of the Harvard TH Chan School of Public Health, the International Institute for Population Sciences (IIPS) in Mumbai, India, and the University of Southern California (USC) [3].

This book deals with self-rated health status, age discrimination, major injuries, recurrent falls, perceived everyday discrimination, elder abuse, hypertension, diabetes, angina pectoris, stroke, arthritis, back pain or problems, oral health problems, cataract, edentulism, hearing loss, tobacco use, alcohol use, loneliness, health care discrimination, weight discrimination, religiosity and well-being. We hope that findings from these papers may aid public policy and programmes for middle-aged and older adults in India.

References

[1] The United Nations Population Fund. India 2018. URL: https://www.unfpa.org/sites/default/files/IN_UNFPA_Results_07_27.pdf.

[2] United Nations Population Fund. Caring for our elders: Early responses - India Ageing Report 2017. New Delhi: UNFPA, 2017.

[3] International Institute for Population Sciences (IIPS), NPHCE, MoHFW, Harvard TH Chan School of Public Health (HSPH) and the University of Southern California (USC). Longitudinal Ageing Study in India (LASI) Wave 1, 2017-18. Mumbai: India Report, International Institute for Population Sciences, 2020.

SECTION I: AGEING ASPECTS

In: Social and Health Issues … ISBN: 978-1-53619-937-6
Editors: S Pengpid, K Peltzer et al.

Chapter 2

PREVALENCE AND PREDICTORS OF SELF-RATED HEALTH STATUS AMONG A NATIONALLY REPRESENTATIVE POPULATION-BASED SAMPLE OF OLDER ADULTS IN INDIA IN 2017-2018

Supa Pengpid[1,2], MPH, DrPH, MBA
and Karl Peltzer[2,3,*], MA Clin Psych, PhD, Dr Habil
[1]ASEAN Institute for Health Development, Mahidol University, Salaya, Phutthamonthon, Nakhon Pathom, Thailand
[2]Department of Research Administration and Development, University of Limpopo, Turfloop, South Africa
[3]Department of Psychology, College of Medical and Health Science, Asia University, Taichung, Taiwan

---

* *Correspondence*: Professor Karl Peltzer, Department of Research Administration and Development, University of Limpopo, Turfloop Campus, Private Bag X1106, Sovenga 0727, South Africa. Email: kfpeltzer@gmail.com.

ABSTRACT

This chapter aimed to determine the prevalence and predictors of self-rated health (SRH) in older adults in India. The cross-sectional sample consisted of 52,393 individuals (≥50 years) from the Longitudinal Ageing Study in India (LASI) Wave 1 in 2017-2018. SRH was assessed with one single item. Results indicate that the prevalence of fair or poor SRH was 43.3%. In adjusted binary and ordered logistic regression analyses, older age, medium level of education, Muslim, Sikh, underweight, arthritis, diabetes, asthma, angina, stroke and functional disability were associated with poorer SRH (poor or fair SRH and poorer SRH as a scale), while subjective socioeconomic status, and vigorous physical activity were negatively associated with poorer SRH (poor or fair SRH and poorer SRH as a scale). In addition, current tobacco use and hypertension were associated with poor or fair SRH, and heart disease was associated with poorer SRH (as scale). Almost one in two older adults in India had fair or poor SRH. Several risk factors were identified, which can be targeted in public health interventions.

INTRODUCTION

"Self rated health, or self-reported health (SRH), is a measure of a respondent's subjective sense of health, and is commonly used to capture a general sense of health from the perspective of the respondent, which is assessed by one simple global question about their overall health" [1] For example, "In general, would you say that your health is excellent, very good, good, fair, or poor?" [1]. "Methodologically, the SRH has been found to be both a reliable and valid measure of a respondent's health status" [1]. SRH tends to deteriorate with age [2-7]. In a study among older adults (≥50 years) in 11 European countries, the prevalence of bad or very bad SRH was 12.4% and fair/bad/very bad SRH was 44.9% [8], in South Africa (≥50 years) 23.2% had bad or very bad SRH [5], in Thailand (≥60 years) 56% had fair or very bad/bad SRH [9], in Cali, Columbia (≥60 years) 40.1% had poor or fair SRH [10], and in four states in India in 2010 (≥45 years) 9% had poor or fair SRH [3]. There is a lack of recent national studies among older adults on the prevalence and predictors of SRH in India.

Sociodemographic factors have been found associated with poor SRH, including older age [2-7], female sex [2, 4-7, 11], less education [5-7], lower wealth [5-7], ethnicity [5, 12], not married [6, 7], widowhood [13], and rural residence [3]. Health risk behaviour factors associated with poor SRH may include underweight [12, 14], physical inactivity [12, 15, 16], smoking [2], former smoker [12], drinking [2], and current drinkers [12]. Health status factors associated with poor SRH may include functional disability [2, 9, 16], number of chronic conditions [9], hypertension [2, 12], arthritis [12], asthma [12], heart disease [2, 12], diabetes [2, 10], depression [10], and frailty syndrome [10]. This study aimed to determine the prevalence and predictors of SRH in older community-dwelling adults in India in 2017-2018.

OUR STUDY

This secondary data analysis utilized data from the cross-sectional and nationally representative Longitudinal Ageing Study in India (LASI) Wave 1, 2017-2018; "the overall household response rate is 96%, and the overall individual response rate is 87%" [17]. In a household survey, "interview, physical measurement and biomarker data were collected from individuals aged 45 and above and their spouses, regardless of age" [17]. We restricted our analysis to those 50 years and older. Specific details on the sampling approach are found elsewhere [17]. The study was approved by the "Indian Council of Medical Research (ICMR) Ethics Committee and written informed consent was obtained from the participants" [17].

Outcome variable

SRH was assessed with one item, "In general, would you say your health is excellent, very good, good, fair, or poor?" [17] SRH was used as a scale ranging from 1 = excellent to 5 = poor, and was dichotomized as fair or poor = 1, and excellent, very good or good = 0, as in previous research in India

[3, 4]. The SRH item used has "satisfactory construct validity in the context of India and may be a reliable indicator of general health of the Indian population" [18].

Covariates

Sociodemographic variables consisted of level of education (none, ≥1 years), age group (50-59, 60-69, 70-79, and 80 or more years), sex (male, female), religion, and residence (rural, urban). Subjective socioeconomic status was assessed with the question, "Please imagine a ten-step ladder, where at the bottom are the people who are the worst off – who have the least money, least education, and the worst jobs or no jobs, and at the top of the ladder are the people who are the best off – those who have the most money, most education, and best jobs. Please indicate the number (1-10) on the rung on the ladder where you would place yourself" [17]. Steps 1 to 3 on the socioeconomic ladder were defined as low, 4-5 as medium, and 6-10 as high socioeconomic status.

Health risk behaviours included underweight, physical activity, tobacco and alcohol use.

Anthropometry: "Height and weight of adults were measured using the Seca 803 digital scale." [17]. "Body Mass Index = BMI was calculated according to Asian criteria: underweight (<18.5 kg/m^2)" [19].

Vigorous physical activity. "For vigorous activity, respondents were asked about their involvement in running or jogging, swimming, going to a health centre/gym, cycling, digging with a spade or shovel, heavy lifting, chopping, farm work, fast bicycling, and cycling with loads every day, more than once a week, once a week, one to three times a month, or hardly ever or never?" [17]. Participants who engaged in vigorous physical activity more than once a week were defined as having sufficient physical activity [20].

Current tobacco use was assessed from 1) "Do you currently smoke any tobacco products (cigarettes, bidis, cigars, hookah, cheroot, etc.)? and 2) Do you use smokeless tobacco (such as chewing tobacco, gutka, pan masala, etc.)?" [17].

Lifetime alcohol use was assessed with the question, "Have you ever consumed any alcoholic beverages such as beer, wine, liquor, country liquor, etc.?" (Yes, No) [17].

Health status variables included arthritis, diabetes, hypertension, asthma, angina, heart disease, stroke and functional disability.

Chronic conditions were sourced from the question, "Has any health professional ever told you that you have…?": 1) Diabetes or high blood sugar; 2) Asthma, 3) "Chronic heart diseases such as Coronary heart disease (heart attack or Myocardial Infarction), congestive heart failure, or other chronic heart problems," and 4) Arthritis or rheumatism (Yes/No)" [17].

Hypertension or raised blood pressure (BP) was defined as "systolic BP ≥140 mm Hg and/or diastolic BP ≥90 mm Hg (based on the last two averaged of three readings) or where the participant is currently on antihypertensive medication." [21].

Angina was assessed with the "World Health Organization's Rose angina questionnaire" [22], defined on the basis of "discomfort at walking uphill or hurrying, or at an ordinary pace on level ground. Furthermore, the pain should be located at the sternum or in the left chest and arm, causing the patient to stop or slow down, and the pain should resolve within 10 minutes when the patient stops or slows down" [23].

Functional disability was assessed with six items of Activities of Daily Living (ADL) and seven items of Instrumental Activities of Daily Living (IADL) (Yes, No) [24, 25]. Cronbach alpha was 0.87 for ADL and 0.90 for IADL in this study. Responses were trichotomized into 0, 1, and ≥2 ADL and IADL items.

Data analysis

Descriptive statistics were applied to describe health status, health risk behaviour, sociodemographic information, and SRH prevalence and means. Adjusted logistic regression was utilized to assess the predictors of poor or fair SRH and ordered logistic regression with SRH (with 1 the highest and 5 the poorest SRH). $P < 0.05$ was accepted as significant, missing values were excluded, and no multi-collinearity was found. Statistical analyses were conducted using STATA software version 15.0 (Stata Corporation, College Station, TX, USA), taking the complex study design into account.

FINDINGS

The sample included 52,393 older adults (50 years and older), with a median age of 62 years (14 years interquartile range), 53.3% were female and 46.7% male. Majority (69.0%) of the participants were residing in rural areas, 82.4% were Hindus, 38.2% had low subjective socioeconomic status and 53.0% had no schooling. Almost half of the participants (45.4%) had hypertension, 23.0% were underweight, 33.0% had current tobacco use, 14.9% had ever engaged in alcohol use, 62.3% did not engage in vigorous physical activity, 14.7% arthritis, 13.4% diabetes, 5.4% asthma, 8.9% angina, 4.2% heart disease, 2.2% stroke and 33.8% multiple functional disability. The prevalence of fair or poor SRH was 43.3% (see Table 1).

Associations with SRH

In adjusted binary and ordered logistic regression analysis, older age, medium level of education, Muslim, Sikh, underweight, arthritis, diabetes, asthma, angina, stroke and functional disability were associated with poorer SRH (poor or fair SRH and poorer SRH as a scale), while subjective socioeconomic status, and vigorous physical activity were negatively associated with poorer SRH (poor or fair SRH and poorer SRH as a scale). In addition, current tobacco use and hypertension were associated with poor or fair SRH, and heart disease was associated with poorer SRH (as a scale) (see Table 2).

Table 1. Sample and self-rated health (SRH) characteristics among older adults in India, 2017-2018

Variable	Sample	Poor or fair SRH	SRH scale (1-5)[1]
	N (%)	%	M (SD)
All	**52393**	**43.3**	**3.3 (1.0)**
Sociodemographic factors			
Age in years			
50-59	20916 (38.1)	34.8	3.1 (1.0)
60-69	18979 (36.2)	44.9	3.3 (1.0)
70-79	9108 (18.7)	51.8	3.5 (1.0)
≥80	3390 (7.0)	59.9	3.7 (1.0)
Sex			
Female	27815 (53.3)	45.5	3.4 (1.0)
Male	24578 (46.7)	40.7	3.3 (1.0)
Marital status			
Not married	15151 (29.9)	49.9	3.5 (1.0)
Married	37236 (70.1)	40.4	3.2 (1.0)
Education in years			
0	25983 (53.0)	46.2	3.4 (1.0)
1-4	6138 (11.0)	47.9	3.4 (1.0)
5-9	11246 (19.5)	43.3	3.3 (1.0)
≥10	9026 (16.5)	30.8	3.0 (1.0)
Subjective socioeconomic status			
Low	17462 (38.2)	51.8	3.5 (1.0)
Medium	20070 (37.4)	42.4	3.3 (1.0)
High	13176 (24.4)	31.6	3.0 (1.0)
Residence			
Rural	34099 (69.0)	46.1	3.4 (1.0)
Urban	18294 (31.0)	36.9	3.2 (1.0)
Religious affiliation			
Hindu	38498 (82.4)	42.3	3.3 (1.0)
Muslim	6186 (11.3)	48.9	3.4 (1.0)
Christian	5206 (2.8)	46.0	3.4 (1.0)
Sikh	1528 (1.8)	51.7	3.4 (1.0)
Other or none	973 (1.7)	42.0	3.3 (1.0)
Health risk behaviour			
Underweight	9428 (23.0)	49.6	3.5 (1.0)
Vigorous physical activity			
Never	32762 (62.3)	48.3	3.4 (1.0)
Once/week	4262 (8.8)	37.9	3.2 (1.0)
>once/week	14930 (28.9)	34.1	3.1 (1.0)
Current tobacco use	16403 (33.0)	44.9	3.4 (1.0)
Ever alcohol use	9346 (14.9)	42.4	3.3 (1.0)
Health status			
Arthritis	6647 (14.7)	58.4	3.7 (0.9)
Diabetes	7423 (13.4)	52.3	3.5 (1.0)
Hypertension	22826 (45.4)	46.7	3.4 (1.0)
Asthma	2292 (5.4)	63.3	3.8(1.0)
Angina	4510 (8.9)	55.6	3.6 (1.0)
Heart disease	2154 (4.2)	63.2	3.8 (1.0)
Stroke	1109 (2.2)	73.8	4.0 (0.9)
Functional disability			
0	31213 (55.5)	32.8	3.1 (1.0)
1	5592 (10.7)	44.7	3.3 (0.9)
2 or more	15318 (33.8)	60.5	3.7 (1.0)

[1]1 the highest and 5 the poorest SRH; M = Mean; SD = Standard Deviation.

Table 2. Associations with poor or fair self-rated health (SRH) and SRH scale among older adults in India, 2017-2018

Variable	Binary logistic regression with poor or fair SRH	Ordered logistic regression with SRH
	Adjusted Odds Ratio (95% CI)	Adjusted Odds Ratio (95% CI)
Sociodemographic factors		
Age in years		
50-59	1 (Reference)	1 (Reference)
60-69	1.20 (1.03, 1.39)*	1.20 (1.08, 1.33)***
70-79	1.27 (1.05, 1.54)*	1.30 (1.12, 1.51)***
≥80	1.48 (1.17, 1.87)***	1.56 (1.27, 1.93)***
Sex		
Female	1 (Reference)	1 (Reference)
Male	1.04 (0.92, 1.18)	1.05 (0.90, 1.22)
Marital status		
Not married	1 (Reference)	1 (Reference)
Married	0.98 (0.90, 1.08)	0.96 (0.89, 1.04)
Education in years		
0	1 (Reference)	1 (Reference)
1-4	1.16 (1.02, 1.31)*	1.06 (0.94, 1.20)
5-9	1.21 (1.09, 1.35)***	1.14 (1.01, 1.30)*
≥10	0.93 (0.76, 1.15)	0.89 (0.75, 1.06)
Subjective socioeconomic status		
Low	1 (Reference)	1 (Reference)
Medium	0.69 (0.63, 0.76)***	0.67 (0.62, 0.72)***
High	0.43 (0.35, 0.53)***	0.43 (0.37, 0.50)***
Residence		
Rural	1 (Reference)	1 (Reference)
Urban	0.75 (0.52, 1.09)	0.77 (0.54, 1.10)
Religious affiliation		
Hindu	1 (Reference)	1 (Reference)
Muslim	1.27 (1.05, 1.53)*	1.23 (1.05, 1.43)**
Christian	1.25 (0.85, 1.82)	1.30 (0.90, 1.88)
Sikh	1.64 (1.27, 2.11)***	1.42 (1.16, 1.74)***
Other or none	0.86 (0.56, 1.31)	0.90 (0.65, 1.24)
Health risk behaviour		
Underweight	1.17 (1.09, 1.26)***	1.18 (1.10, 1.26)***
Vigorous physical activity		
Never	1 (Reference)	1 (Reference)
Once/week	0.77 (0.67, 0.88)***	0.80 (0.69, 0.91)**
>once/week	0.64 (0.58, 0.71)***	0.68 (0.61, 0.75)***
Current tobacco use	1.12 (1.02, 1.23)*	1.08 (0.97, 1.21)
Ever alcohol use	0.98 (0.87, 1.11)	1.00 (0.90, 1.12)
Health status		
Arthritis	1.66 (1.37, 2.03)***	1.61 (1.39, 1.87)***
Diabetes	1.63 (1.44, 1.88)***	1.66 (1.51, 1.82)***
Hypertension	1.09 (1.01, 1.18)*	1.06 (0.99, 1.14)
Asthma	1.82 (1.39, 2.39)***	2.29 (1.94, 2.70)***
Angina	1.44 (1.25, 1.67)***	1.38 (1.22, 1.57)***
Heart disease	1.59 (0.98, 2.58)	1.67 (1.26, 2.22)***
Stroke	2.30 (1.89, 2.79)***	2.22 (1.80, 2.74)***
Functional disability		
0	1 (Reference)	1 (Reference)
1	1.49 (1.30, 1.72)***	1.41 (1.26, 1.59)***
2 or more	2.36 (2.05, 2.71)***	2.30 (1.99, 2.66)***

CI = Confidence Interval; ***$p < 0.001$; ** $p < 0.01$; *$p < 0.05$.

Discussion

In this nationally representative sample of older adults (≥50 years) in India in 2017-2018, the prevalence of fair or poor SRH was 43.3%, which seems to be higher than in four states in India in 2010 (≥45 years) (9% poor or fair SRH) [3], similar to a study among older adults (≥50 years) in 11 European countries (44.9% fair/bad/very bad SRH) [8], and among older adults (≥60 years) in Cali, Columbia (40.1% poor or fair SRH) [10], but lower than in Thailand (≥60 years) (56% fair/very bad/bad SRH) [9]. It is not clear why there is such a drastic increase in poor SRH in India in 2010 to 2017-2018, especially because the same SRH measure was used. More detailed research is needed to explain these differences.

Consistent with previous research [2-7, 15], this study found that older age, lower socioeconomic status and ethnicity (Muslims and Sikhs) were associated with poorer SRH. The relationship between older age and poor SRH may be related to the biological processes of ageing [16] and due to a decline in mobility and activity [9]. Having a lower socioeconomic status may negatively impact on health outcomes by less access to health care, lessor ability to fulfil one's basic needs, and less participation in social activities [16]. In addition, the link between low socioeconomic status and the development of physical and mental morbidity has been well established [26]. It is possible that Muslims and Sikhs had a higher rate of poor SRH than Hindus, which may be related to differences in the perception of health status [12]. Income insecurity should be addressed among older adults in India. Some studies [5-7] found that less education was associated with poorer SRH, this study showed that medium level education was associated with poorer SRH. While previous studies found an association between female sex [2, 4-7, 11], not married [6, 7, 13], rural residence [3] and poorer SRH, this study did not find a significant association in adjusted analyses. This may mean that health prevention strategies among older adults in India should be directed at both older men and women, both oral rural and urban residents, as well as married and not married or widowed older adults [10].

Furthermore, in line with previous findings [2, 12, 14-16], this study found that underweight, physical inactivity and current tobacco use were associated with poorer SRH. The prevalence of current tobacco use among older adults in India was high (33.0%) in this study, and the government should reinforce policies of tobacco use cessation to reverse the harmful effects and improve health [16]. Furthermore, the prevalence of underweight was high (23.0%) in this study, calling for programmes that alleviate food insecurity. Physical activity has been recognized as an important behaviour to improve physical and mental health among older adults [12, 15, 16]. However, while some research [2, 12] found an association between alcohol use and poorer SRH. This result may be related to the low prevalence of alcohol use in India.

Largely in agreement with previous investigations [2, 9, 10, 12, 16], chronic conditions (hypertension, arthritis, asthma, heart disease, angina, stroke, diabetes) and functional disability increased the odds of poorer SRH in this study. There is consistent evidence that chronic diseases impact negatively on SRH, be it through pain or disability [12]. The onset of chronic conditions should be reduced by health promotion activities, screening and effective control of non-communicable diseases [16]. By doing so functional disabilities can also be reduced.

Study limitations include the cross-sectional design, the assessment of some variables by self-report. Another limitation was that only subjective socioeconomic status was assessed and not a more objective measure of wealth or economic status. The study only included community-dwelling older adults and did not include institutionalized older adults, which could have provided different rates of SRH.

CONCLUSION

Almost one in two older adults in India had fair or poor SRH. Several potential risk factors for poor SRH, such as older age, lower subjective socioeconomic status, medium level of education, Muslim, Sikh, underweight, physical inactivity, current tobacco use, arthritis, diabetes, asthma, angina, hypertension, heart disease, stroke and functional disability were identified, which can be targeted in public health interventions.

ACKNOWLEDGMENTS

The Longitudinal Aging Study in India Project is funded by the Ministry of Health and Family Welfare, Government of India, the National Institute on Aging (R01 AG042778, R01 AG030153), and United Nations Population Fund, India.

REFERENCES

[1] Snead MC. Health, self-rated. In: Ritzer G, ed. The Blackwell Encyclopedia of Sociology 2007: 2085-6. URL: http://philosociology.com/UPLOADS/_PHILOSOCIOLOGY.ir_Blackwell%20Encyclopedia%20of%20Sociology_George%20Ritzer.pdf.

[2] Dong W, Wan J, Xu Y, Chen C, Bai G, Fang L, et al. Determinants of self-rated health among shanghai elders: a cross-sectional study. BMC Public Health 2017;17(1):307. doi: 10.1186/s12889-017-4718-5.

[3] Cramm JM, Bornscheuer L, Selivanova A, Lee J. The health of India's elderly population: A comparative assessment using subjective and objective health outcomes. J Popul Ageing 2015;8(4):245-9. doi: 10.1007/s12062-015-9122-2.

[4] Cramm JM, Lee J. Smoking, physical activity and healthy aging in India. BMC Public Health 2014;14:526. doi: 10.1186/1471-2458-14-526.

[5] Phaswana-Mafuya N, Peltzer K, Chirinda W, Kose Z, Hoosain E, Ramlagan S, et al. Self-rated health and associated factors among older South Africans: evidence from the study on global ageing and adult health. Glob Health Action 2013;6(1):19880. doi: 10.3402/gha.v6i0.19880.

[6] Ng N, Hakimi M, Byass P, Wilopo S, Wall S. Health and quality of life among older rural people in Purworejo District, Indonesia. Glob Health Action 2010;3. doi: 10.3402/gha.v3i0.2125.

[7] Xavier Gómez-Olivé F, Thorogood M, Clark BD, Kahn K, Tollman SM. Assessing health and well-being among older people in rural South Africa. Glob Health Action 2010;3. doi: 10.3402/gha.v3i0.2126.

[8] Verropoulou G. Determinants of change in self-rated health among older adults in Europe: a longitudinal perspective based on SHARE data. Eur J Ageing 2012;9(4):305-18. doi: 10.1007/s10433-012-0238-4.

[9] Haseen F, Adhikari R, Soonthorndhada K. Self-assessed health among Thai elderly. BMC Geriatr 2010;10:30. doi: 10.1186/1471-2318-10-30.

[10] Ocampo-Chaparro JM, Zapata-Ossa Hde J, Cubides-Munévar AM, Curcio CL, Villegas Jde D, Reyes-Ortiz CA. Prevalence of poor self-rated health and associated risk factors among older adults in Cali, Colombia. Colomb Med 2013;44(4):224-31.

[11] Pandey A, Ladusingh L. Socioeconomic correlates of gender differential in poor health status among older adults in India. J Appl Gerontol 2015;34(7):879-905. doi: 10.1177/0733464813481850.

[12] Chan YY, Teh CH, Lim KK, Lim KH, Yeo PS, Kee CC, et al. Lifestyle, chronic diseases and self-rated health among Malaysian adults: results from the 2011 National Health and Morbidity Survey (NHMS). BMC Public Health 2015;15:754. doi: 10.1186/s12889-015-2080-z.

[13] Sudha S, Suchindran C, Mutran EJ, Rajan SI, Sarma PS. Marital status, family ties, and self-rated health among elders in South India. J Cross Cult Gerontol 2006;21(3-4):103-20. doi: 10.1007/s10823-006-9027-x.

[14] Selvamani Y, Singh P. Socioeconomic patterns of underweight and its association with self-rated health, cognition and quality of life among older adults in India. PLoS One 2018;13(3):e0193979. doi: 10.1371/journal.pone.0193979.

[15] Yaya S, Bishwajit G. Patterns of physical activity and self-rated health among adult populations in South Asia. Cent Asian J Glob Health 2020;9(1):e347. doi: 10.5195/cajgh.2020.347.

[16] Fonta CL, Nonvignon J, Aikins M, Nwosu E, Aryeetey GC. Predictors of self-reported health among the elderly in Ghana: a cross sectional study. BMC Geriatr 2017;17(1):171. doi: 10.1186/s12877-017-0560-y.

[17] International Institute for Population Sciences (IIPS), NPHCE, MoHFW, Harvard T. H. Chan School of Public Health (HSPH) and the University of Southern California (USC). Longitudinal Ageing Study in India (LASI) Wave 1, 2017-18, India Report. Mumbai: International Institute for Population Sciences, 2020.

[18] Cullati S, Mukhopadhyay S, Sieber S, Chakraborty A, Burton-Jeangros C. Is the single self-rated health item reliable in India? A construct validity study. BMJ Glob Health 2018;3(6):e000856. doi: 10.1136/bmjgh-2018-000856.

[19] Wen CP, David Cheng TY, Tsai SP, Chan HT, Hsu HL, Hsu CC, et al. Are Asians at greater mortality risks for being overweight than Caucasians? Redefining obesity for Asians. Public Health Nutr 2009;12(4):497-506. doi: 10.1017/S136898 0008002802.

[20] Lübs L, Peplies J, Drell C, Bammann K. Cross-sectional and longitudinal factors influencing physical activity of 65 to 75-year-olds: a pan European cohort study based on the survey of health, ageing and retirement in Europe (SHARE). BMC Geriatr 2018;18(1):94. doi: 10.1186/s12877-018-0781-8.

[21] Chobanian AV, Bakris GL, Black HR, Cushman WC, Green LA, Izzo Jr JL, et al. The seventh report of the joint national committee on prevention, detection, evaluation, and treatment of high blood pressure: the JNC 7 report. JAMA 2003;289(19):2560–71.

[22] Rose GA. The diagnosis of ischaemic heart pain and intermittent claudication in field surveys. Bull World Health Organ 1962;27:645–58.

[23] Achterberg S, Soedamah-Muthu SS, Cramer MJ, Kappelle LJ, van der Graaf Y, Algra A; SMART Study Group. Prognostic value of the Rose questionnaire: a validation with future coronary events in the SMART study. Eur J Prev Cardiol 2012;19(1):5-14. doi: 10.1177/1741826710391117.

[24] Katz S, Ford AB, Moskowitz RW, Jackson BA, Jaffe MW. Studies of illness in the aged. the index of ADL: a standardized measure of biological and psychosocial function. JAMA 1963;185:914-9. doi: 10.1001/jama.1963.03060120024016.

[25] Lawton MP, Brody EM. Assessment of older people: self-maintaining and instrumental activities of daily living. Gerontologist 1969;9(3):179-86.

[26] Kivimäki M, Batty GD, Pentti J, Shipley MJ, Sipilä PN, Nyberg ST, et al. Association between socioeconomic status and the development of mental and physical health conditions in adulthood: a multi-cohort study. Lancet Public Health 2020;5(3):e140-9. doi: 10.1016/S2468-2667(19)30248-8.

In: Social and Health Issues ... ISBN: 978-1-53619-937-6
Editors: S Pengpid, K Peltzer et al.

Chapter 3

PREVALENCE AND CORRELATES OF MAJOR INJURIES AMONG MIDDLE-AGED AND OLDER ADULTS IN INDIA: RESULTS OF A NATIONAL CROSS-SECTIONAL SURVEY IN 2017-2018

Karl Peltzer[1,2], MA Clin Psych, PhD, Dr Habil and Supa Pengpid[1,3,*], MPH, DrPH, MBA

[1]Department of Research Administration and Development, University of Limpopo, Turfloop, South Africa

[2]Department of Psychology, College of Medical and Health Science, Asia University, Taichung, Taiwan

[3]ASEAN Institute for Health Development, Mahidol University, Salaya, Phutthamonthon, Nakhon Pathom, Thailand

* *Correspondence*: Professor Supa Pengpid, ASEAN Institute for Health Development, Mahidol University, 25/25 Phutthamonthon Road 4, Salaya, Phutthamonton, Nakhon Pathom 73170, Thailand. Email: supaprom@yahoo.com.

Abstract

In this chapter we examine the prevalence and correlates of injury among middle-aged and older adults in India. The study included 72,262 individuals (45 years and older) from the cross-sectional 2017-2018 Longitudinal Ageing Study in India (LASI) Wave 1. Results indicate that 12.9% had a major injury in the past two years, 2.3% had a road traffic injury, 9.4% had a fall injury and 1.9% had other injuries in the past two years. In adjusted logistic regression analysis, having 5-9 years education (Adjusted Odds Ratio-AOR: 1.14, 95% Confidence Interval-CI: 1.01-1.79), having sleep problems (AOR: 1.39, 95% CI: 1.23-1.57), having two or more chronic conditions (AOR: 1.21, 95% CI: 1.05-1.39), functional disability (AOR: 1.19, 95% CI: 1.04-1.35), pain (AOR: 1.81, 95% CI: 1.63-2.02), binge drinking (AOR: 1.27, 95% CI: 1.03-1.55), tobacco use (AOR: 1.22, 95% CI: 1.10-1.36), poor near vision (AOR: 1.17, 95% CI: 1.03-1.33), and hearing problems (AOR: 1.30, 95% CI: 1.11-1.52) were positively associated with past two years major injury. Compared to scheduled tribes, scheduled castes (AOR: 0.65, 95% CI: 0.54-0.78), and other backward classes (AOR: 0.85, 95% CI: 0.76-0.96), having high subjective socioeconomic status (AOR: 0.85, 95% CI: 0.75-0.97), and urban residence (AOR: 0.82, 95% CI: 0.73-0.93) were negatively associated with past two years major injury. Younger age and male sex were associated with road traffic injury, and older age and female sex with were associated with fall injury. Rural residence was associated with fall and other injury. Poor grip strength was positively associated with fall and other injury. Having depressive symptoms and vigorous physical activity were associated with other injuries. More than one in ten participants (12.9%) had a major injury in the past two years, and several risk factors were found that can be utilized in injury prevention strategies in India.

Introduction

"Unintentional injuries are typically classified according to the means of their occurrence: poisoning, burns and scalds, drowning, falls and transport-related" [1]. Low- and middle-income countries, such as in India, experiencing an increase in the older population, rapid motorization, urbanization, and industrialization, which may contribute to an increase of injuries [2-5]. Older adults may be more vulnerable to injury because of a reduction in muscle mass, loss of mineral bone density, dietary calcium deficiency, a decrease in physical activity, and increase in functional disability [6, 7]. To monitor the prevalence and risk factors of unintentional non-fatal injury among middle-aged and older adults is vital to inform intervention strategies [8].

In a national study among older adults (≥50 years) in India in 2007, the prevalence of past-year unintentional injury was 9.1%, past-year fall-related injuries 6.6% [9], past-year road traffic injury 2.4%, and other bodily injury (except falls) 2.6% [10]. In India, 11% of all deaths are caused by injury [11]. There is a lack of a more recent national study on the prevalence and correlates of injury among middle-aged and older adults in India.

In other low- and middle-income countries, among older adults (≥50 years), the prevalence of past-year unintentional injury was 5.1% in China, 5.7% in Ghana, 4.2% in Mexico and 1.3% in South Africa, and the prevalence of past-year fall-related injury was 3.1% in China, 2.6% in Ghana, 2.8% in Mexico and 1.0% in South Africa [9]. The prevalence of past-year road traffic injury was 1.8% in China, 1.7% in Ghana, 1.7% in Mexico, and 1.8% in South Africa, and the prevalence of other bodily injury (except falls) was 2.1% in China, 2.8% in Ghana, 1.4% in Mexico and 0.9% in South Africa [10]. In Indonesia, among older adults (≥50 years), the past 2-years prevalence of fall related injuries was 12.8% [12], in the Philippines among older adults (≥60 years), the prevalence of self-reported injuries was 1.2% [13], in Ecuador among persons (≥60 years) the prevalence of past-year fall-related injury was 11.4% [14], and in a review on falls among older adults in various regions in India, Joseph et al. [15] found that the prevalence of falls ranged from 26% to 37%.

Risk factors among older adults for injuries, including fall-related injury, may include lower socioeconomic status, older age, female sex, residing in rural areas, mutimorbidity, pain, low grip strength, poor cognitive functioning, functional disability, pain, imbalance, vision problems, hearing problems, sleeping problems, depressive symptoms, physical inactivity, tobacco use, alcohol use and obesity [9, 10, 12, 15-17]. The aim of the study was to assess the prevalence and correlates of nonfatal injury among persons aged 45 years and older in India.

OUR STUDY

Cross-sectional data from the nationally representative Longitudinal Ageing Study in India (LASI) Wave 1, 2017-2018 were analyzed (the overall household response rate is 96%, and the overall individual response rate is 87%) [18]. Interview, physical measurement and biomarker data were collected from individuals aged 45 and above and their spouses, regardless of age, in a household survey. Details of the sampling strategy have been described elsewhere [18]. The study was approved by the Indian Council of Medical Research (ICMR) Ethics Committee, which conforms to the provisions of the Declaration of Helsinki (as revised in Brazil 2013), and written informed consent was obtained from participants [18].

Outcome measure

Major injury was assessed with the question, "In the past two years, have you sustained any major injury?" (Yes/No) "What was the cause of that injury? [Multiple answers are allowed]" ("Traffic accident, Struck by person or object, c. Fire, flames, burn, electric Shock, Drowning, Poisoning, Animal attack or bite, Fall, and Others") [18]. We grouped these injury causes into 1) road traffic injuries, 2) fall injuries, and 3) other injury.

Sociodemographic information included age (years), sex (male, female), education (none, <5 years, 5-9 years, and ≥10 years), caste or tribe (scheduled tribe, scheduled caste, other backward classes, none of these), residence (rural, urban) and subjective socioeconomic status. The latter was sourced from the item, "Please imagine a ten-step ladder, where at the bottom are the people who are the worst off – who have the least money, least education, and the worst jobs or no jobs, and at the top of the ladder are the people who are the best off – those who have the most money, most education, and best jobs. Please indicate the number given (1-10) on the rung on the ladder where you would place yourself" [18]. Socioeconomic steps 1 to 3 were classified as poor, 4-5 as medium, and 5-10 as high socioeconomic status.

Sleep problems were assessed with four questions: 1) "How often do you have trouble falling asleep?" 2) "How often do you have trouble with waking up during the night?" 3) "How often do you have trouble with waking up too early and not being able to fall asleep again?" 4) "How often do you feel really rested when you wake up in the morning?" Responses options were "never, rarely (1-2 nights per week), occasionally (3-4 nights per week), and frequently (5 or more nights per week)" [18]. Participants who reported any of these four symptoms frequently were classified as having sleep problems [19].

Depressive symptoms were assessed with a modified Centre for Epidemiological Studies Depression Scale (CES-D-10) [20]. The 10 items included seven negative symptoms (trouble concentrating, feeling depressed, low energy, fear of something, feeling alone, bothered by things, and everything is an effort), and three positive symptoms (feeling happy, hopeful, and satisfied). Response options included rarely or never (< 1 day), sometimes (1 or 2 days), often (3 or 4 days), and most or all of the time (5-7 days) in a week prior to the interview. For negative symptoms, rarely or never (< 1 day), and sometimes (1 or 2 days) were scored zero, and often (3 or 4 days) and most or all of the time (5-7 days) categories were scored one. Scoring was reversed for positive symptoms. The overall score ranges from zero to 10 and scores of four or more were indicative for depressive symptoms [21]. The Cronbach α of the CES-D-10 in this study was 0.79.

Chronic conditions were assessed with the question, "Has any health professional ever told you that you have…?": 1) "Hypertension or high blood pressure (Yes/No); 2) Diabetes or high blood sugar; 3) Cancer or malignant tumor; 4) Chronic lung disease such as asthma, chronic obstructive pulmonary disease/Chronic bronchitis or other chronic lung problems; 5) Chronic heart diseases such as Coronary heart disease (heart attack or Myocardial Infarction), congestive heart failure, or other chronic heart problems; 6) Stroke; 7) Arthritis or rheumatism, Osteoporosis or other bone/joint diseases; 8) Any neurological, or psychiatric problems such as depression, Alzheimer's/Dementia, unipolar/bipolar disorders, convulsions, Parkinson's etc.; and 9) High cholesterol (Yes/No)." [18]. Responses for the nine chronic conditions were summed and trichotomized into 0,1, or ≥2 chronic conditions.

Functional disability was sourced from Activities of Daily Living (ADL) (6 items) and Instrumental Activities of Daily Living (IADL) (7 items) [22, 23]. Cronbach alpha for the ADL and IADL scale was 0.89. Responses were "Yes/No" and were trichotomized into 0,1, or ≥2 ADL/IADL items.

Hand grip strength (HGS) was measured with a "Baseline Smedley Spring type dynamometer" on "each hand twice, beginning with the dominant hand, alternating hands in between measurements" [18]. A mean HGS (kg) variable was calculated from all four measurements [24]. HGS <30 kg for men and <20 kg for women using the average value of the four handgrip assessments were defined as "weak" [25].

Symptom-based pain was defined as troubled by pain and required some form of medication or treatment for relief of pain [18].

Anthropometry: "Height and weight of adults were measured using the Seca 803 digital scale." [18]. "BMI was calculated according to Asian criteria: underweight (<18.5 kg/m^2), normal weight (18.5-22.9 kg/m^2), overweight (23.0-24.9 kg/m^2), class I obesity (25.0-29.9 kg/m^2), and class II obesity (≥30.0 kg/m^2)" [26].

Binge drinking was assessed with the question, "In the last 3 months, how frequently on average, have you had at least 5 or more drinks on one occasion?" [18] and defined as "one to three days per month, one to four days per week, five or more days per week, or daily."

Current tobacco use was sourced from two items, 1) "Do you currently smoke any tobacco products (cigarettes, bidis, cigars, hookah, cheroot, etc.)? and 2) Do you use smokeless tobacco (such as chewing tobacco, gutka, pan masala, etc.)?" [18].

Vigorous physical activity. "For vigorous activity, respondents were asked about their involvement in running or jogging, swimming, going to a health centre/gym, cycling, digging with a spade or shovel, heavy lifting, chopping, farm work, fast bicycling, and cycling with loads everyday, more than once a week, once a week, one to three times a month, or hardly ever or never?" [18]. Participants who engaged in vigorous physical activity more than once a week were defined as having sufficient physical activity [27].

Vision was assessed with two questions, 1) "How good is your eyesight for seeing things at a distance, like recognizing a person across the street (or 20 meters away), whether or not you wear glasses, contacts, or corrective lenses?" and 2) "How good is your eyesight for seeing things up close, like reading an ordinary newspaper print whether or not you wear glasses, contacts, or corrective lenses?" [18]. Response options ranged from 1=Very good to 5=Very poor, and poor near or far vision was defined as "poor or very poor."

Cognitive functioning measures in the LASI were derived from the cognition module of the Health and Retirement Study (HRS), including memory (immediate and delayed word recall), orientation (time and place), arithmetic function (backward counting, serial 7, computation), executive function (paper folding and Pentagon drawing), and object naming. A composite cognitive index is created with the lowest 10th percentile as a proxy measure of poor cognitive functioning [18].

Hearing problem was measured with the item. "Have you ever been diagnosed with any hearing or ear-related problem or condition?" (Yes/No) [18].

Inadequate balance was defined as <10 seconds or no attempt [18].

Data analysis

Descriptive statistics were used to describe sociodemographic, health, and injury variables. Adjusted logistic regression was used to estimate the prevalence of past 2-years major injuries, road traffic injuries, fall-related injuries, and other injuries. No multi-collinearity was detected. $P < 0.05$ was considered significant, and missing values were discarded. All statistical operations were conducted with STATA software version 13.0 (Stata Corporation, College Station, TX, USA), taking the multistage sample design into account.

FINDINGS

The study sample included 72,262 persons aged 45 years and older (female spouse, any age) from India. Table 1 describes the sample characteristics. More than one in ten participants (12.9%) had a major injury in the past two years, 2.3% had a road traffic injury, 9.4% had a fall injury and 1.9% had other injuries in the past two years (see Table 1).

Table 1. Sample characteristics and prevalence of type of injury

Variable	Sample	Major injury	Road traffic injury	Fall injury	Other injury
	%	%	%	%	%
All	**72262**	**12.9**	**2.0**	**9.4**	1.9
Age (years)					
45-59 (female spouse: any age)	40785 (54.1)	11.1	2.3	7.4	1.6
≥60	31477 (45.9)	15.1	1.6	11.7	2.1
Sex					
Female	41685 (58.0)	13.1	1.2	10.5	1.6
Male	30577 (42.0)	12.7	3.1	7.8	2.2
Education					
No schooling	33213 (49.5)	13.4	1.5	10.2	2.0
<5 years	8056 (10.8)	14.4	2.1	10.8	2.1
5-9 years	16911 (21.1)	13.9	2.8	9.3	2.1
≥10 years	14079 (18.5)	9.8	2.4	6.4	1.1
Caste/tribe					
Scheduled tribe	12047 (19.7)	15.0	2.4	10.9	2.1
Scheduled caste	12509 (8.8)	10.5	1.1	7.5	2.1
Other backward class	27185 (46.7)	12.3	1.9	8.9	1.7
None of the above	17893 (24.9)	13.5	2.2	9.8	2.0
Subjective socioeconomic status					
Low	23625 (37.2)	14.3	2.0	10.7	2.0
Medium	28380 (38.7)	12.8	2.1	9.0	2.0
High	18134 (24.1)	11.0	1.7	7.9	1.5
Residence					
Rural	46539 (68.2)	13.9	2.0	10.1	2.3
Urban	25723 (31.8)	10.8	2.0	7.9	1.0
Sleep problems	8367 (12.7)	20.0	3.2	14.8	2.7
Depressive symptoms	17650 (27.6)	15.5	2.4	11.3	2.3

Variable	Sample	Major injury	Road traffic injury	Fall injury	Other injury
	%	%	%	%	%
All	**72262**	**12.9**	**2.0**	**9.4**	1.9
Chronic conditions					
0	39715 (55.0)	11.1	1.9	7.5	1.9
1	19336 (26.9)	14.3	2.2	10.6	1.9
2 or more	12991 (18.1)	16.5	1.9	13.3	1.6
Functional disability					
0	46762 (60.7)	10.7	2.1	7.2	1.6
1	7425 (10.5)	12.2	2.0	8.3	2.0
2 or more	17700 (28.8)	17.9	1.8	14.3	2.3
Grip strength (men: <30 kg, women: <20 kg)	41981 (69.7)	13.4	1.7	9.9	2.1
Symptom-based pain	19145 (27.7)	19.9	2.6	14.8	2.9
Obesity (≥25 kg/m^2)	19636 (28.0)	12.4	2.3	9.0	1.2
Past month binge drinking	2600 (2.9)	15.3	2.7	10.9	2.2
Current tobacco use	21071 (30.4)	15.0	2.5	10.5	2.4
Vigorous physical activity	22210 (32.0)	12.2	2.3	8.0	2.2
Poor near vision	11866 (16.8)	17.6	2.4	13.3	2.3
Poor distant vision	9756 (14.2)	17.9	2.0	14.0	2.3
Poor cognitive functioning	5980 (11.3)	14.7	1.3	11.7	1.9
Hearing problem	4874 (6.6)	20.6	2.4	15.8	3.0
Balance (no/<10s)	2129 (3.9)	16.0	1.3	13.8	1.1

Cause of injury

Majority of participants (72.6%) had a fall, followed by traffic accident (15.4%), struck by a person or object (7.6%), animal attack or bite (4.9%), fire, flames, burn or electric shock (1.1%), and drowning (0.1%). The younger age group (45-59 years) had more traffic injuries than the older age group (≥60 years), while the older age group had more fall injuries than the younger age group ($p<0.001$). Women had more often a fall than men and men had more traffic and struck by person or object injuries than women ($p<0.001$). Traffic injuries were more prevalent in participants residing in urban than rural areas, while struck by a person or object and animal attack or bites were more common in rural than urban areas ($p<0.001$) (see Table 2).

Table 2. Cause of major injury in the past 2 years (N=8,019)

Variable	Total	45-59 years	60 years and more	Male	Female	Urban	Rural
	N (%)	%	%	%	%	%	%
Traffic accident	1298 (15.4)	20.7*	10.8	24.5*	9.0	19.1*	14.1
Struck by person or object	608 (7.6)	8.1	7.2	9.7*	6.2	5.7*	8.3
Fire, flames, burn, electric shock	65 (1.1)	1.1	1.1	1.5	0.9	1.1	1.1
Drowning	10 (0.1)	0.1	0.1	0.0	0.2	0.1	0.1
Poisoning	4 (0.0)	0.1	0.0	0.1	0.0	0.0	0.1
Animal attack or bite	371 (4.9)	5.0	4.9	5.4	4.6	1.7*	6.1
Fall	5782 (72.6)	66.7*	77.8	61.3*	80.6	73.5	72.3
Other	66 (0.7)	0.6	0.8	0.8	0.7	0.3	0.9

*$p<0.001$.

Associations with injury types

In adjusted logistic regression analysis, having 5-9 years education (Adjusted Odds Ratio-AOR: 1.14, 95% Confidence Interval-CI: 1.01-1.79), having sleep problems (AOR: 1.39, 95% CI: 1.23-1.57), having two or more chronic conditions (AOR: 1.21, 95% CI: 1.05-1.39), functional disability (AOR: 1.19, 95% CI: 1.04-1.35), pain (AOR: 1.81, 95% CI: 1.63-2.02),, binge drinking (AOR: 1.27, 95% CI: 1.03-1.55), tobacco use (AOR: 1.22, 95% CI: 1.10-1.36), poor near vision (AOR: 1.17, 95% CI: 1.03-1.33), and hearing problems (AOR: 1.30, 95% CI: 1.11-1.52) were positively associated with past two years major injury. Compared to scheduled tribes, scheduled castes (AOR: 0.65, 95% CI: 0.54-0.78), and other backward classes (AOR: 0.85, 95% CI: 0.76-0.96), having high subjective socioeconomic status (AOR: 0.85, 95% CI: 0.75-0.97), and urban residence (AOR: 0.82, 95% CI: 0.73-0.93) were negatively associated with past two years major injury. Younger age and male sex were associated with road traffic injury, and older age and female sex were associated with fall injuries. Rural residence was associated with fall and other injuries. Poor grip strength was positively associated with fall and other injuries. Having depressive symptoms and vigorous physical activity were associated with other injuries (see Table 3).

Table 3. Associations with injury

Variable	Major injury	Road traffic injury	Fall injury	Other injury
	AOR (95% CI)	AOR (95% CI)	AOR (95% CI)	AOR (95% CI)
Age (years)				
45-59 (female spouse: any age)	1 (Reference)	1 (Reference)	1 (Reference)	1 (Reference)
≥60	1.10 (0.98, 1.23)	0.68 (0.52, 0.90)**	1.23 (1.08, 1.41**	1.11 (0.91, 1.37)
Sex				
Female	1 (Reference)	1 (Reference)	1 (Reference)	1 (Reference)
Male	0.99 (0.88, 1.12)	3.04 (2.29, 4.04)***	0.70 (0.60, 0.80)***	1.32 (1.00, 1.74)
Education				
No schooling	1 (Reference)	1 (Reference)	1 (Reference)	1 (Reference)
<5 years	1.05 (0.90, 1.23)	1.05 (0.74, 1.48)	1.14 (0.95, 1.37)	0.89 (0.66, 1.20)
5-9 years	1.14 (1.01, 1.29)*	1.35 (1.01, 1.79)*	1.09 (0.95, 1.26)	1.10 (0.82, 1.49)
≥10 years	0.88 (0.75, 1.05)	1.10 (0.81, 1.50)	0.85 (0.68. 1.07)	0.72 (0.52, 1.00)
Caste/tribe				
Scheduled tribe	1 (Reference)	1 (Reference)	1 (Reference)	1 (Reference)
Scheduled caste	0.65 (0.54, 0.78)***	0.48 (0.32, 0.73)***	0.67 (0.54, 0.84)***	0.88 (0.58, 1.35)
Other backward class	0.85 (0.76, 0.96)**	0.77 (0.57, 1.05)	0.86 (0.76, 0.99)*	0.93 (0.72, 1.20)
None of the above	0.98 (0.87, 1.12)	0.91 (0.67, 1.25)	0.98 (0.84, 1.11)	1.33 (1.01, 1.73)*
Subjective socioeconomic status				
Low	1 (Reference)	1 (Reference)	1 (Reference)	1 (Reference)
Medium	0.99 (0.89, 1.10)	1.03 (0.79, 1.33)	0.92 (0.82. 1.04)	1.25 (0.99, 1.57)
High	0.85 (0.75, 0.97)*	0.78 (0.59, 1.02)	0.82 (0.70, 0.96)*	1.12 (0.88, 1.44)
Residence				
Rural	1 (Reference)	1 (Reference)	1 (Reference)	1 (Reference)
Urban	0.82 (0.73, 0.93)**	1.06 (0.79, 1.42)	0.81 (0.70, 0.93)**	0.61 (0.47, 0.80)***
Sleep problems	1.39 (1.23, 1.57)***	1.71 (1.31, 2.22)***	1.33 (1.16, 1.53)***	1.20 (0.93, 1.56)

Table 3. (Continued)

Variable	Major injury	Road traffic injury	Fall injury	Other injury
	AOR (95% CI)	**AOR (95% CI)**	**AOR (95% CI)**	**AOR (95% CI)**
Depressive symptoms	1.12 (1.00, 1.24)	1.33 (0.96, 1.83)	1.03 (0.92, 1.15)	1.35 (1.09, 1.67)**
Chronic conditions				
0	1 (Reference)	1 (Reference)	1 (Reference)	1 (Reference)
1	1.19 (1.06, 1.33)**	1.13 (0.83, 1.54)	1.23 (1.09, 1.40)***	1.07 (0.83, 1.39)
2 or more	1.21 (1.05, 1.39)**	0.94 (0.70, 1.26)	1.37 (1.16, 1.62)***	0.89 (0.68, 1.16)
Functional disability				
0	1 (Reference)	1 (Reference)	1 (Reference)	1 (Reference)
1	0.94 (0.82, 1.09)	0.91 (0.65, 1.29)	0.94 (0.79, 1.11)	0.93 (0.70, 1.25)
or more	1.19 (1.04, 1.35)**	0.92 (0.71, 1.19)	1.22 (1.05, 1.42)**	1.25 (0.92, 1.70)
Grip strength (men: <30 kg, women: <20 kg)	1.05 (0.94, 1.17)	0.71 (0.55, 0.92)**	1.14 (1.00, 1.29)*	1.27 (1.03, 1.57)*
Symptom-based pain	1.81 (1.63, 2.02)***	1.59 (1.28, 1.97)***	1.75 (1.54, 1.98)***	1.85 (1.45, 2.32)***
Obesity (≥25 kg/m^2)	0.99 (0.87, 1.11)	1.26 (0.94, 1.71)	0.97 (0.84, 1.11)	0.66 (0.51, 0.85)***
Past month binge drinking	1.27 (1.03, 1.55)*	0.90 (0.61, 1.34)	1.51 (1.20, 1.89)***	0.88 (0.49, 1.59)
Current tobacco use	1.22 (1.10, 1.36)***	0.92 (0.68, 1.24)	1.33 (1.18, 1.50)***	1.08 (0.84, 1.38)
Vigorous physical activity	1.08 (0.97, 1.22)	1.02 (0.81, 1.30)	1.03 (0.89, 1.19)	1.35 (1.09, 1.67)**
Poor near vision	1.17 (1.03, 1.33)*	1.25 (0.86, 1.81)	1.16 (1.01, 1.34)*	0.90 (0.70, 1.15)
Poor distant vision	1.12 (0.98, 1.29)	0.89 (0.62, 1.28)	1.15 (0.99, 1.35)	1.12 (0.85, 1.48)
Poor cognitive functioning	0.91 (0.78, 1.05)	0.98 (0.60, 1.59)	0.89 (0.75, 1.05)	0.79 (0.58, 1.08)
Hearing problem	1.30 (1.11, 1.52)***	1.14 (0.75, 1.74)	1.30 (1.08, 1.56)**	1.53 (1.12, 2.09)**
Balance (no/<10s)	0.86 (0.66, 1.11)	0.71 (0.29, 1.77)	0.91 (0.69, 1.21)	0.67 (0.39, 1.16)

AOR=Adjusted Odds Ratio; CI=Confidence Interval; ***p<0.001; **p<0.01; *p<0.05.

Discussion

The study found in a national population-based survey among middle-aged and older adults (≥45 years) in India in 2017-2018, a prevalence of 12.9% major injuries in the past two years, 2.3% road traffic injuries, 9.4% had a fall injury and 1.9% had other injuries in the past two years, which are similar to past-year prevalence rates of 9.1% injury, 6.6% fall-related injury, 2.4% road traffic injuries, and other bodily injury (except falls) in the India 2007 national survey among older adults (≥50 years) [9, 10]. The prevalence of injury (12.9% past two years) in this study seems higher than in China (5.1% past year), in Ghana (5.7% past year), in Mexico (4.2%) and in South Africa (1.3%) [9], while the prevalence of fall-related injury (9.4%) is higher than in China (3.1%), Ghana (2.6%), Mexico (2.8%) and South Africa (1.0%) [9], but lower than in Indonesia (12.8% past 2 years) [12], and Ecuador (11.4% past year) [14]. The prevalence of road traffic injury (2.3%) and other injuries (1.9%) in the past two years in this study were similar to previous studies, ranging from 1.7% in China and Mexico to 1.8% in China and South Africa in terms of road traffic injuries (past year) and ranging from 0.9% in South Africa to 2.8% in Ghana in terms of other injury [9, 10].

In line with previous research [4, 10], the most common non-road traffic injuries in this study were falls, struck by a person or object and animal attacks or bite. The latter two were significantly more common in rural areas in this study. The high proportion of interpersonal violence (struck by a person or objects) was also found in the previous 2007 study among older adults in India [10], which should be addressed in interventions to reduce injuries in middle-aged and older adults [10]. As found in a six country study [9], the majority of injuries were fall-related, confirming that the most common cause of injury among middle-aged and older adults is falls [28].

Among older women in this study the prevalence of fall injuries was higher than in younger men, which is consistent with previous findings [9, 29-32]. Among younger men and those living in urban areas, the prevalence of road traffic injuries was higher than in younger women and those living in rural areas in this study. In a multi-country study among persons aged 35-70 years, younger age, males, residing in low-income countries, and urban residence were associated with road traffic injuries [32]. In a study on road traffic injury in a tertiary care hospital in India, urban residence also outnumbered rural residents [33]. The gender differences in terms of higher fall injury rates among women than men may be attributed to "differences in higher levels of physical activity, muscle strength, bone density, and fatal fall rates in men than in women" [34]. In terms of gender differences regarding road traffic injury, this may be related to higher risk-taking behaviour among men than women [35]. Fall injuries were significantly higher in rural than urban areas in this study. It is possible that environmental factors such as "open street gutters, poor quality footpaths, and unsafe walking areas" in rural areas contribute to this [9, 36].

In agreement with previous research [9, 27, 38], higher socioeconomic status reduced the odds of injury, including fall injuries. In relation to the different caste groups, compared to members of scheduled tribes, members of scheduled castes and other backward classes had lower odds of injury, including fall injury. Among all caste groups, schedule tribes had the lowest income, followed by scheduled castes and other backward classes [18]. Compared to other backward classes, scheduled castes and scheduled tribes have experienced the largest deprivation within the Indian social hierarchy [39]. This seems to partially confirm that castes at the higher social hierarchy and higher economic status have decreased odds of injury. Regarding educational status, compared to persons with no formal schooling, persons with five to nine years education had a higher likelihood of having had a major injury, including road traffic injuries.

In agreement with previous research [9, 10, 16, 17, 40-43], pain and sleeping problems were associated with both road traffic and fall injury. Sleep problems may increase drowsiness, increasing the risk of road traffic and fall injuries [42, 43]. To target interventions, further research should establish the type of sleep problems that increase the risk of injury [10]. While some studies [9, 12, 44] found that depressive symptoms were associated with injurous falls and unintentional injury in general, this study only found a positive association between depressive symptoms and other injuries.

In line with previous research [9, 12, 37, 38, 46, 47], this study found an association between functional disability, visual difficulties, hearing problems, and injurious falls and/or injury in general. In addition, multimorbidity was found associated with fall injuries, as found in previous studies [9, 12, 44]. Having functional disability and multimorbidity may compromise one's mobility, increasing the risk of falls [12]. Vision problems and/or hearing problems may increase the risk for falling because of poor perception of spatial distances and relationships [48, 49]. Unlike some former findings [44], this study did not find a significant association between inadequate standing balance and injury, including fall-related injury.

In agreement with previous research [50], low hand grip strength was positively associated with fall and other injuries. While some studies showed an association between poor cognitive functioning [9, 12, 37] and injury, we did not find any significant association with any injury indicator. In this study, heavy episodic drinking and current tobacco use were associated with injury in general, including fall injury but not road traffic injury. In a study among emergency department patients in India alcohol was found to be involved in various types of injuries, including road traffic injuries [51]. Vigorous physical activity increased the odds of other injury in this study, while among middle-aged and older adults in the USA, leisure-time physical activity increased the risk of fall injuries [52]. In a study in a high-income setting (Texas, USA) [53], obesity increased the odds of fall injury among persons 45 years and older, while in this study it was not fall but other injuries.

Study limitations include the cross-sectional design and self-report of the data. The reference period for injury was the past two years, which may have introduced a recall bias. Some variables were not assessed, such as the impact of injuries, which should be included in future research.

CONCLUSION

Among older adults in India, more than one in ten participants (12.9%) had a major injury in the past two years, and several risk factors, such as lower subjective socioeconomic status, scheduled tribe, rural residence, sleep problems, chronic conditions, functional disability, pain, binge drinking, current tobacco use, poor near vision and hearing problems, were identified that can help in guiding injury prevention efforts in India.

ACKNOWLEDGMENTS

The Longitudinal Aging Study in India Project is funded by the Ministry of Health and Family Welfare, Government of India, the National Institute on Aging (R01 AG042778, R01 AG030153), and United Nations Population Fund, India.

REFERENCES

[1] World Health Organization. Injuries and violence: The facts. Geneva: WHO, 2010.

[2] Chandran A, Hyder AA, Peek-Asa C. The global burden of unintentional injuries and an agenda for progress. Epidemiol Rev 2010;32(1):110-20. doi: 10.1093/epirev/mxq009.

[3] Nakahara S, Ichikawa M. Injuries are growing public health concern in low- and middle-income countries (LMICs). J Trauma 2006;61(3):768. doi: 10.1097/01.ta.0000236033.25861.aa.

[4] Moncatar TJR, Nakamura K, Siongco KL, Rahman M, Seino K. Prevalence and determinants of self-reported injuries among community-dwelling older adults in the Philippines: A 10-Year Pooled Analysis. Int J Environ Res Public Health 2020;17(12):4372. doi: 10.3390/ijerph17124372.

[5] Gururaj G. Injuries in India: A national perspective. URL: https://nimhans.ac.in/wp-content/uploads/2019/02/BD_7-India-Injury-Report_0.pdf.

[6] India State-Level Disease Burden Initiative Road Injury Collaborators. Mortality due to road injuries in the states of India: the Global Burden of Disease Study 1990-2017. Lancet Public Health 2020;5(2):e86-98. doi: 10.1016/S2468-2667(19)30246-4.

[7] Navaratnarajah A, Jackson SHD. The physiology of ageing. Medicine in Older Adults. 2017;45(1):6-10. doi: https://doi.org/10.1016/j.mpmed.2016.10.008.

[8] Udofia EA, Aheto JM, Mensah G, Biritwum R, Yawson AE. Prevalence and risk factors associated with non-traffic related injury in the older population in Ghana:

Wave 2 of the WHO Study on Global AGEing and adult health (SAGE). Prev Med Rep 2019;15:100934. doi: 10.1016/j.pmedr.2019.100934.

[9] Jagnoor J, Ponnaiah M, Varghese M, Ivers R, Kumar R, Prinja S, et al. Potential for establishing an injury surveillance system in India: A review of data sources and reporting systems. BMC Public Health 2020;20(1):1909. doi: 10.1186/s12889-020-09992-9.

[10] Stewart Williams J, Kowal P, Hestekin H, O'Driscoll T, Peltzer K, Yawson A, et al. Prevalence, risk factors and disability associated with fall-related injury in older adults in low- and middle-incomecountries: Results from the WHO Study on global Ageing and adult health (SAGE). BMC Med 2015;13:147. doi: 10.1186/s12916-015-0390-8.

[11] Peltzer K, Phaswana-Mafuya N, Arokiasamy P, Biritwum R, Yawson A, Minicuci N, et al. Prevalence, circumstances and consequences of non-fatal road traffic injuries and other bodily injuries among older people in China, Ghana, India, Mexico, Russia and South Africa. Afr Saf Promot 2015;13(2):59-77.

[12] World Health Organization. Noncommunicable diseases (NCD) country profiles, India 2018. URL: https://www.who.int/nmh/countries/2018/ind_en.pdf?ua=1.

[13] Pengpid S, Peltzer K. Prevalence and risk factors associated with injurious falls among community-dwelling older adults in Indonesia. Curr Gerontol Geriatr Res 2018;2018:5964305. doi: 10.1155/2018/5964305.

[14] Orces CH. Prevalence and Determinants of Fall-Related Injuries among Older Adults in Ecuador. Curr Gerontol Geriatr Res 2014;2014:863473. doi: 10.1155/2014/863473.

[15] Joseph A, Kumar D, Bagavandas M. A review of epidemiology of fall among elderly in India. Indian J Commun Med 2019;44(2):166-8. doi: 10.4103/ijcm.IJCM_201_18.

[16] Almegbel FY, Alotaibi IM, Alhusain FA, Masuadi EM, Al Sulami SL, Aloushan AF, et al. Period prevalence, risk factors and consequent injuries of falling among the Saudi elderly living in Riyadh, Saudi Arabia: A cross-sectional study. BMJ Open 2018;8(1):e019063. doi: 10.1136/bmjopen-2017-019063.

[17] Bekibele CO, Gureje O. Fall incidence in a population of elderly persons in Nigeria. Gerontology 2010;56(3):278-83. doi: 10.1159/000236327.

[18] International Institute for Population Sciences (IIPS), NPHCE, MoHFW, Harvard T. H. Chan School of Public Health (HSPH) and the University of Southern California 2020. Longitudinal Ageing Study in India (LASI) Wave 1, 2017-18, India Report. Mumbai: International Institute for Population Sciences, 2020.

[19] Cho E, Chen TY. The bidirectional relationships between effort-reward imbalance and sleep problems among older workers. Sleep Health 2020;6(3):299-305. doi: 10.1016/j.sleh.2020.01.008.

[20] Andresen EM, Malmgren JA, Carter WB, Patrick DL. Screening for depression in well older adults: evaluation of a short form of the CES-D (Center for Epidemiologic Studies Depression Scale). Am J Prev Med 1994;10(2):77-84.

[21] Kumar S, Nakulan A, Thoppil SP, Parassery RP, Kunnukattil SS. Screening for depression among community-dwelling elders: Usefulness of the Center for

Epidemiologic Studies Depression Scale. Indian J Psychol Med 2016;38(5):483-5. doi: 10.4103/0253-7176.191380.

[22] Katz S, Ford AB, Moskowitz RW, Jackson BA, Jaffe MW. Studies of illness in the aged. the index of adl: a standardized measure of biological and psychosocial function. JAMA 1963;185:914-9. doi: 10.1001/jama.1963.03060120024016.

[23] Lawton MP, Brody EM. Assessment of older people: self-maintaining and instrumental activities of daily living. Gerontologist 1969;9(3):179-86.

[24] Roberts HC, Denison HJ, Martin HJ, Patel HP, Syddall H, Cooper C, et al. A review of the measurement of grip strength in clinical and epidemiological studies: towards a standardised approach. Age Ageing 2011;40(4):423-9. doi: 10.1093/ageing/afr051.

[25] Cruz-Jentoft AJ, Baeyens JP, Bauer JM, Boirie Y, Cederholm T, Landi F, et al. Sarcopenia: European consensus on definition and diagnosis: Report of the European Working Group on Sarcopenia in Older People. Age Ageing 2010;39(4):412-23. doi: 10.1093/ageing/afq034.

[26] Wen CP, David Cheng TY, Tsai SP, Chan HT, Hsu HL, Hsu CC, et al. Are Asians at greater mortality risks for being overweight than Caucasians? Redefining obesity for Asians. Public Health Nutr 2009;12(4):497-506. doi: 10.1017/S1368980008002802.

[27] Lübs L, Peplies J, Drell C, Bammann K. Cross-sectional and longitudinal factors influencing physical activity of 65 to 75-year-olds: a pan European cohort study based on the survey of health, ageing and retirement in Europe (SHARE). BMC Geriatr 2018;18(1):94. doi: 10.1186/s12877-018-0781-8.

[28] Karlsson MK, Vonschewelov T, Karlsson C, Cöster M, Rosengen BE. Prevention of falls in the elderly: a review. Scand J Public Health 2013;41(5):442-54. doi: 10.1177/1403494813483215.

[29] Chan KM, Pang WS, Ee CH, Ding YY, Choo P. Epidemiology of falls among the elderly community dwellers in Singapore. Singapore Med J 1997;38(10):427-31.

[30] D'souza SA, Shringarpure A, Karol J. Circumstances and consequences of falls in Indian older adults. Indian J Occup Therapy 2008;40(1):3–11.

[31] Mitchell RJ, Watson WL, Milat A, Chung AZ, Lord S. Health and lifestyle risk factors for falls in a large population-based sample of older people in Australia. J Safety Res 2013;45:7-13. doi: 10.1016/j.jsr.2012.11.005.

[32] Raina P, Sohel N, Oremus M, Shannon H, Mony P, Kumar R, et al. Assessing global risk factors for non-fatal injuries from road traffic accidents and falls in adults aged 35-70 years in 17 countries: a cross-sectional analysis of the Prospective Urban Rural Epidemiological (PURE) study. Inj Prev 2016;22(2):92-8. doi: 10.1136/injuryprev-2014-041476.

[33] Singh R, Singh HK, Gupta SC, Kumar Y. Pattern, severity and circumtances of injuries sustained in road traffic accidents: A tertiary care hospital-based study. Indian J Commun Med 2014;39(1):30-4. doi: 10.4103/0970-0218.126353.

[34] Stevens JA, Sogolow ED. Gender differences for non-fatal unintentional fall related injuries among older adults. Inj Prev 2005;11(2):115-9. doi: 10.1136/ip.2004.005835.

[35] El Tayeb S, Abdalla S, Mørkve O, Heuch I, Van den Bergh G. Injuries in Khartoum state, the Sudan: a household survey of incidence and risk factors. Int J Inj Contr Saf Promot 2014;21(2):144-53. doi: 10.1080/17457300.2013.792283.

[36] Krishnaswamy B, Gnanasambandam U. Falls in older people: national/regional review of India. Chennai, Tamil Nadu, India: WHO background paper to the global report on falls among older persons, 2007

[37] Zhang D, He Y, Liu M, Yang HB, Wu L, Wang JH, et al. Study on incidence and risk factors of fall in the elderly in a rural community in Beijing. Zhonghua Liu Xing Bing Xue Za Zhi 2016;37(5):624-8. doi: 10.3760/cma.j.issn.0254-6450.2016.05.007.

[38] Yiengprugsawan V, Stephan K, McClure R, Kelly M, Seubsman S, Bain C, et al. Risk factors for injury in a national cohort of 87,134 Thai adults. Public Health 2012;126(1):33-9. doi: 10.1016/j.puhe.2011.09.027.

[39] Subramanian SV, Nandy S, Irving M, Gordon D, Lambert H, Davey Smith G. The mortality divide in India: the differential contributions of gender, caste, and standard of living across the life course. Am J Public Health 2006;96(5):818-25. doi: 10.2105/AJPH.2004.060103.

[40] Papalia L, Goldoni M, Spaggiari MC, Roscelli F, Corradi M, Mutti A. Sleep disorders, risk of accidents and traffic accidents in a group of drivers of public transport. G Ital Med Lav Ergon 2012;34(3 Suppl):353-6.

[41] Brassington GS, King AC, Bliwise DL. Sleep problems as a risk factor for falls in a sample of community-dwelling adults aged 64-99 years. J Am Geriatr Soc 2000;48(10):1234-40. doi: 10.1111/j.1532-5415.2000.tb02596.x.

[42] Gureje O, Kola L, Ademola A, Olley BO. Profile, comorbidity and impact of insomnia in the Ibadan study of ageing. Int J Geriatr Psychiatry 2009;24(7):686-93. doi: 10.1002/gps.2180.

[43] Ebrahimi MH, Sadeghi M, Dehghani M, Niiat KS. Sleep habits and road traffic accident risk for Iranian occupational drivers. Int J Occup Med Environ Health 2015;28(2):305-12. doi: 10.13075/ijomeh.1896.00360.

[44] Gale CR, Cooper C, Aihie Sayer A. Prevalence and risk factors for falls in older men and women: The English Longitudinal Study of Ageing. Age Ageing 2016;45(6):789-794. doi: 10.1093/ageing/afw129.

[45] Korniloff K, Häkkinen A, Koponen HJ, Kautiainen H, Järvenpää S, Peltonen M, et al. Relationships between depressive symptoms and self-reported unintentional injuries: the cross-sectional population-based FIN-D2D survey. BMC Public Health 2012;12:516. doi: 10.1186/1471-2458-12-516.

[46] Yamashita T, Noe DA, Bailer AJ. Risk factors of falls in community-dwelling older adults: logistic regression tree analysis. Gerontologist 2012;52(6):822-32. doi: 10.1093/geront/gns043.

[47] Lukaszyk C, Harvey L, Sherrington C, Keay L, Tiedemann A, Coombes J, et al. Risk factors, incidence, consequences and prevention strategies for falls and fall-injury within older indigenous populations: a systematic review. Aust NZ J Public Health 2016;40(6):564-8. doi: 10.1111/1753-6405.12585.

[48] Chang VC, Do MT. Risk factors for falls among seniors: implications of gender. Am J Epidemiol 2015;181(7):521-31. doi: 10.1093/aje/kwu268.

[49] Lord SR, Smith ST, Menant JC. Vision and falls in older people: risk factors and intervention strategies. Clin Geriatr Med 2010;26(4):569-81. doi: 10.1016/j.cger.2010.06.002.

[50] Stalenhoef PA, Diederiks JP, Knottnerus JA, Kester AD, Crebolder HF. A risk model for the prediction of recurrent falls in community-dwelling elderly: a prospective cohort study. J Clin Epidemiol 2002;55(11):1088-94. doi: 10.1016/s0895-4356(02)00502-4.

[51] Benegal V. India: alcohol and public health. Addiction 2005;100(8):1051–6.

[52] Li W, Keegan TH, Sternfeld B, Sidney S, Quesenberry CP Jr, Kelsey JL. Outdoor falls among middle-aged and older adults: a neglected public health problem. Am J Public Health 2006;96(7):1192-200. doi: 10.2105/AJPH.2005.083055.

[53] Ren J, Waclawczyk A, Hartfield D, Yu S, Kuang X, Zhang H, et al. Analysis of fall injuries by body mass index. South Med J 2014;107(5):294-300. doi: 10.1097/SMJ.0000000000000097.

In: Social and Health Issues … ISBN: 978-1-53619-937-6
Editors: S Pengpid, K Peltzer et al.

Chapter 4

NATIONAL DATA ON THE PREVALENCE AND CORRELATES OF RECURRENT FALLS AMONG COMMUNITY-DWELLING OLDER ADULTS IN INDIA IN 2017-2018

Supa Pengpid*[1,2]*, MPH, DrPH, MBA
and Karl Peltzer*[2,3,*]*, MA Clin Psych, PhD, Dr Habil
[1]ASEAN Institute for Health Development, Mahidol University, Salaya, Phutthamonthon, Nakhon Pathom, Thailand
[2]Department of Research Administration and Development, University of Limpopo, Turfloop, South Africa
[3]Department of Psychology, College of Medical and Health Science, Asia University, Taichung, Taiwan

* *Correspondence*: Professor Karl Peltzer, Department of Research Administration and Development, University of Limpopo, Turfloop Campus, Private Bag X1106, Sovenga 0727, South Africa. Email: kfpeltzer@gmail.com.

ABSTRACT

In this chapter we examine the prevalence and correlates of occasional and recurrent falls among older adults in India. The sample included 31,477 older adults (≥60 years) from the cross-sectional 2017-2018 Longitudinal Ageing Study in India (LASI) Wave 1. Results indicate that 12.9% of participants had an occasional fall (1 time) and 9.8% had recurrent falls (≥2 times) in the past two years. In adjusted multinomial logistic regression analysis, factors positively associated with recurrent falls included older age (≥80 years) (Adjusted Relative Risk Ratio-ARRR: 1.29, 95% Confidence Interval-CI: 1.05-1.59), live event stressors (ARRR: 1.64, 95% CI: 1.34-2.01), poor or fair self-rated health status (ARRR: 1.39, 95% CI: 1.08-1.80), insomnia symptoms (ARRR: 1.33, 95% CI: 1.11-1.50), major depressive disorder (ARRR: 1.38, 95% CI: 1.13-1.69), diabetes (ARRR: 1.39, 95% CI: 1.01-1.89), angina (ARRR: 1.49, 95% CI: 1.21-1.85), stroke (ARRR: 1.52, 95% CI: 1.09-2.12), arthritis or rheumatism, osteoporosis or other bone/joint diseases (ARRR: 1.34, 95% CI: 1.06-1.69), high functional disability (ARRR: 1.27, 95% CI: 1.04-1.55), pain (ARRR: 1.30, 95% CI: 1.08-1.57), hearing problem (ARRR: 1.72, 95% CI: 1.09-2.70) and incontinence (ARRR: 1.91, 95% CI: 1.45-2.52). Factors negatively associated with recurrent falls were male sex (ARRR: 0.65, 95% CI: 0.54-0.79), and urban residence (ARRR: 0.82, 95% CI: 0.68-0.97). In addition, food insecurity increased and no schooling decreased the odds of occasional falls. One in ten participants had recurrent falls in the past two years, and several factors associated with recurrent falls were identified that can be used in designing falls prevention programmes in India.

INTRODUCTION

"A fall is defined as an event which results in a person coming to rest inadvertently on the ground or floor or other lower level" [1] "Falls are the second leading cause of accidental or unintentional injury deaths worldwide, and adults older than 65 years of age suffer the greatest number of fatal falls" [1]. "Falls in older adults are a reasonably common occurrence and about 10% of these experience recurrent falls annually" [2] In a national community dwelling survey among older adults (≥60 years) in Mexico, 16% had one fall and 30% had recurrent falls in the past two years [3]. Compared to falling once, older adults with recurrent falls have a higher risk or more severe health consequences [4]. In order to inform falls prevention strategies, it is important to assess the prevalence and risk factors of recurrent falls among older adults [5, 6]. In a study among older adults (N=2049 (≥60 years) in Mumbai and Maharashtra, India, the prevalence of past-year falls was 25.0% [7]. There is a lack of national studies investigating recurrent falls among older adults in India.

Factors associated with recurrent falls among older adults include sociodemographic factors, such as older age [3, 4], being female [4], rural residence [3], life stressors or polyvictimization [8], poor self-rated health status [3, 4], poor mental health, such as depression [3, 4, 9, 10], sleep disturbances [4], poor physical health, such as higher number of diseases [11], hearing problems [3], visual impairment [12], diabetes [3], rheumatoid arthritis [3], urinary incontinence [3, 4, 11], activity-limiting pain [3], and functional disability [3, 4]. The aim of the study was to assess the prevalence and correlates of recurrent falls in a national study among community-dwelling older adults in India.

OUR STUDY

Nationally representative and cross-sectional data of the Longitudinal Ageing Study in India (LASI) Wave 1, 2017-2018 were analyzed; the individual response rate was 87% [13]. "Interview, physical measurement and biomarker data were collected from individuals aged 45 and above and their spouses, regardless of age, in a household survey" [13]. We restricted our analysis to persons aged 60 years and older in this analysis. More methodological details, such as the sampling approach have been described previously [13]. The study was approved by the "Indian Council of Medical Research (ICMR) Ethics Committee and written or oral informed consent was obtained from participants" [13].

MEASURES

Falls were assessed with the question, "How many times have you fallen in the last 2 years?" (Number of times:…) [13]. Responses were coded into 0, 1 (occasional), and 2 or more (recurrent) falls [3].

Sociodemographic variables included age, sex, years of education, and residence status [13].

Food insecurity was assessed with four questions, 1) "In the last 12 months, did you ever reduce the size of your meals or skip meals because there was not enough food at your household? (Yes/No) 2) In the last 12 months, were you hungry but didn't eat because there was not enough food at your household? (Yes/No) 3) In the past 12 months, did you ever not eat for a whole day because there was not enough food at your household? 4) Do you think that you have lost weight in the last 12 months because there was not enough food in your household?" [13]. Any positive response to the four questions was scored as one.

Life event stressors were assessed with four items: 1) ill-treatment ("Have you felt that you were ill-treated in the past year?" Yes/No), 2) victim of violent crime ("In the last 12 months, have you been the victim of a violent crime, such as assault/mugging/threat to life/others?" (Yes/No), 3) disaster exposure causing health effects ("In the last five years, has your health been severely affected by disasters such as floods, landslides, extreme cold and hot weather, cyclone/typhoons, droughts, earthquakes, tsunamis, or any other natural calamities?" (Yes/No), 4) man-made incident causing health effects ("In the last five years, has your health been severely affected by man-made incidents such as riots, terrorism, building collapses, fires, traffic accidents or any other man-made incidents?" (Yes/No) [13]. Any affirmative response was coded with one.

Self-rated health status was sourced from the question, "In general, would you say your health is excellent, very good, good, fair, or poor?" [13] Responses were dichotomized into 1= 1=poor or fair, and 0=good, very good or excellent."

Insomnia symptoms were assessed with four questions: 1) "How often do you have trouble falling asleep?" 2) "How often do you have trouble with waking up during the night?" 3) "How often do you have trouble with waking up too early and not being able to fall asleep again?" 4) "How often did you feel unrested during the day, no matter how many hours of sleep you had?" Responses options were "never, rarely (1-2 nights per week), occasionally (3-4 nights per week), and frequently (5 or more nights per week)" [13]. Insomnia symptoms were coded as "frequently" for the any of the four symptoms as one [14].

Major depressive disorder (MDD) in the past 12 months was assessed with the Health and Retirement Study (HRS) Composite International Diagnostic Interview short form (CIDI-SF) [15], using criteria of the Diagnostic and Statistical Manual of Mental Disorders (DSM; 16). Study respondents were required to "endorse either anhedonia or depressed mood for most of the day for most of a 2-week period or more," and those who fulfilled this criterion "completed an additional seven symptoms: lost interest, feeling tired, change in weight, trouble with sleep, trouble concentrating, feeling down, and thoughts of death." [17]. "Those with a score ≥3 were considered to meet the criteria for having MDD in the previous 12 months; MDD symptomology scores ranged from 0 to 7." [17].

Chronic conditions were assessed as follows: "Has any health professional ever told you that you have…?": 1) "Diabetes or high blood sugar; 2) Chronic lung disease such as asthma, chronic obstructive pulmonary disease/Chronic bronchitis or other chronic lung problems; 3) Stroke; 4) Arthritis or rheumatism, Osteoporosis or other bone/joint diseases, and [5] Incontinence (Yes/No)." [13].

Hypertension or raised blood pressure (BP) was defined as "systolic BP ≥140 mm Hg and/or diastolic BP ≥90 mm Hg (based on the last two averaged of three readings) or where the participant is currently on antihypertensive medication." [18]

Angina was assessed with the "World Health Organization's Rose angina questionnaire" [19], defined on the basis of "discomfort at walking uphill or hurrying, or at an ordinary pace on level ground. Furthermore, the pain should be located at the sternum or in the left chest and arm, causing the patient to stop or slow down, and the pain should resolve within 10 minutes when the patient stops or slows down." [20].

Functional disability was assessed with six items of Activities of Daily Living (ADL) and seven items of Instrumental Activities of Daily Living (IADL) (Yes, No) [21, 22]; Cronbach alpha 0.89 in this study. Responses were summed and trichotomized into 0,1, or ≥2 functional disability (ADL/IADL) items.

Symptom-based pain was classified as "troubled by pain and required some form of medication or treatment for relief of pain" [13].

Vision was sourced from two items, 1) "How good is your eyesight for seeing things at a distance, like recognizing a person across the street (or 20 meters away), whether or not you wear glasses, contacts, or corrective lenses?" And 2) " How good is your eyesight for seeing things up close, like reading an ordinary newspaper print whether or not you wear glasses, contacts, or corrective lenses?" (1=very good to 5=very poor) [13]. Poor near vision and poor far vision were defined as "poor or very poor."

Hearing problem was sourced from the question, "Have you ever been diagnosed with any hearing or ear-related problem or condition?" (Yes/No) [18].

Data analysis

Descriptive statistics were utilised to describe sample and fall characteristics. Adjusted multinomial logistic regression was used to estimate the prevalence of occasional (1 time) and recurrent falls (≥2 times) in the past two years, with no falls in the past 2-years as the reference category. Missing values were excluded from the analysis and $p < 0.05$ was accepted as significant. Considering the multistage sample design into account, STATA software version 13.0 (Stata Corporation, College Station, TX, USA), was utilized for statistical procedures.

OUR FINDINGS

Table 1. Sample characteristics and falls frequency

Variable	Sample	No fall	Occasional falls	Recurrent falls
	%	%	%	%
All	**31477**	**77.3**	**12.9**	**9.8**
Age (years)				
60-69	18979 (58.5)	78.4	12.8	8.8
70-79	9108 (30.2)	76.6	12.5	10.9
≥80	3390 (11.3)	72.5	14.7	12.7
Sex				
Female	16371 (52.5)	74.5	13.9	11.5
Male	15106 (47.5)	80.3	11.8	7.9
Education				
≥1 years	14583 (43.5)	78.1	12.6	9.2
No schooling	16894 (56.5)	76.6	13.1	10.3
Food insecurity				
No	28355 (89.5)	78.1	12.4	9.5
Yes	2747 (10.5)	69.5	17.5	13.0
Residence				
Rural	20730 (70.5)	76.1	13.7	10.2
Urban	10747 (29.5)	80.0	10.9	9.1
Life event stressors	2421 (9.2)	67.2	16.8	16.0
Self-rated health (poor or fair)	14379 (48.6)	72.6	14.7	12.7
Insomnia symptoms	4357 (14.8)	67.3	18.0	14.7
Major depressive disorder	2029 (8.2)	65.4	18.4	16.1
Hypertension	15037 (49.8)	76.6	12.6	10.8
Diabetes	4862 (14.3)	75.2	11.9	12.9
Lung disease	2371 (8.5)	71.5	11.9	16.6
Angina	2805 (9.2)	67.4	17.2	15.4
Stroke	842 (2.7)	66.1	16.9	17.2
Arthritis or rheumatism, osteoporosis or other bone/joint diseases	5586 (19.7)	71.1	14.3	14.6
Functional disability				
0	16361 (48.0)	81.4	11.2	7.4
1	4467 (10.6)	79.5	12.1	8.4
2 or more	11571 (41.4)	61.6	15.2	13.2
Symptom-based pain	3858 (13.9)	67.4	17.5	15.1
Poor near vision	6479 (21.2)	73.6	14.4	12.1
Poor distant vision	6424 (20.7)	72.1	15.1	12.8
Hearing problem	3155 (9.6)	69.9	13.4	16.7
Incontinence	1185 (4.1)	62.3	16.7	21.0

The study subsample consisted of 31,477 older adults (≥60 years) from India. Details of the sample and fall characteristics are shown in table 1. Among older adults in India, 12.9% had an occasional fall (1 time) and 9.8% had recurrent falls (≥2 times) in the past two years (see Table 1).

Associations with occasional and recurrent falls

In adjusted multinomial logistic regression analysis, factors positively associated with recurrent falls included older age (≥80 years) (Adjusted Relative Risk Ratio-ARRR: 1.29, 95% Confidence Interval-CI: 1.05-1.59), live event stressors (ARRR: 1.64, 95% CI: 1.34-2.01), poor or fair self-rated health status (ARRR: 1.39, 95% CI: 1.08-1.80), insomnia symptoms (ARRR: 1.33, 95% CI: 1.11-1.50), major depressive disorder (ARRR: 1.38, 95% CI: 1.13-1.69), diabetes (ARRR: 1.39, 95% CI: 1.01-1.89), angina (ARRR: 1.49, 95% CI: 1.21-1.85), stroke (ARRR: 1.52, 95% CI: 1.09-2.12), arthritis or rheumatism, osteoporosis or other bone/joint diseases (ARRR: 1.34, 95% CI: 1.06-1.69), high functional disability (ARRR: 1.27, 95% CI: 1.04-1.55), pain (ARRR: 1.30, 95% CI: 1.08-1.57), hearing problem (ARRR: 1.72, 95% CI: 1.09-2.70) and incontinence (ARRR: 1.91, 95% CI: 1.45-2.52). Factors negatively associated with recurrent falls were male sex (ARRR: 0.65, 95% CI: 0.54-0.79), and urban residence (ARRR: 0.82, 95% CI: 0.68-0.97). In addition, food insecurity increased and no schooling decreased the odds of occasional falls (see Table 2).

Table 2. Associations with occasional and recurrent falls

Variable	Occasional fall	Recurrent falls
	ARRR (95% CI)	ARRR (95% CI)
Age (years)		
60-69	1 (Reference)	1 (Reference)
70-79	0.95 (0.82, 1.10)	1.10 (0.88, 1.37)
≥80	1.15 (0.87, 1.52)	1.29 (1.05, 1.59)*
Sex		
Female	1 (Reference)	1 (Reference)
Male	0.77 (0.67, 0.88)***	0.65 (0.54, 0.79)***

Table 2. (Continued)

Variable	Occasional fall	Recurrent falls
	ARRR (95% CI)	**ARRR (95% CI)**
Education		
Some	1 (Reference)	1 (Reference)
No schooling	0.86 (0.74, 0.99)*	0.91 (0.75, 1.10)
Food insecurity		
No	1 (Reference)	1 (Reference)
Yes	1.24 (1.05, 1.47)*	1.16 (0.94, 1.42)
Residence		
Rural	1 (Reference)	1 (Reference)
Urban	0.81 (0.67, 0.98)*	0.82 (0.68, 0.97)*
Life event stressors	1.28 (1.08, 1.52)**	1.64 (1.34, 2.01)***
Self-rated health (poor or fair)	1.20 (1.04, 1.38)*	1.39 (1.08, 1.80)*
Insomnia symptoms	1.36 (1.18, 1.58)***	1.33 (1.11, 1.58)***
Major depressive disorder	1.24 (1.03, 1.50)*	1.38 (1.13, 1.69)***
Hypertension	0.95 (0.82, 1.10)	1.04 (0.91, 1.18)
Diabetes	0.96 (0.77, 1.20)	1.39 (1.01, 1.89)*
Lung disease	0.89 (0.71, 1.11)	1.51 (0.88, 2.57)
Angina	1.47 (1.14, 1.88)**	1.49 (1.21, 1.85)***
Stroke	1.36 (1.00, 1.86)	1.52 (1.09, 2.12)*
Arthritis or rheumatism, osteoporosis or other bone/joint diseases	1.04 (0.89, .21)	1.34 (1.06, 1.69)*
Functional disability		
0	1 (Reference)	1 (Reference)
1	1.02 (0.84, 1.24)	1.00 (0.80, 1.25)
2 or more	1.22 (1.01, 1.46)*	1.27 (1.04, 1.55)*
Symptom-based pain	1.25 (1.07, 1.46)**	1.30 (1.08, 1.57)**
Poor near vision	0.96 (0.81, 1,13)	0.96 (0.80, 1.15)
Poor distant vision	1.09 (0.91, 1.29)	1.04 (0.87, 1.24)
Hearing problem	1.07 (0.88, 1.28)	1.72 (1.09, 2.70)*
Incontinence	1.35 (1.05, 1.75)*	1.91 (1.45, 2.52)***

ARRR=Adjusted Relative Risk Ratio; CI=Confidence Interval; ***$p<0.001$; **$p<0.01$; *$p<0.05$.

DISCUSSION

The study found in a national study among community-dwelling older adults (≥60 years) in India in 2017-2018, a prevalence of 12.9% occasional fall (1 time) and 9.8% had recurrent falls (≥2 times) in the past two years, which is lower than in a study among community dwelling older adults (≥60 years) in Mexico (16% had one fall and 30% had recurrent falls in the past two years) [3], and among older adults (≥60 years) in Mumbai, and Maharashtra, India (25.0% falls in the past year) [7].

Consistent with previous research [3, 4], older age, being female and rural residence were associated with higher odds of recurrent falls. The sex differences may be attributed to "differences in higher levels of physical activity, muscle strength, bone density, and fatal fall rates in men than in women" [23]. The higher proportion of recurrent falls in rural than urban areas in this study may be attributed to poorer environmental factors, poorer health status and higher functional disability in rural areas [3, 24, 25].

As found in a previous study among older adults in Ecuador [8], exposure to life stressors or polyvictimization was associated with a higher likelihood of recurrent falls. In agreement with previous studies [3, 4, 9, 10, 26], poor self-rated health status, and poor mental health (depression and sleep disturbances) increased the odds of recurrent falls. It is possible that exposure to life stressors increases depressive symptoms, which in turn may be associated with recurrent falls [8]. In this case, assessing life stressors, sleep problems, and depression in older adults with recurrent falls and stress management and treatment of depression and sleep disturbances may reduce the risk of further falls [8, 26].

In line with a number of previous studies [3, 4, 11], having a number of chronic conditions (hearing problems, diabetes, arthritis or rheumatism, osteoporosis or other bone/joint diseases, urinary incontinence, physical pain, and functional disability were associated with recurrent falls in this study. The risk of falls may be increased because of lower mobility due to having chronic conditions and/or functional disability [27]. "Urge urinary incontinence, but not stress urinary incontinence, is associated with a modest increase in falls." [28]. Unlike some previous research among community-dwelling older adults in Brazil [12], this study did not find a significant association between poor vision and recurrent falls. Furthermore, the findings of this study that compared to occasional fallers, recurrent fallers had a greater number of variables, especially chronic conditions, associated with recurrent falls [3, 10], supporting the notion that recurrent fallers may have a more complex, multifactorial risk profile, increasing the possibility of falling several times [3, 10, 12]. Therefore, multifactorial strategies may be indicated in the prevention of recurrent falls [3].

Study limitations constitute self-reported data and the cross-sectional study design, which may have biased results and no causative conclusions can be drawn. Some studies investigating falls use a shorter reference period as in this study (2 years), which may reduce recall bias.

Conclusion

In this nationally representative sample of older adults in India, one in ten had recurrent falls in the past two years, and several associated factors, such as older age, female sex, rural residence, life event stressors, poor or fair self-rated health, insomnia symptoms, major depressive disorder, diabetes, were identified that can be utilized in targeting falls prevention programmes among older adults in India.

Acknowledgments

The Longitudinal Aging Study in India Project is funded by the Ministry of Health and Family Welfare, Government of India, the National Institute on Aging (R01 AG042778, R01 AG030153), and United Nations Population Fund, India.

References

[1] World Health Organization. Falls, 2018. URL: https://www.who.int/news-room/fact-sheets/detail/falls#:~:text=A%20fall%20is%20defined%20as,though%20most%20are%20non%2Dfatal.

[2] Vaishya R, Vaish A. Falls in older adults are serious. Indian J Orthop 2020;54(1):69-74. doi: 10.1007/s43465-019-00037-x.

[3] Agudelo-Botero M, Giraldo-Rodríguez L, Murillo-González JC, Mino-León D, Cruz-Arenas E. Factors associated with occasional and recurrent falls in Mexican community-dwelling older people. PLoS One 2018;13(2):e0192926. doi: 10.1371/journal.pone.0192926.

[4] Deandrea S, Lucenteforte E, Bravi F, Foschi R, La Vecchia C, Negri E. Risk factors for falls in community-dwelling older people: a systematic review and meta-analysis. Epidemiology 2010;21(5):658-68. doi: 10.1097/EDE.0b013e3181e89905.

[5] Jagnoor J, Ponnaiah M, Varghese M, Ivers R, Kumar R, Prinja S, et al. Potential for establishing an injury surveillance system in India: a review of data sources and reporting systems. BMC Public Health 2020;20(1):1909. doi: 10.1186/s12889-020-09992-9.

[6] Pitchai P, Dedhia HB, Bhandari N, Krishnan D, D'Souza NRJ, Bellara JM. Prevalence, risk factors, circumstances of falls and level of functional independence among geriatric population - A descriptive study. Indian J Public Health 2019;63(1):21-6. doi: 10.4103/ijph.IJPH_332_17.

[7] Reyes-Ortiz CA, Perez-Zepeda MU, Ocampo-Chaparro JM, Campo-Arias A, Borda MG, Holmes HM, et al. Polyvictimization and recurrent falling in older Ecuadorian adults: The mediation role of depressive symptoms. J Aging Health 2021;33(1-2):27-38. doi: 10.1177/0898264320952916.

[8] Launay C, De Decker L, Annweiler C, Kabeshova A, Fantino B, Beauchet O. Association of depressive symptoms with recurrent falls: a cross-sectional elderly population based study and a systematic review. J Nutr Health Aging 2013;17(2):152-7. doi: 10.1007/s12603-012-0370-z.

[9] Stalenhoef PA, Diederiks JP, Knottnerus JA, Kester AD, Crebolder HF. A risk model for the prediction of recurrent falls in community-dwelling elderly: A prospective cohort study. J Clin Epidemiol 2002;55(11):1088-94. doi: 10.1016/s0895-4356(02)00502-4.

[10] Immonen M, Haapea M, Similä H, Enwald H, Keränen N, Kangas M, et al. Association between chronic diseases and falls among a sample of older people in Finland. BMC Geriatr 2020;20(1):225. doi: 10.1186/s12877-020-01621-9.

[11] Abreu DR, Azevedo RC, Silva AM, Reiners AA, Abreu HC. Factors associated with recurrent falls in a cohort of older adults. Cien Saude Colet 2016;21(11):3439-46. doi: 10.1590/1413-812320152111.21512015.

[12] International Institute for Population Sciences (IIPS), NPHCE, MoHFW, Harvard TH Chan School of Public Health (HSPH) and the University of Southern California (USC). Longitudinal Ageing Study in India (LASI) Wave 1, 2017-18, India Report. Mumbai: International Institute for Population Sciences, 2020.

[13] Cho E, Chen TY. The bidirectional relationships between effort-reward imbalance and sleep problems among older workers. Sleep Health 2020;6(3):299-305. doi: 10.1016/j.sleh.2020.01.008.

[14] Kessler RC, Andrews A, Mroczek D, Ustun B, Wittchen HU. The World Health Organization Composite International Diagnostic Interview Short-Form (CIDI-SF). Int J Methods Psychiatr Res 1998;7:171–85.

[15] American Psychiatric Association. Diagnostic and statistical manual of mental disorders (DSM-5), 5th ed. Washington, DC: American Psychiatric Publishing, 2013.

[16] Steffick D. Documentation of affective functioning measures in the health and retirement study, 2000. URL: http://hrsonline. isr.umich.edu/sitedocs/userg/dr-005.pdf.

[17] Chobanian AV, Bakris GL, Black HR, Cushman WC, Green LA, Izzo JL Jr, et al. Seventh report of the Joint National Committee on Prevention, Detection, Evaluation, and Treatment of High Blood Pressure. Hypertension 2003;42(6):1206-52. doi: 10.1161/01.HYP.0000107251.49515.c2.

[18] Rose GA. The diagnosis of ischaemic heart pain and intermittent claudication in field surveys. Bull World Health Organ 1962;27:645–58.

[19] Achterberg S, Soedamah-Muthu SS, Cramer MJ, Kappelle LJ, van der Graaf Y, Algra A; SMART Study Group. Prognostic value of the Rose questionnaire: a validation with future coronary events in the SMART study. Eur J Prev Cardiol 2012;19(1):5-14. doi: 10.1177/1741826710391117.

[20] Katz S, Ford AB, Moskowitz RW, Jackson BA, Jaffe MW. Studies of illness in the aged. the index of adl: A standardized measure of biological and psychosocial function. JAMA 1963;185:914-9. doi: 10.1001/jama.1963.03060120024016.

[21] Lawton MP, Brody EM. Assessment of older people: self-maintaining and instrumental activities of daily living. Gerontologist 1969;9(3):179-86.

[22] Stevens JA, Sogolow ED. Gender differences for non-fatal unintentional fall related injuries among older adults. Inj Prev 2005;11(2):115-9. doi: 10.1136/ip.2004.005835.

[23] Krishnaswamy B, Gnanasambandam U. Falls in older people: national/ regional review of India. Chennai, Tamil Nadu, India: WHO background paper to the global report on falls among older persons, 2007.

[24] Stewart Williams J, Kowal P, Hestekin H, O'Driscoll T, Peltzer K, Yawson A, et al. Prevalence, risk factors and disability associated with fall-related injury in older adults in low- and middle-incomecountries: results from the WHO Study on global AGEing and adult health (SAGE). BMC Med 2015;13:147. doi: 10.1186/s12916-015-0390-8.

[25] Gureje O, Kola L, Ademola A, Olley BO. Profile, comorbidity and impact of insomnia in the Ibadan study of ageing. Int J Geriatr Psychiatry 2009;24(7):686-93. doi: 10.1002/gps.2180.

[26] Pengpid S, Peltzer K. Prevalence and risk factors associated with injurious falls among community-dwelling older adults in Indonesia. Curr Gerontol Geriatr Res 2018;2018:5964305. doi: 10.1155/2018/5964305.

[27] Chiarelli PE, Mackenzie LA, Osmotherly PG. Urinary incontinence is associated with an increase in falls: a systematic review. Aust J Physiother 2009;55(2):89-95. doi: 10.1016/s0004-9514(09)70038-8.

In: Social and Health Issues … ISBN: 978-1-53619-937-6
Editors: S Pengpid, K Peltzer et al.

Chapter 5

PERCEIVED EVERYDAY DISCRIMINATION AMONG OLDER ADULTS IN INDIA: NATIONAL PREVALENCE AND ASSOCIATED FACTORS IN 2017-2018

Karl Peltzer[1,2], MA Clin Psych, PhD, Dr Habil and Supa Pengpid[1,3,*], MPH, DrPH, MBA

[1]Department of Research Administration and Development, University of Limpopo, Turfloop, South Africa

[2]Department of Psychology, College of Medical and Health Science, Asia University, Taichung, Taiwan

[3]ASEAN Institute for Health Development, Mahidol University, Salaya, Phutthamonthon, Nakhon Pathom, Thailand

---

* *Correspondence*: Professor Supa Pengpid, ASEAN Institute for Health Development, Mahidol University, 25/25 Phutthamonthon Road 4, Salaya, Phutthamonton, Nakhon Pathom 73170, Thailand. Email: supaprom@yahoo.com.

Abstract

In this chapter we estimate the prevalence and correlates of perceived everyday discrimination (PED) among older adults in a national population survey in India. The sample included 52,933 older adults (≥50 years) from a cross-sectional national community-dwelling survey in India in 2017-2018. PED was assessed with the Everyday Discrimination Scale (short version). Results indicate that the prevalence of PED was 17.3%, 17.0% among women, and 17.8% among men. In the adjusted logistic regression analysis, food insecurity, scheduled tribes, other backward classes, and functional disability were positively associated with PED, while higher subjective socioeconomic status, Christians and Sikhs were negatively associated with PED. In addition, in unadjusted analysis, no schooling and having a chronic condition were positively associated with PED. Age, sex, marital status and residence status were not associated with PED. Almost one in five older adults in India experienced PED, and several associated factors were identified that may be targeted to reduce PED.

Introduction

"Everyday discrimination refers to acts of interpersonal discrimination that can happen repeatedly over the life course, in a variety of contexts, and includes events such as being treated with disrespect and being given poor services" [1]. Most studies investigating perceived everyday discrimination (PED) have been conducted in high-income countries, such as in the United States, and there has been a lack of studies in low- and middle-income countries, such as in India. In a study among adult Muslim Americans the prevalence of PED was 36.3% [2], among adult American Latinos 30% [3], and among racial/ethnic minorities in the USA PED was 79.6% [4]. In two national studies among adults in Canada, the prevalence of PED was 22.7% [5], and 46.2% [6], respectively. In persons aged 50 years and older in Brazil, the prevalence PED was 16.8% [7], and among pregnant women in rural Gujarat in India, 67.6% reported PED [8]. In older adults (≥50 years) in USA the prevalence of PED was 71.5% [9] in the UK 39.3% (≥60 years) [10].

Older adults may be at higher risk of being discriminated against due to their decreasing social and financial status [11]. Factors associated with PED in adults and older adults include older age [6, 12], younger age [5], younger than 80 years [7], women [5, 6], higher education [6, 7, 12], lower household income [6], not married [5], ethnic minority groups [5, 6, 12], specific ethnic groups [7, 13], urban residence [7], some or many health problems (chronic conditions) [7], functional disability [14], and lack of social trust [7].

To better understand and respond to PED in India, it is necessary to identify these experiences at the national level. The objective of our study was to characterize PED in a nationally representative sample of the Indian older adult population in terms of prevalence and correlates of PED.

OUR STUDY

National cross-sectional data from the Longitudinal Aging Study in India (LASI) Wave 1, 2017-2018 were analyzed (individual response rate 87%) [11]. Face-to-face interviews were conducted by male and female trained research teams with individuals aged 45 and above and their female spouses, regardless of age, in a household survey from 35 states and union territories of India (excluding Sikkim). In this paper, we restricted our sample to 50 years and above. Field teams input responses directly into a laptop computer. Details of the sampling strategy have been described elsewhere [11].The study was approved by the Indian Council of Medical Research (ICMR) Ethics Committee and written or oral informed consent was attained from participants [11].

Measures

PED was assessed with the Everyday Discrimination Scale (short version), including six different social situations, such as less courtesy, service setting, less clever, harassed, afraid, and medical setting [15]. Response options ranged from 1="never" to 6="almost every day," and were dichotomised to 'never'=0 and 'ever' (collapsing those reporting 'less than once a year' or greater into one category)=1.

Covariates consisted of education, age, sex, caste/tribe, religious affiliation, urban and rural residence [11]. Scheduled tribes, scheduled castes, and other backward classes have been historically disadvantaged due to various socio-economic factors like wealth or traditional occupation and are given reservation by the government of India [16]. Subjective socioeconomic status was assessed with the question, "Please imagine a ten-step ladder, where at the bottom are the people who are the worst off – who have the least money, least education, and the worst jobs or no jobs, and at the top of the ladder are the people who are the best off – those who have the most money, most education, and best jobs. Please indicate the number (1-10) on the rung on the ladder where you would place yourself." [11]. Steps 1 to 3 on the socioeconomic ladder were defined as low, 4-5 as medium, and 6-10 as high.

Food insecurity was assessed with four questions, 1) "In the last 12 months, did you ever reduce the size of your meals or skip meals because there was not enough food at your household? (Yes/No) 2) In the last 12 months, were you hungry but didn't eat because there was not enough food at your household? (Yes/No) 3) In the past 12 months, did you ever not eat for a whole day because there was not enough food at your household? 4) Do you think that you have lost weight in the last 12 months because there was not enough food in your household?" [11]. Any positive response to the four questions was scored as one.

Functional disability was measured with 6 items of Activities of Daily Living (ADL) and 7 items of Instrumental Activities of Daily Living (IADL) [17, 18]. Cronbach alpha for the ADL measure was 0.86 and for the IADL measure 0.88. Responses were "Yes/No." Responses were dichotomized into 0 and ≥1 ADL and IADL items.

Chronic conditions were sourced from the question, "Has any health professional ever told you that you have…?": 1) " Hypertension or high blood pressure (Yes/No); 2) Diabetes or high blood sugar; 3) Cancer or malignant tumor; 4) Chronic lung disease such as asthma, chronic obstructive pulmonary disease/Chronic bronchitis or other chronic lung problems; 5) Chronic heart diseases such as Coronary heart disease (heart attack or Myocardial Infarction), congestive heart failure, or other chronic heart problems; 6) Stroke; 7) Arthritis or rheumatism, Osteoporosis or other bone/joint diseases, and 8) High cholesterol (Yes/No)." [11]. Summed responses were trichotomized into 0, 1, or 2 or more chronic conditions.

Data analysis

Considering the clustered study design, data analyses were conducted with "STATA software version 15.0 (Stata Corporation, College Station, TX, USA)." Unadjusted and adjusted logistic regression analyses were used to calculate associations between independent variables and PED. Variables with a significance level of <0.05 in univariate analyses were subsequently included in the multivariable model. Covariates were selected based on previous literature review [5-6, 12-14]. *P*-values of below 0.05 were accepted as significant and missing values were excluded from the analysis.

FINDINGS

The sample included 52,933 older adults (50 years and older), 53.3% were female and 46.7% male. More than half of the participants (53.0%) had no formal education, and 69.0% were residing in rural areas. One in ten participants (9.9%) had food insecurity, 38.2% had low subjective socioeconomic status, and 70.1% were married. Majority were Hindus (82.4%) and 46.7% belonged to other backward classes. More than one in five participants (21.2%) had multiple chronic conditions, and 33.8% had two or more functional disabilities. The prevalence of PED was 17.3%, 17.0% among women, and 17.8% among men (see Table 1).

Table 1. Sample characteristics of older adults (≥50 years) in India, 2017-2018 (N=52,933)

Variable	Variable specification	Sample	Perceived everyday discrimination
		%	%
All			**17.3**
Age in years	50-59	38.1	16.8
	60-69	36.2	18.1
	70-79	18.7	17.2
	80 or more	7.0	16.7
Sex	Female	53.3	17.0
	Male	46.7	17.8
Education	≥1 years	47.0	14.9
	No schooling	53.0	19.5
Subjective socioeconomic status	Low	38.2	21.8
	Medium	37.4	15.2
	High	24.4	13.6
Food insecurity	No	90.1	15.3
	Yes	9.9	35.5
Marital status	Not married	29.9	18.4
	Married	70.1	16.9
Caste/tribe	None of the below	25.1	14.4
	Scheduled tribe	19.4	19.5
	Scheduled caste	8.8	15.8
	Other backward class	46.7	18.7
Religious affiliation	Hindu	82.4	17.7
	Muslim	11.3	17.7
	Christian	2.8	12.6
	Sikh	1.8	7.2
	Other or none	1.7	15.2
Residence	Rural	69.0	18.2
	Urban	31.0	15.3
Functional disability	0	55.5	14.7
	1	10.7	17.0
	2 or more	33.8	21.9
Chronic conditions	0	50.4	16.3
	1	28.4	18.0
	2-8	21.2	18.9

Frequency distribution of everyday discrimination

Table 2 shows the frequency distributions for the six types of PED measured in this study. The highest any PED was for less courtesy (12.9%), followed by not smart (7.9%), service access (6.8%), harassed (6.3%), medical setting (6.1%) and afraid (5.2%) (see Table 2).

Table 2. Frequency distribution of everyday discrimination

Everyday discrimination items	**Almost every day**	**At least once a week**	**A few times a month**	**A few times a year**	**Less than once a year**	**Never**
	%	%	%	%	%	%
[Less courtesy] "You are treated with less courtesy or respect than other people."	2.0	0.9	2.4	2.5	4.3	87.9
[Service access] "You receive poorer service than other people at restaurants or stores."	0.4	0.5	1.0	2.0	2.8	93.2
[Not smart] "People act as if they think you are not smart."	0.5	0.7	1.3	2.2	3.1	92.1
[Afraid] "People act as if they are afraid of you."	0.4	0.4	1.0	1.5	1.8	94.8
[Harassed] "You are threatened or harassed."	0.4	0.5	1.0	1.7	2.7	93.7
[Medical setting] "You receive poorer service or treatment than other people from doctors or hospitals."	0.3	0.4	1.0	1.7	2.7	93.9

Associations with everyday discrimination

In the adjusted logistic regression analysis, food insecurity, scheduled tribes, other backward classes, and functional disability were positively associated with PED, while higher subjective socioeconomic status, Christians, and Sikhs were negatively associated with PED. In addition, in unadjusted analysis, no schooling and having a chronic condition were positively associated with PED. Age, sex, marital status and residence status were not associated with PED (see Table 3).

Table 3. Associations with perceived everyday discrimination

Variable	Variable specification	COR (95% CI)	AOR (95% CI)
Age in years	50-59	1 (Reference)	---
	60-69	1.09 (0.93, 1.27)	
	70-79	1.02 (0.87, 1.20)	
	80 or more	0.99 (0.82, 1.20)	
Sex	Female	1 (Reference)	---
	Male	1.06 (0.93, 1.20)	
Education	≥1 years	1 (Reference)	1 (Reference)
	No schooling	1.39 (1.21, 1.59)***	1.13 (0.98, 1.30)
Subjective socioeconomic status	Low	1 (Reference)	1 (Reference)
	Medium	0.64 (0.57, 0.72)***	0.71 (0.63, 0.82)***
	High	0.56 (0.46, 0.69)***	0.65 (0.52, 0.81)***
Food insecurity	No	1 (Reference)	1 (Reference)
	Yes	3.05 (2.70, 3.45)***	2.67 (2.35, 3.04)***
Marital status	Not married	1 (Reference)	---
	Married	0.90 (0.78, 1.03)	
Caste/tribe	None of the below	1 (Reference)	1 (Reference)
	Scheduled tribe	1.45 (1.29, 1.62)***	1.19 (1.04, 1.35)**
	Scheduled caste	1.12 (0.97, 1.30)	0.97 (0.82, 1.16)
	Other backward class	1.37 (1.19, 1.58)***	1.25 (1.07, 1.46)**
Religious affiliation	Hindu	1 (Reference)	1 (Reference)
	Muslim	1.00 (0.76, 1.32)	0.99 (0.75, 1.31)
	Christian	0.67 (0.55, 0.83)***	0.68 (0.55. 0.84)***
	Sikh	0.36 (0.29, 0.46)***	0.38 (0.30, 0.48)***
	Other or none	0.83 (0.61, 1.14)	0.82 (0.58, 1.14)
Residence	Rural	1 (Reference)	---
	Urban	0.81 (0.66, 1.00)	
Functional disability	0	1 (Reference)	1 (Reference)
	1	1.19 (1.04, 1.36)*	1.10 (0.96, 1.26)
	2 or more	1.63 (1.42, 1.88)***	1.37 (1.20, 1.56)***
Chronic conditions	0	1 (Reference)	1 (Reference)
	1	1.13 (1.01, 1.25)*	1.11 (1.00, 1.25)
	2-8	1.19 (0.96, 1.48)	1.21 (0.99, 1.49)

COR=Crude Odds Ratio; AOR=Adjusted Odds ratio; CI=Confidence Interval; *$p<0.05$;**$p<0.01$; ***$p<0.001$.

DISCUSSION

The study aimed to estimate the prevalence and correlates of PED in older adults in a national population survey in India in 2017-2018. Results show for the first time that the prevalence of PED was 17.3% in India, which is similar to a study among older adults (≥50 years) in Brazil (16.8%) [7], and lower than among adult populations, e.g., among pregnant women in rural Gujarat in India (67.6%) [8], studies in USA (Muslim Americans 36.3% [2], American Latinos 30% [3], and among racial/ethnic minorities 79.6% [4], and Canada (22.7% [5] and 46.2% [6], and in studies among older adults (≥50 years) in USA (71.5%) [9] and in the UK (39.3%, ≥60 years) [10]. Some of these differences may be related to different assessment modalities. For example, this study measured PED with six types, the Brazil study with five types [7], the UK study five types [10] and some of the North American studies with nine or ten types [3, 12]. However, it appears PED among older adults is less common in India than in high-income countries. It is possible that older adults in middle-income countries, such as in India and Brazil, enjoy more respect than in high-income countries [19] thereby reducing PED.

In consistence with some studies [6], this study showed an association between lower socioeconomic status (subjective socioeconomic status, food insecurity, and no education) and PED. Compared to people with lower socioeconomic status, people with higher socioeconomic status (having some education, not having food insecurity, and higher subjective socioeconomic status) may be less likely to experience PED due to lower exposure to discriminatory situations [20]. Compared to general castes, participants belonging to lower castes (scheduled tribes and other backward classes) were more likely to report PED. Similar results were found in a study among rural pregnant women in India [8], emphasising the negative role of the caste system in India on discrimination [8].

While some studies found age, sex, marital status and residence status differences in the prevalence of PED [5-7, 12], we did not find significant differences. While some previous studies found a higher prevalence of PED in racial or ethnic minority groups [5-7], this study found lower odds of PED in religious minorities (Christians and Sikhs) in India. Consistent with former research [7, 14], this study found a positive association between functional disability and PED and in an unadjusted analysis between having a chronic condition and PED. It is possible that a stigmatization process that devalues a person's identity, in particular in those with functional disability, leads to higher interpersonal mistreatment and PED [14, 21].

Strength and limitations of the study

Study strengths included the use of standardized measures adapted from the Health and Retirement Study and a large, nationally representative sample of older adults in India. The self-report of most data may have their limitations. It is possible that participants underreported PED. Due to the cross-sectional design of the study, we were unable to determine the direction of the assessed associations.

CONCLUSION

Almost one in five older adults in India experienced PED, and several associated factors were identified. Factors associated with PED were food insecurity, lower subjective socioeconomic status, lower castes (scheduled tribes, and other backward classes), and functional disability and not Christians and Sikhs. These associated factors may be targeted to reduce PED.

ACKNOWLEDGMENTS

The Longitudinal Aging Study in India Project is funded by the Ministry of Health and Family Welfare, Government of India, the National Institute on

Aging (R01 AG042778, R01 AG030153), and United Nations Population Fund, India.

REFERENCES

[1] Essed P. Understanding everyday racism: an interdisciplinary theory. Thousand Oaks, CA: Sage, 1991.

[2] Zainiddinov H. Racial and ethnic differences in perceptions of discrimination among Muslim Americans. Ethnic Racial Stud 2016; 39:15, 2701-21. doi: 10.1080/01419870.2016.1164877.

[3] Pérez DJ, Fortuna L, Alegria M. Prevalence and Correlates of Everyday Discrimination among U.S. Latinos. J Commun Psychol 2008;36(4):421-33. doi:10.1002/jcop.20221.

[4] Gong F, Xu J, Takeuchi DT. Racial and ethnic differences in perceptions of everyday discrimination. Sociol Race Ethnicity 2017;3(4):506–21.

[5] Godley J. Everyday discrimination in Canada: Prevalence and patterns. CJS 2018;43(2) 111-42.

[6] Hyman I, O'Campo P, Ansara DL, Siddiqi A, Forte T, Smylie J et al. Prevalence and predictors of everyday discrimination in Canada: Findings from the Canadian Community Health Survey, 2019. URL: https://www.wellesleyinstitute.com/wp-content/uploads/2019/10/Prevalence-and-Predictors.pdf.

[7] Braga LS, Caiaffa WT, Ceolin APR, de Andrade FB, Lima-Costa MF. Perceived discrimination among older adults living in urban and rural areas in Brazil: a national study (ELSI-Brazil). BMC Geriatr 2019;19(1):67. doi: 10.1186/s12877-019-1076-4.

[8] Khubchandani J, Soni A, Fahey N, Raithatha N, Prabhakaran A, Byatt N, et al. Caste matters: perceived discrimination among women in rural India. Arch Womens Ment Health 2018;21(2):163-70. doi: 10.1007/s00737-017-0790-1.

[9] Ayalon L, Gum AM. The relationships between major lifetime discrimination, everyday discrimination, and mental health in three racial and ethnic groups of older adults. Aging Ment Health 2011;15(5):587-94. doi: 10.1080/13607863.2010.543664.

[10] Shankar A, Hinds P. Perceived discrimination: Associations with physical and cognitive function in older adults. Health Psychol 2017;36(12):1126-34. doi: 10.1037/hea0000522.

[11] International Institute for Population Sciences (IIPS), NPHCE, MoHFW, Harvard TH Chan School of Public Health (HSPH) and the University of Southern California (USC). Longitudinal Ageing Study in India (LASI) Wave 1, 2017-18. India Report. Mumbai: International Institute for Population Sciences, 2020.

[12] Mouzon DM, Taylor RJ, Nguyen AW, Ifatunji MA, Chatters LM. Everyday discrimination typologies among older African Americans: Gender and

socioeconomic status. J Gerontol B Psychol Sci Soc Sci 2020;75(9):1951-60. doi: 10.1093/geronb/gbz088.

[13] Keys HM, Noland GS, De Rochars MB, Taylor TH, Blount S, Gonzales M. Perceived discrimination in Bateyes of the Dominican Republic: Results from the Everyday Discrimination Scale and implications for public health programs. BMC Public Health 2019;19(1):1513. doi: 10.1186/s12889-019-7773-2.

[14] Namkung EH, Carr D. Perceived interpersonal and institutional discrimination among persons with disability in the US: Do patterns differ by age? Soc Sci Med 2019;239:112521. doi: 10.1016/j.socscimed.2019.112521.

[15] Sternthal M, Slopen N, Williams DR. Racial disparities in health: how much does stress really matter? Du Bois Review 2011;8:95-113.

[16] Legal Affairs. Issues of social justice: Scheduled castes and scheduled tribes and other backward classes: An unfinished national agenda. URL: https://legalaffairs.gov.in/sites/default/files/IX.ISSUESOF%20SOCIAL%20JUSTICE%20%20SCHEDULED%20CASTES%20%20AND%20SCHEDULED%20TRIBES%20AND%20OTHER%20BACKWARD%20CLASSESAN%20UNFINISHED%20NATION.pdf.

[17] Katz S, Ford AB, Moskowitz RW, Jackson BA, Jaffe MW. Studies of illness in the aged. the index of ADL: a standardized measure of biological and psychosocial function. JAMA 1963;185:914-9. doi: 10.1001/jama.1963.03060120024016.

[18] Lawton MP, Brody EM. Assessment of older people: self-maintaining and instrumental activities of daily living. Gerontologist 1969;9(3):179-86.

[19] Van den Heuvel W. Discrimination against older people. Rev Clin Gerontol 2012; 22(4):293-300. doi:10.1017/S095925981200010X

[20] Rippon I, Kneale D, de Oliveira C, Demakakos P, Steptoe A. Perceived age discrimination in older adults. Age Ageing 2014;43(3):379-86. doi: 10.1093/ageing/aft146.

[21] Link BG, Phelan JC. Conceptualizing stigma. Annual Rev Sociol 2001;27(1):363-85.

In: Social and Health Issues ... ISBN: 978-1-53619-937-6
Editors: S Pengpid, K Peltzer et al.

Chapter 6

ELDER ABUSE AMONG COMMUNITY DWELLING OLDER ADULTS IN INDIA: PREVALENCE AND CORRELATES OF A NATIONAL SURVEY IN 2017-2018

Supa Pengpid[1,2], MPH, DrPH, MBA
and Karl Peltzer[2,3,*], MA Clin Psych, PhD, Dr Habil
[1]ASEAN Institute for Health Development, Mahidol University, Salaya, Phutthamonthon, Nakhon Pathom, Thailand
[2]Department of Research Administration and Development, University of Limpopo, Turfloop, South Africa
[3]Department of Psychology, College of Medical and Health Science, Asia University, Taichung, Taiwan

* *Correspondence:* Professor Karl Peltzer, Department of Research Administration and Development, University of Limpopo, Turfloop Campus, Private Bag X1106, Sovenga 0727, South Africa. Email: kfpeltzer@gmail.com.

Abstract

In this chapter we estimate the prevalence and correlates of elder abuse in community-dwelling older adults in India. The study sample included 31,477 older adults (≥60 years) from a cross-sectional national population-based survey in India in 2017-2018. Results indicate that the prevalence of elder abuse in the past 12 months was 5.2%. In the adjusted logistic regression analysis, food insecurity, functional disability, loneliness, depressive symptoms, and current tobacco use were positively associated with elder abuse, while higher subjective socioeconomic status, Christian and Sikh were negatively associated with elder abuse. In addition, in unadjusted analysis, no schooling, belonging to the Scheduled castes, and poor cognition were positively and urban residence was negatively associated with elder abuse. One in twenty older adults in India experienced elder abuse, and several associated factors were identified which could be targeted in elder abuse prevention efforts.

Introduction

According to the World Health Organization "elder abuse is a single or repeated act, or lack of appropriate action, occurring within any relationship where there is an expectation of trust, which causes harm or distress to an older person. This type of violence constitutes a violation of human rights and includes physical, sexual, psychological, and emotional abuse; financial and material abuse; abandonment; neglect; and serious loss of dignity and respect [1]." Elder abuse constitutes a major public health problem [1], and has been associated with premature mortality, mental and physical morbidity [2], Globally, in a systematic review of 52 studies of community dwelling older adults (≥60 years), 15.7% reported some form of abuse in the past 12 months, including "psychological abuse 11.6%, financial abuse 6.8%, neglect 4.2%, physical abuse 2.6%, and sexual abuse 0.9%" [3]. In seven states in India in 2011, the prevalence of elder abuse was 11.4% [4], in a rural area of West Bengal (2015-2017), 25.6% had experienced abuse [5], among non-institutionalised older adults (≥65 years) 14% reported mistreatment [6], among 541 community-dwelling older adults (≥60 years) in several states in India in 2010, 28.8% experienced elder abuse [7], and in rural Puducherry, India, 50.2% of 243 older adults reported elder abuse [8]. There is a lack of recent national data on elder abuse in India.

According to a systematic review [9], factors associated with elder abuse include "age, sex, marital status, educational level, income, family arrangement, social support, solitude, mental disorder, depression, suicide attempt, dependence on others in daily activities, cognitive function, chronic diseases, alcohol or drug abuse, among others." In studies in India, multimorbidity [4], functional disability [5, 10], low social cohesion [6, 7], lower education, and older age [8] were associated with elder abuse. In studies from China, "younger age, lower income levels, depression, cognitive impairment, and lack of social support" [11], depression [12] and loneliness [13] were associated with elder abuse. This study aimed to estimate the prevalence and correlates of elder abuse in a national community-dwelling older adult population in India.

OUR STUDY

National cross-sectional data from the Longitudinal Aging Study in India (LASI) Wave 1, 2017-2018 were analyzed (individual response rate 87%) [14]. Face-to-face interviews were conducted by male and female trained research teams with persons aged 45 and older and their female spouses, regardless of age, in a household survey from 35 states and union territories of India (excluding Sikkim). Field teams input responses directly into a laptop computer [14]. We restricted our sample to those who were 60 years and older. Details of the sampling strategy have been described elsewhere [14]. The Indian Council of Medical Research (ICMR) Ethics Committee approved the study and written/oral informed consent was attained from participants [14].

Measures

Elder abuse was assessed with the question, "Have you felt that you were ill-treated in the past year? (Yes, No) [14]. This measure was found to be valid in estimating the overall prevalence of elder abuse [7, 15, 16]. A follow-up question measured the frequency and type of ill treatment experienced the past year. Response options were 1) Physical, 2) Verbal/Disrespect, 3) Economic exploitation, 4) Emotional/Psychological, and 5) Neglect (Within household: Yes, No; outside household: Yes, No) [14].

Sociodemographic variables

Covariates consisted of education (none and ≥1 years), age, sex (male, female), marital status (currently married vs. widowed/divorced/separated/deserted/live-in relationship/never married), caste, urban and rural residence [14]. Subjective socioeconomic status was assessed with the question, "Please imagine a ten-step ladder, where at the bottom are the people who are the worst off – who have the least money, least education, and the worst jobs or no jobs, and at the top of the ladder are the people who are the best off – those who have the most money, most education, and best jobs. Please indicate the number (1-10) on the rung on the ladder where you would place yourself" [14]. Steps 1 to 3 on the socioeconomic ladder were defined as low, 4-5 as medium, and 6-10 as high.

Food insecurity was assessed with four questions, 1) "In the last 12 months, did you ever reduce the size of your meals or skip meals because there was not enough food at your household? (Yes/No) 2). In the last 12 months, were you hungry but didn't eat because there was not enough food at your household? (Yes/No) 3) In the past 12 months, did you ever not eat for a whole day because there was not enough food at your household? 4) Do you think that you have lost weight in the last 12 months because there was not enough food in your household?" [14]. Any positive response to the four questions was scored as one.

Protective factor variables

Protective factor variables included religion, organized religiosity, and social network.

Organizational religiosity was assessed with the question, "In the past year, how often have you attended religious services (at a temple/mosque/church, etc.)?" Response options were grouped into 1 (low) = not at all, 2 (medium) = 1-3 times a month or 1 or more times a year, and 3(high) = once a week or more than once a week or every day [14].

Social network was measured with 11 items, e.g., "Eat-out-of-house (restaurant/hotel)" [14]. Responses were coded 1 = daily to at least once a month and 0 = rarely/once a year or never (Cronbach's alpha 0.67).

Health status variables

Functional disability was assessed with six items of Activities of Daily Living (ADL) and seven items of Instrumental Activities of Daily Living (IADL) (Yes, No) [17, 18]. Cronbach alpha was 0.87 for ADL and 0.90 for IADL in this study. Responses were trichotomized into 0, 1, and ≥2 ADL and IADL items.

Chronic conditions were sourced from the question, "Has any health professional ever told you that you have…?": 1) " Hypertension or high blood pressure (Yes/No); 2) Diabetes or high blood sugar; 3) Cancer or malignant tumor; 4) Chronic lung disease such as asthma, chronic obstructive pulmonary disease/Chronic bronchitis or other chronic lung problems; 5) Chronic heart diseases such as Coronary heart disease (heart attack or Myocardial Infarction), congestive heart failure, or other chronic heart problems; 6) Stroke; 7) Arthritis or rheumatism, Osteoporosis or other bone/joint diseases, 8) neurological or psychiatric problems, and 9) High cholesterol (Yes/No)." [14]. Summed responses were trichotomized into 0, 1, or 2 or more chronic conditions.

Depressive symptoms were measured with the Centre for Epidemiological Studies Depression Scale (CES-D-10) [19]. The overall scores ranged from zero to 10 and scores of four or more were classified as having depressive symptoms [20]. (Cronbach α was 0.79 in this study).

Loneliness was sourced from one item of the CES-D-10 [19]: "How often did you feel lonely in the past week?" Response options were coded into no loneliness: "0 = rarely or none of the time (<1 day) or sometimes or 1–2 days/week and 1 = severe loneliness: 3 = occasionally or all the time or 3–7 days/week)."

Current tobacco use was sourced from two items, 1) "Do you currently smoke any tobacco products (cigarettes, bidis, cigars, hookah, cheroot, etc.)? and 2) Do you use smokeless tobacco (such as chewing tobacco, gutka, pan masala, etc.)?" (Yes, No) [14].

Heavy episodic alcohol use was measured with the item, "In the last 3 months, how frequently on average, have you had at least 5 or more drinks on one occasion?" [14], and defined as "one to three days per month, one to four days per week, five or more days per week, or daily."

Cognitive functioning was assessed with tests for immediate and delayed word recall, serial 7s, and orientation [21]. Poor cognitive functioning was defined as the lowest quintile.

Data analysis

Considering the clustered study design, data analyses were conducted with "STATA software version 15.0 (Stata Corporation, College Station, TX, USA)." Unadjusted and adjusted logistic regression analyses were used to calculate the predictors (sociodemographic, protective, and health variables) of elder abuse. Variables that were significant in the univariate analysis were subsequently included in the multivariable logistic regression model. *P*-values of below 0.05 were accepted as significant and missing values were excluded from the analysis.

FINDINGS

The sample included 31,477 older adults (60 years and older), 52.5% were female and 47.5% male. More than half of the participants (56.5%) had no formal education, 61.6% were married, and 70.5% were residing in rural areas. One in ten participants (10.5%) had food insecurity, 82.2% were Hindus, 26.2% attended at least weekly religious services, and 27.4% had a high social network. In terms of health status variables, 55.0% had at least one functional disability, 53.4% had at least one chronic condition, 14.9% had loneliness, 30.2% depressive symptoms, 33.7% current tobacco use, 2.6% heavy episodic alcohol use and 18.5% poor cognitive functioning. The overall prevalence of elder abuse in the past 12 months was 5.2% (see Table 1). Among those who reported to have been abused, 14.4% were abused

Table 1. Sample characteristics of older adults (≥60 years) in India, 2017-2018

Variable	Sample	Elder abuse
	N (%)	%
Sociodemographic factors		
All	**31477**	**5.2**
Age in years		
60-69	18979 (58.5)	5.1
70-79	9108 (30.2)	5.8
80 or more	3390 (11.3)	4.2
Sex		
Female	16371 (52.5)	5.6
Male	15106 (47.5)	4.8
Education		
≥1 years	14583 (43.5)	4.3
No schooling	16894 (56.5)	5.9
Subjective socioeconomic status		
Low	10664 (39.1)	6.9
Medium	11757 (36.7)	4.6
High	7836 (24.2)	3.4
Caste/tribe		
None of below	8224 (25.8)	4.4
Scheduled caste	5141 (19.4)	6.7
Scheduled tribe	5173 (8.3)	4.5
Other backward class	11887 (46.4)	5.2

Table 1. (Continued)

Variable	Sample	Elder abuse
	N (%)	%
Food insecurity		
No	28355 (89.5)	4.3
Yes	2747 (10.5)	13.0
Marital status		
Married	19926 (61.6)	4.9
Widowed/separated/never married	11545 (38.4)	5.8
Residence		
Rural	20730 (70.5)	5.8
Urban	10747 (29.5)	3.8
Protective factors		
Religion		
Hindu	23047 (82.2)	5.5
Muslim	3732 (11.3)	5.1
Christian	3151 (2.9)	1.7
Sikh	979 (1.9)	1.9
Other or none	567 (1.7)	3.3
Organizational religiosity		
None	8711 (29.3)	5.0
<weekly	13447 (44.4)	5.6
≥weekly	9262 (26.2)	4.8
Social network		
Low	13047 (44.4)	5.1
Medium	9096 (28.2)	5.3
High	8871 (27.4)	5.4
Health status		
Functional disability		
0	16361 (48.0)	3.7
1	3367 (10.6)	4.5
2 or more	11571 (41.4)	7.2
Chronic conditions		
0	14336 (46.6)	5.0
1	9242 (29.3)	5.6
2 or more	7799 (24.1)	5.2
Loneliness	4078 (14.9)	9.7
Depressive symptoms	8506 (30.2)	8.7
Current tobacco use	9845 (33.7)	6.1
Heavy episodic alcohol use	1022 (2.6)	5.5
Poor cognitive functioning	4545 (18.5)	6.4

frequently, 52.8% occasionally and 32.8% a few times. Among those participants who elder abuse, 13.3% and 13.1% reported physical abuse within household and outside household, respectively, 53.4% and 39.6% had verbal abuse, 17.8% and 13.7% had economic exploitation, 29.4% and 21.0% emotional/psychological abuse, and 38.1% and 25.7% neglect within household and outside household, respectively.

Associations between elder abuse

In the adjusted logistic regression analysis, food insecurity, functional disability, loneliness, depressive symptoms, and current tobacco use were positively associated with elder abuse, while higher subjective socioeconomic status, Christian and Sikh were negatively associated with elder abuse. In addition, in unadjusted analysis, no schooling, belonging to the scheduled castes, and poor cognition were positively and urban residence was negatively associated with elder abuse (see Table 2).

Table 2. Associations with elder abuse

Variable	COR (95% CI)	AOR (95% CI)
Sociodemographic factors		
Age in years		
60-69	1 (Reference)	---
70-79	1.13 (0.93, 1.38)	
80 or more	0.82 (0.63, 1.06)	
Sex (Male)	0.87 (0.73, 1.03)	---
Education (No schooling)	1.39 (1.16, 1.68)***	1.03 (0.83, 1.27)
Subjective socioeconomic status		
Low	1 (Reference)	1 (Reference)
Medium	0.66 (0.54, 0.80)***	0.79 (0.64, 0.98)*
High	0.48 (0.35, 0.65)***	0.64 (0.43, 0.94)*
Caste/tribe		
None of below	1 (Reference)	1 (Reference)
Scheduled caste	1.54 (1.23, 1.93)***	1.18 (0.90, 1.55)
Scheduled tribe	1.00 (0.72, 1.39)	0.88 (0.60, 1.30)
Other backward class	1.18 (0.94, 1.47)	1.02 (0.79, 1.31)
Food insecurity	3.34 (2.78, 3.99)***	2.58 (2.09, 3.18)***
Marital status (Married)	0.84 (0.70, 1.01)	---
Residence (Urban)	0.64 (0.49, 0.83)***	0.87 (0.61, 1.24)

Table 2. (Continued)

Variable	COR (95% CI)	AOR (95% CI)
Protective factors		
Religion		
Hindu	1 (Reference)	1 (Reference)
Muslim	0.92 (0.73, 1.16)	0.98 (0.74, 1.29)
Christian	0.29 (0.16, 0.52)***	0.23 (0.12, 0.41)***
Sikh	0.34 (0.21, 0.56)***	0.45 (0.27, 0.75)**
Other or none	0.58 (0.26, 1.32)	0.47 (0.17, 1.31)
Organizational religiosity		
None	1 (Reference)	---
<weekly	1.12 (0.91, 1.38)	
≥weekly	0.95 (0.77, 1.17)	
Social network		
Low	1 (Reference)	---
Medium	1.06 (0.87, 1.29)	
High	1.07 (0.85, 1.34)	
Health status		
Functional disability		
0	1 (Reference)	1 (Reference)
1	1.23 (0.93, 1.63)	1.02 (0.73, 1.42)
2 or more	2.03 (1.69, 2.43)***	1.66 (1.32, 2.08)***
Chronic conditions		
0	1 (Reference)	---
1	1.11 (0.90, 1.38)	
2 or more	1.03 (0.84, 1.27)	
Loneliness	2.31 (1.84, 2.89)***	1.35 (1.02, 1.78)*
Depressive symptoms	2.44 (2.05, 2.91)***	1.58 (1.27, 1.97)***
Current tobacco use	1.28 (1.08, 1.52)**	1.25 (1.03, 1.52)*
Heavy episodic alcohol use	1.07 (0.70, 1.63)	---
Poor cognitive functioning	1.37 (1.04, 1.80)*	1.00 (0.98, 1.03)

CI = Confidence Interval; ***$p < 0.001$;**$p < 0.01$; *$p < 0.05$; COR = Crude Odds Ratio; AOR = Adjusted Odds Ratio

DISCUSSION

The study aimed to estimate the prevalence and correlates of elder abuse in older adults in a national population survey in India in 2017-2018. Results show for the first time that the national prevalence of elder abuse was 5.2% in the past 12 months in India, which seems to be lower than global estimates (15.7% in the past 12 months) [3], and various local studies in India (11.4%

in seven states in 2011) [4], (25.6% in rural area of West Bengal, 2015-2017) [5], (14%, ≥65 years, non-institutionalised in Chennai) [6], (28.8%, ≥60 years, non-institutionalised, in several states in 2010) [7], and (50.2% in rural Puducherry) [8]. Some of the differences in the prevalence rates of elder abuse may be related to the measurements used. If multiple item measures, e.g., in the Puducherry study [8] were used to assess elder abuse, it appears higher elder abuse rates were found than in single item measures, as in this study and in the seven states India study [4,10]. Further research is, however, needed to explain the lower prevalence of elder abuse in this national study compared to various local studies.

Consistent with some previous research [8, 9, 11], lower socioeconomic status (lower subjective socioeconomic status, food insecurity, and in univariate analysis, no schooling). This may indicate that older adults with less access to financial resources may be more vulnerable to elder abuse [9]. Contrary to expectation, religious minority groups (Christians and Sikhs) had lower odds of elder abuse than Hindus (religious majority). Unlike some previous investigations [8, 9, 11, 16], this survey did not find age, sex and marital status differences in the prevalence of elder abuse.

Some studies have shown protective factors, such as social support and social cohesion [6, 7, 9, 11], against elder abuse, but this study only showed that Christian and Sikh religion and not social support and social cohesion was protective against elder abuse. Consistent with several studies [5, 10, 11-13], this study showed that functional disability, loneliness, depressive symptoms, and current tobacco use were associated with elder abuse. Older adults with functional disabilities may increase caregiver stress, thereby increasing the vulnerability to elder abuse [10]. Regarding loneliness and depressive symptoms, it is also possible that older adults became depressed and/or lonely as a consequence of elder abuse. Longitudinal research is needed to clarify the direction of the relationship between poor mental health and elder abuse. Some studies [4, 9, 11] found an association between chronic conditions, multimorbidity, poor cognition and elder abuse, while this study only found an association between poor cognition and elder abuse in univariate analysis.

Strength and limitations of the study

Study strengths included the use of standardized measures adapted from the Health and Retirement Study and a large, nationally representative sample of older adults in India. The self-report of most data may have their limitations. It is possible that participants underreported elder abuse, and some chronic conditions were not verified by clinical diagnosis. Due to the cross-sectional design of the study, we were unable to determine the direction of the assessed associations. Some variables, such as past abuse (beyond the past 12 months), such as childhood abuse and sexual abuse, were not assessed and should be included in future studies.

Conclusion

One in twenty older adults in India experienced elder abuse. Factors associated with elder abuse included food insecurity, functional disability, loneliness, depressive symptoms, and current tobacco, lower subjective socioeconomic status, not Christian and not Sikh that can be targeted in elder abuse prevention efforts.

Acknowledgments

The Longitudinal Aging Study in India Project is funded by the Ministry of Health and Family Welfare, Government of India, the National Institute on Aging (R01 AG042778, R01 AG030153), and United Nations Population Fund, India.

References

[1] World Health Organization. Elder abuse, 2020. URL: https://www.who.int/news-room/fact-sheets/detail/elder-abuse#:~:text=Around%201%20in%206%20people, abuse%20in%20the%20past%20year.

[2] Yunus RM, Hairi NN, Choo WY. Consequences of elder abuse and neglect: A systematic review of observational studies. Trauma Violence Abuse 2019;20(2):197-213. doi: 10.1177/1524838017692798.

[3] Yon Y, Mikton CR, Gassoumis ZD, Wilber KH. Elder abuse prevalence in community settings: a systematic review and meta-analysis. Lancet Glob Health 2017;5(2):e147-56. doi: 10.1016/S2214-109X(17)30006-2.

[4] Sathya T, Nagarajan R, Selvamani Y. Multimorbidity as a risk factor of elder abuse/mistreatment in India: A cross-sectional study. J Interpers Violence 2020:886260520980391. doi: 10.1177/0886260520980391.

[5] Sembiah S, Dasgupta A, Taklikar CS, Paul B, Bandyopadhyay L, Burman J. Elder abuse and its predictors: a cross-sectional study in a rural area of West Bengal, eastern part of India. Psychogeriatrics 2020;20(5):636-44. doi: 10.1111/psyg.12550.

[6] Chokkanathan S, Lee AE. Elder mistreatment in urban India: a community-based study. J Elder Abuse Negl 2005;17:45–61.

[7] Chang E-S, Levy BR. Protective effects of neighborhood community factors on elder abuse in India. J Elder Abuse Negl 2021;33:1-16, doi: 10.1080/08946566.2020.1864695

[8] Ramalingam A, Sarkar S, Premarajan KC, Rajkumar RP, Subrahmanyam DK. Prevalence and correlates of elder abuse: A cross-sectional, community-based study from rural Puducherry. Natl Med J India 2019;32(2):72-6. doi: 10.4103/0970-258X.275344.

[9] Santos MABD, Moreira RDS, Faccio PF, Gomes GC, Silva VL. Factors associated with elder abuse: A systematic review of the literature. Cien Saude Colet 2020;25(6):2153-75. doi: 10.1590/1413-81232020256.25112018.

[10] Sathya T, Premkumar R. Association of functional limitations and disability with elder abuse in India: a cross-sectional study. BMC Geriatr 2020;20(1):220. doi: 10.1186/s12877-020-01619-3.

[11] Dong X. Elder abuse in Chinese populations: a global review. J Elder Abuse Negl 2015;27(3):196-232. doi: 10.1080/08946566.2015.1039154.

[12] Dong X, Simon MA, Odwazny R, Gorbien M: Depression and elder abuse and neglect among a community-dwelling Chinese elderly population. J Elder Abuse Negl 2008; 20:25–41.

[13] Dong X, Simon MA, Gorbien M, Percak J, Golden R: Loneliness in older Chinese adults: a risk factor for elder mistreatment. J Am Geriatr Soc 2007;55:1831–5.

[14] International Institute for Population Sciences (IIPS), NPHCE, MoHFW, Harvard TH Chan School of Public Health (HSPH) and the University of Southern California

(USC). Longitudinal Ageing Study in India (LASI) Wave 1, 2017-18, India Report. Mumbai: International Institute for Population Sciences, 2020.

[15] Berkman LS, Capistrant TV, Zheng Y. Social networks, family, and care giving among older adults in India. In: Smith JM, ed. Aging in Asia. Washington, DC: National Research Council of the National Academies, 2012:261-78.

[16] Rudra A. Ill-treatment an evolving form of elderly abuse: Evidence from LASI pilot study. International Journal of Innovative Research and Advanced Studies, Int J Innov Res Adv Stud 2016;3:93–6.

[17] Katz S, Ford AB, Moskowitz RW, Jackson BA, Jaffe MW. Studies of illness in the aged. the index of ADL: A standardized measure of biological and psychosocial function. JAMA 1963;185:914-9. doi: 10.1001/jama.1963.03060120024016.

[18] Lawton MP, Brody EM. Assessment of older people: self-maintaining and instrumental activities of daily living. Gerontologist 1969;9(3):179-86.

[19] Andresen EM, Malmgren JA, Carter WB, Patrick DL. Screening for depression in well older adults: evaluation of a short form of the CES-D (Center for Epidemiologic Studies Depression Scale). Am J Prev Med 1994;10(2):77-84.

[20] Kumar S, Nakulan A, Thoppil SP, Parassery RP, Kunnukattil SS. Screening for depression among community-dwelling elders: Usefulness of the Center for Epidemiologic Studies Depression Scale. Indian J Psychol Med 2016;38(5):483-5. doi: 10.4103/0253-7176.191380.

[21] Lee J, Smith JP. Regional disparities in adult height, educational attainment and gender difference in late- life cognition: Findings from the Longitudinal Aging Study in India (LASI). J Econ Ageing 2014;4:26-34. doi: 10.1016/j.jeoa.2014.02.002.

In: Social and Health Issues … ISBN: 978-1-53619-937-6
Editors: S Pengpid, K Peltzer et al.

Chapter 7

PREVALENCE AND CORRELATES OF HYPERTENSION AMONG A NATIONALLY REPRESENTATIVE POPULATION-BASED SAMPLE OF OLDER ADULTS IN INDIA IN 2017-2018

Karl Peltzer[1,2], MA Clin Psych, PhD, Dr Habil and Supa Pengpid[1,3,*], MPH, DrPH, MBA

[1]Department of Research Administration and Development, University of Limpopo, Turfloop, South Africa,

[2]Department of Psychology, College of Medical and Health Science, Asia University, Taichung, Taiwan

[3]ASEAN Institute for Health Development, Mahidol University, Salaya, Phutthamonthon, Nakhon Pathom, Thailand

* *Correspondence*: Professor Supa Pengpid, ASEAN Institute for Health Development, Mahidol University, 25/25 Phutthamonthon Road 4, Salaya, Phutthamonton, Nakhon Pathom 73170, Thailand. Email: supaprom@yahoo.com.

Abstract

In this study we aimed to determine the prevalence and correlates of hypertension in older adults in India. The cross-sectional sample consisted of 52,393 individuals (≥50 years) from the Longitudinal Ageing Study in India (LASI) Wave 1 in 2017-2018. Hypertension was defined as "systolic BP ≥140 mm Hg and/or diastolic BP ≥90 mm Hg or where the participant is currently on antihypertensive medication." Results indicate that the prevalence of hypertension was 45.4%, 48.0% among women and 42.3% among men. In adjusted logistic regression analysis, older age, higher education, urban residence, Muslims and Sikhs, overweight/obesity, arthritis, diabetes, angina and heart disease were positively associated with hypertension, while male sex, underweight, and vigorous physical activity were negatively associated with hypertension. In addition, in unadjusted analysis, higher subjective socioeconomic status, Muslims, and high cholesterol were positively and current tobacco use negativey associated with hypertension. Almost one in two older adults in India had hypertension. Several risk factors were identified, which can be targeted in public health interventions.

Introduction

"Hypertension - or elevated blood pressure - is a serious medical condition that significantly increases the risk of heart, brain, kidney, and other diseases, and is a major cause of premature death worldwide. An estimated 1.13 billion people worldwide have hypertension, most (two-thirds) living in low- and middle-income countries. In 2015, 1 in 4 men and 1 in 5 women had hypertension" [1]. "Modifiable risk factors hypertension include unhealthy diets (excessive salt consumption, a diet high in saturated fat and trans fats, low intake of fruits and vegetables), physical inactivity, consumption of tobacco and alcohol, and being overweight or obese. Non-modifiable risk factors include a family history of hypertension, age over 65 years and co-existing diseases such as diabetes or kidney disease" [1]. In a study among older adults (≥50 years) in six low- and middle-income countries, the prevalence of hypertension was 52.9%, and in India in 2007 32.3% [2], and in South Africa 77.3% [3]. In a study of a total of 420 persons aged 60 years and above from a rural area of Ballabgarh, Haryana, India, the prevalence of hypertension was 50.3% [4]. There is a lack of recent national studies among older adults on the prevalence and associated factors of hypertension in India.

As reviewed in Boateng et al. [5] risk factors for hypertension include sociodemographic factors (age, sex, socioeconomic status, residence status) and health factors (unhealthy diet, physical inactivity, obesity, substance use, diabetes, arthritis, angina, asthma, and depression). In a prospective of 573 families (and 997 participants aged 30 years and above) in India, "the prevalence of hypertension was higher among persons with comorbidities (diabetes 64.5%, transient ischemic attack 54.7%, and heart disease 64.4%) and lower among persons who did regular vigorous intensity exercise versus those who did moderate intensity exercise (32% vs. 45.7%) and among nonsmokers versus smokers (42.2% vs. 46.6%)" [6]. This study aimed to determine the prevalence and correlates of hypertension in older community-dwelling adults in India in 2017-2018.

OUR STUDY

This secondary data analysis utilized data from the cross-sectional and nationally representative Longitudinal Ageing Study in India (LASI) Wave 1, 2017-2018; "the overall household response rate is 96%, and the overall individual response rate is 87%" [7]. In a household survey, "interview, physical measurement and biomarker data were collected from individuals aged 45 and above and their spouses, regardless of age" [7]. We restricted our analysis to those 50 years and older. Specific details on the sampling approach are found elsewhere [7]. The study was approved by the "Indian Council of Medical Research (ICMR) Ethics Committee and written informed consent was obtained from the participants" [7].

Measures

Hypertension or raised blood pressure (BP) was defined as "systolic BP ≥140 mm Hg and/or diastolic BP ≥90 mm Hg (based on the last two averaged of three BP readings) or where the participant is currently on antihypertensive medication" [8].

Covariates

Sociodemographic variables consisted of level of education (none, ≥1 years), age group (50-59, 60-69, 70-79, and 80 or more years), sex (male, female), religion, and residence (rural, urban). Subjective socioeconomic status was assessed with the question, "Please imagine a ten-step ladder, where at the bottom are the people who are the worst off – who have the least money, least education, and the worst jobs or no jobs, and at the top of the ladder are the people who are the best off – those who have the most money, most education, and best jobs. Please indicate the number (1-10) on the rung on the ladder where you would place yourself" [7]. Steps 1 to 3 on the socioeconomic ladder were defined as low, 4-5 as medium, and 6-10 as high socioeconomic status.

Health factors

Anthropometry. "Height and weight of adults were measured using the Seca 803 digital scale." [7]. "Body Mass Index=BMI was calculated according to Asian criteria: underweight (<18.5 kg/m^2), normal weight (18.5-22.9 kg/m^2), overweight (23.0-24.9 kg/m^2), class I obesity (25.0-29.9 kg/m^2), and class II obesity (≥30.0 kg/m^2)" [9].

Vigorous physical activity. "For vigorous activity, respondents were asked about their involvement in running or jogging, swimming, going to a health centre/gym, cycling, digging with a spade or shovel, heavy lifting, chopping, farm work, fast bicycling, and cycling with loads." [7]. Participants, "who more than once a week engaged in vigorous physical activity were defined as having sufficient physical activity." [10].

Current tobacco use was assessed from 1) "Do you currently smoke any tobacco products (cigarettes, bidis, cigars, hookah, cheroot, etc.)? and 2) Do you use smokeless tobacco (such as chewing tobacco, gutka, pan masala, etc.)?" (Yes, No) [7].

Lifetime alcohol use was assessed with the question, "Have you ever consumed any alcoholic beverages such as beer, wine, liquor, country liquor etc.? (Yes, No) [7].

Chronic conditions were sourced from the question, "Has any health professional ever told you that you have…?": 1) "Diabetes or high blood sugar; 2) Asthma, 3) Chronic heart diseases such as Coronary heart disease (heart attack or Myocardial Infarction), congestive heart failure, or other chronic heart problems; 4) Arthritis or rheumatism; and 5) High cholesterol." (Yes/No) [7].

Angina was assessed with the "World Health Organization's Rose angina questionnaire" [11], defined on the basis of "discomfort at walking uphill or hurrying, or at an ordinary pace on level ground. Furthermore, the pain should be located at the sternum or in the left chest and arm, causing the patient to stop or slow down, and the pain should resolve within 10 minutes when the patient stops or slows down." [12].

Major depressive disorder in the past 12 months was assessed with the Health and Retirement Study (HRS) Composite International Diagnostic Interview short form (CIDI-SF) [13], using criteria of the Diagnostic and Statistical Manual of Mental Disorders (DSM) [14]. Study respondents were required to "endorse either anhedonia or depressed mood for most of the day for most of a 2-week period or more," and those who fulfilled this criterion "completed an additional seven symptoms: lost interest, feeling tired, change in weight, trouble with sleep, trouble concentrating, feeling down, and thoughts of death" [15]. "Those with a score ≥3 were considered to meet the criteria for having MDD in the previous 12 months; MDD symptomology scores ranged from 0 to 7" [15].

Data analysis

Descriptive statistics were applied to describe health status, sociodemographic information, and hypertension prevalence. Unadjusted and adjusted logistic regression was utilized to assess the predictors of hypertension; variables found significant in univariate analyses were included in the adjusted model. $P < 0.05$ was accepted as significant, missing values were excluded, and no multi-collinearity was found. Statistical analyses were conducted using STATA software version 15.0 (Stata Corporation, College Station, TX, USA), taking the complex study design into account.

FINDINGS

The sample included 52,393 older adults (50 years and older), with a median age of 62 years (14 years interquartile range), 53.3% were female and 46.7% male. Majority (69.0%) of the participants were residing in rural areas, 82.4% were Hindus, 38.2% had low subjective socioeconomic status and 53.0% had no schooling. Almost half of the participants (45.4%) had hypertension, 6.4% obesity class II (≥30 kg/m^2), 33.0% had current tobacco use, 14.9% had ever engaged in alcohol use, 62.3% did not engage in vigorous physical activity, 14.7% arthritis, 13.4% diabetes, 5.4% asthma, 8.9% angina, 4.2% heart disease, and 2.4% had high cholesterol (see Table 1).

Table 1. Sample and diabetes characteristics among older adults in India, 2017-2018

Variable	Sample	Hypertension
	N (%)	%
All	**52393**	**45.4**
Sociodemographic factors		
Age in years		
50-59	20916 (38.1)	38.1
60-69	18979 (36.2)	47.9
70-79	9108 (18.7)	52.9
≥80	3390 (7.0)	52.2
Sex		
Female	27815 (53.3)	48.0
Male	24578 (46.7)	42.3
Education		
No schooling	25983 (53.0)	41.6
1-4 years	6138 (11.0)	47.0
5-9 years	11246 (19.5)	47.6
≥10 years	9026 (16.5)	53.8

Variable	Sample	Hypertension
	N (%)	%
Subjective socioeconomic status		
Low	17462 (38.2)	42.3
Medium	20070 (37.4)	45.8
High	13176 (24.4)	49.7
Residence		
Rural	34099 (69.0)	40.5
Urban	18294 (31.0)	57.0
Religious affiliation		
Hindu	38498 (82.4)	44.2
Muslim	6186 (11.3)	49.5
Christian	5206 (2.8)	51.4
Sikh	1528 (1.8)	61.0
Other or none	973 (1.7)	48.1
Health factors		
Body mass index		
Normal	17179 (37.2)	40.3
Underweight	9428 (23.0)	30.2
Overweight	6922 (13.7)	50.7
Obesity class I	9846 (19.7)	60.5
Obesity class II	3271 (6.4)	67.8
Vigorous physical activity		
Never	32762 (62.3)	49.5
Once/week	4262 (8.8)	37.0
>once/week	14930 (28.9)	39.3
Current tobacco use	16403 (33.0)	39.3
Ever alcohol use	9346 (14.9)	44.7
Arthritis	6647 (14.7)	51.9
Diabetes	7423 (13.4)	70.6
High cholesterol	1946 (2.4)	66.8
Asthma	2292 (5.4)	44.1
Angina	4510 (8.9)	49.9
Heart disease	2154 (4.2)	69.7
Major depressive disorder	3263 (8.0)	45.4

Associations with hypertension

In the adjusted logistic regression analysis, older age, higher education, urban residence, Muslims and Sikhs, overweight/obesity, arthritis, diabetes, angina, and heart disease were positively associated with hypertension, while male sex, underweight, and vigorous physical activity were negatively associated with hypertension. In addition, in unadjusted analysis, higher subjective socioeconomic status, Muslims, and high cholesterol were positively and current tobacco use negatively associated with hypertension (see Table 2).

Table 2. Associations with hypertension among older adults in India, 2017-2018

Variable	Unadjusted Odds Ratio (95% CI)	Adjusted Odds Ratio (95% CI)
Sociodemographic factors		
Age in years		
50-59	1 (Reference)	1 (Reference)
60-69	1.49 (1.36, 1.64)***	1.60 (1.44, 1.77)***
70-79	1.82 (1.64, 2.02)***	2.09 (1.88, 2.31)***
≥80	1.77 (1.51, 2.08)***	2.35 (2.02, 2.73)***
Sex		
Female	1 (Reference)	1 (Reference)
Male	0.79 (0.73, 0.86)***	0.81 (0.76, 0.87)***
Education		
No schooling	1 (Reference)	1 (Reference)
1-4 years	1.26 (1.05, 1.47)**	1.20 (1.05, 1.36)**
5-9 years	1.27 (1.15, 1.41)***	1.14 (1.06, 1.23)***
≥10 years	1.63 (1.49, 1.78)***	1.26 (1.13, 1.40)***
Subjective socioeconomic status		
Low	1 (Reference)	1 (Reference)
Medium	1.15 (1.03, 1.29)*	0.96 (0.86, 1.07)
High	1.35 (1.18, 1.55)***	0.92 (0.83, 1.02)
Residence		
Rural	1 (Reference)	1 (Reference)
Urban	1.95 (1.51, 2.51)***	1.32 (1.04, 1.67)*
Religious affiliation		
Hindu	1 (Reference)	1 (Reference)
Muslim	1.24 (1.06, 1.44)**	1.18 (1.04, 1.34)**
Christian	1.33 (1.05, 1.69)*	1.26 (0.97, 1.63)
Sikh	1.97 (1.59, 2.45)***	1.70 (1.35, 2.13)***
Other or none	1.18 (0.96, 1.44)	1.13 (0.98, 1.30)
Health factors		
Body mass index (BMI)		
Normal	1 (Reference)	1 (Reference)
Underweight	0.64 (0.56, 0.73)***	0.64 (0.56, 0.73)***
Overweight/obesity	2.07 (1.87, 2.28)***	1.77 (1.66, 1.88)***
Vigorous physical activity		
Never	1 (Reference)	1 (Reference)
Once/week	0.60 (0.51, 0.71)***	0.82 (0.74, 0.91)***
>once/week	0.66 (0.60, 0.73)***	0.89 (0.82, 0.96)**
Current tobacco use	0.69 (0.63, 0.76)***	0.98 (0.91, 1.05)
Ever alcohol use	0.97 (0.84, 1.11)	---
Arthritis	1.36 (1.17, 1.58)***	1.11 (1.00, 1.23)*
Diabetes	3.38 (2.91, 3.92)***	2.29 (2.07, 2.54)***
High Cholesterol	2.47 (1.46, 4.19)***	1.18 (0.65, 2.13)
Asthma	1.07 (0.95, 1.21)	---
Angina	1.22 (1.08, 1.39)**	1.18 (1.02, 1.53)*
Heart disease	2.89 (2.20, 3.80)***	1.90 (1.52, 2.38)***
Major depressive disorder	1.00 (0.89, 1.12)	---

CI = Confidence Interval; ***$p < 0.001$; ** $p < 0.01$; *$p < 0.05$.

Discussion

In this nationally representative sample of older adults (≥50 years) in India in 2017-2018, the prevalence of hypertension was 45.4%, which is lower than in a study among older adults (≥50 years) in six low- and middle-income countries (52.7%) [2] and in South Africa (77.3%) [3], but higher than in a national survey of older adults (≥50 years) in India in 2007 (32.3%) [2]. India, being in a rapid epidemiological transition [16], has seen an increase in the prevalence of hypertension in the adult population from 1980 to 2014 in men from 24.5% to 26.6% and in women from 22.7% to 24.7% [17].

Consistent with previous research in Ghana, India, and Columbia, older age [18, 19], female sex [5], higher education [18], higher socioeconomic status [5, 18], urban residence [5, 18] were associated with hypertension in this study. It is possible that older adults with higher education, higher socioeconomic status, and urban residence increasingly adopted sedentary lifestyles, engaged in jobs requiring less physical activity and changed their dietary behaviour [16], increasing the risk for the development of hypertension [18]. This study found a higher prevalence of hypertension in religious minorities, including Muslims, Sikhs, and in unadjusted analysis in Christians, compared to Hindus. Similar results were found in a study among adults in Maharashtra in India, with Muslims and Christians having a higher prevalence of hypertension than the main stream, Hindus [18]. Results seem to support behaviour change education, such as reduction of salt intake, regular exercise, lower fat intake, and increase in whole grains, fruits, and vegetables, in particular targeting the growing middle class to prevent and control high blood pressure in India [5].

While some previous studies showed an association between physical inactivity [5, 6], tobacco use [6, 18] and alcohol users [18], this study only found a positive association between physical inactivity and hypertension. Current tobacco use was negatively associated with hypertension in unadjusted analysis and alcohol use was not associated with hypertension. Similar results were found among older adults in Columbia [19]. It is possible that as a result of health care providers' advice on lifestyle changes, older adults may have reduced tobacco use [19]. Physical activity may decrease the risk of weight again and obesity and thereby reducing the risk of developing hypertension [20].

In line with previous findings, we found positive associations between generalised obesity [1, 18], arthritis [5], diabetes [1, 5, 6, 18, 19], angina [5], and heart disease [6, 19] with hypertension. We did not find an association between asthma and hypertension, as found in some previous research [5, 21]. Similar to a national study in Indonesia [22], this study found that underweight was negatively associated with hypertension. This combination of various medical conditions calls for a multiple rather than a single risk intervention approach in this population. [19]. This study did not find an association between depression and hypertension, while in a study among older adults in Ghana a positive association between depression and hypertension was found [5]. "Interventions programmes operating at multiple levels are urgently needed that can increase awareness of hypertension, access to high blood pressure treatment, and community wide health behaviour interventions that were identified and known to be effective in reducing high blood pressure levels" [22].

Study limitations include the cross-sectional design, the assessment of some variables by self-report. Some variables that may affect hypertension, such as dietary behaviour, were not assessed and should be included in future studies.

CONCLUSION

Almost one in two older adults in India had hypertension. Several potential risk factors for hypertension, such as older age, female, sex, higher education, urban residence, Muslims and Sikhs, overweight/obesity, arthritis, diabetes, angina, heart disease and physical inactivity were identified, which can be targeted in public health interventions.

ACKNOWLEDGMENTS

The Longitudinal Aging Study in India Project is funded by the Ministry of Health and Family Welfare, Government of India, the National Institute on Aging (R01 AG042778, R01 AG030153), and United Nations Population Fund, India.

REFERENCES

[1] World Health Organization. Fact sheet hypertension, 2021. URL: https://www.who.int/news-room/fact-sheets/detail/hypertension.

[2] Lloyd-Sherlock P, Beard J, Minicuci N, Ebrahim S, Chatterji S. Hypertension among older adults in low- and middle-income countries: prevalence, awareness and control. Int J Epidemiol 2014;43(1):116-28. doi: 10.1093/ije/dyt215.

[3] Peltzer K, Phaswana-Mafuya N. Hypertension and associated factors in older adults in South Africa. Cardiovasc J Afr 2013;24(3):67-71. doi: 10.5830/CVJA-2013-002.

[4] Gupta S, Kumar R, Kalaivani M, Nongkynrih B, Kant S, Gupta SK. Prevalence, awareness, treatment, and control of diabetes and hypertension among elderly persons in a rural area of Ballabgarh, Haryana. J Family Med Prim Care 2020;9(2):777-82. doi: 10.4103/jfmpc.jfmpc_1057_19.

[5] Boateng GO, Luginaah IN, Taabazuing MM. Examining the risk factors associated with hypertension among the elderly in Ghana. J Aging Health 2015;27(7):1147-69. doi: 10.1177/0898264315577588.

[6] Saju MD, Allagh KP, Scaria L, Joseph S, Thiyagarajan JA. Prevalence awareness, treatment, and control of hypertension and its associated risk factors: Results from baseline survey of SWADES Family Cohort Study. Int J Hypertens 2020;2020:4964835. doi: 10.1155/2020/4964835. PMID: 32351729; PMCID: PMC7178468.

[7] International Institute for Population Sciences (IIPS), NPHCE, MoHFW, Harvard TH Chan School of Public Health (HSPH) and the University of Southern California (USC). Longitudinal Ageing Study in India (LASI) Wave 1, 2017-18, India Report. Mumbai: International Institute for Population Sciences, 2020.

[8] Chobanian AV, Bakris GL, Black HR, Cushman WC, Green LA, Izzo Jr JL, et al. The seventh report of the joint national committee on prevention, detection, evaluation, and treatment of high blood pressure: the JNC 7 report. JAMA 2003;289(19):2560–71.

[9] Wen CP, David Cheng TY, Tsai SP, Chan HT, Hsu HL, Hsu CC, Eriksen MP. Are Asians at greater mortality risks for being overweight than Caucasians? Redefining obesity for Asians. Public Health Nutr 2009;12(4):497-506. doi: 10.1017/S1368980008002802.

[10] Lübs L, Peplies J, Drell C, Bammann K. Cross-sectional and longitudinal factors influencing physical activity of 65 to 75-year-olds: a pan European cohort study based on the survey of health, ageing and retirement in Europe (SHARE). BMC Geriatr 2018;18(1):94. doi: 10.1186/s12877-018-0781-8.

[11] Rose GA. The diagnosis of ischaemic heart pain and intermittent claudication in field surveys. Bull World Health Organ 1962;27:645–58.

[12] Achterberg S, Soedamah-Muthu SS, Cramer MJ, Kappelle LJ, van der Graaf Y, Algra A; SMART Study Group. Prognostic value of the Rose questionnaire: a validation with future coronary events in the SMART study. Eur J Prev Cardiol 2012;19(1):5-14. doi: 10.1177/1741826710391117.

[13] Kessler RC, Andrews A, Mroczek D, Ustun B, Wittchen HU. The World Health Organization Composite International Diagnostic Interview Short-Form (CIDI-SF). Int J Methods Psychiatr Res 1998;7: 171–185.

[14] American Psychiatric Association. Diagnostic and statistical manual of mental disorders (DSM-5), 5th ed. Washington, DC: American Psychiatric Publishing, 2013.

[15] Steffick D. Documentation of affective functioning measures in the health and retirement study. URL: http://hrsonline. isr.umich.edu/sitedocs/userg/dr-005.pdf.

[16] Geldsetzer P, Manne-Goehler J, Theilmann M, Davies JI, Awasthi A, Vollmer S, et al. Diabetes and hypertension in India: A nationally representative study of 1.3 million adults. JAMA Intern Med 2018;178(3):363-72. doi: 10.1001/jamainternmed.2017.8094.

[17] NCD Risk Factor Collaboration (NCD-RisC). Worldwide trends in diabetes since 1980: a pooled analysis of 751 population-based studies with 4.4 million participants. Lancet 2016;387(10027):1513-30. doi: 10.1016/S0140-6736(16)00618-8.

[18] Bhise MD, Patra S. Prevalence and correlates of hypertension in Maharashtra, India: A multilevel analysis. PLoS One 2018;13(2):e0191948. doi: 10.1371/journal.pone.0191948.

[19] Cano-Gutierrez C, Reyes-Ortiz CA, Samper-Ternent R, Gélvez-Rueda JS, Borda MG. Prevalence and factors associated with hypertension among older adults in Bogotá, Colombia. J Aging Health 2015;27(6):1046-65. doi: 10.1177/0898264315573518.

[20] Hu G, Barengo NC, Tuomilehto J, Lakka TA, Nissinen A, Jousilahti P. Relationship of physical activity and body mass index to the risk of hypertension: a prospective study in Finland. Hypertension 2004;43(1):25-30. doi: 10.1161/01.HYP.0000107400.72456.19. Patel MR, Janevic MR, Heeringa SG, Baptist AP, Clark NM. An examination of adverse asthma outcomes in US adults with multiple morbidities. Ann Am Thorac Soc 2013;10(5):426-31. doi: 10.1513/AnnalsATS.201302-032OC.

[21] Peltzer K, Pengpid S. The prevalence and social determinants of hypertension among adults in Indonesia: A cross-sectional population-based national survey. Int J Hypertens 2018;2018:5610725. doi: 10.1155/2018/5610725.

In: Social and Health Issues … ISBN: 978-1-53619-937-6
Editors: S Pengpid, K Peltzer et al.

Chapter 8

PREVALENCE AND CORRELATES OF SELF-REPORTED DIABETES AMONG A NATIONALLY REPRESENTATIVE POPULATION-BASED SAMPLE OF OLDER ADULTS IN INDIA IN 2017-2018

Supa Pengpid[1,2], MPH, DrPH, MBA
and Karl Peltzer[2,3,*], MA Clin Psych, PhD, Dr Habil
[1]ASEAN Institute for Health Development, Mahidol University, Salaya, Phutthamonthon, Nakhon Pathom, Thailand
[2]Department of Research Administration and Development, University of Limpopo, Turfloop, South Africa
[3]Department of Psychology, College of Medical and Health Science, Asia University, Taichung, Taiwan

* *Correspondence*: Professor Karl Peltzer, Department of Research Administration and Development, University of Limpopo, Turfloop Campus, Private Bag X1106, Sovenga 0727, South Africa. Email: kfpeltzer@gmail.com.

Abstract

In this chapter we aim to determine the prevalence and correlates of self-reported diabetes in older adults in India. The cross-sectional sample consisted of 52,393 individuals (≥50 years) from the Longitudinal Ageing Study in India (LASI) Wave 1 in 2017-2018. Results indicate that the prevalence of self-reported diabetes was 13.4% diabetes, 13.2% among women and 13.8% among men. In adjusted logistic regression analysis, older age, higher childhood economic status, urban residence, overweight and obesity, hypertension and high cholesterol were positively associated with self-reported diabetes, while vigorous physical activity, and current tobacco use were negatively associated with diabetes. In addition, in unadjusted analysis, higher subjective socioeconomic status was positively and lifetime alcohol use was negatively associated with self-reported diabetes. One in eight older adults in India reported having been diagnosed with diabetes. Several risk factors were identified, which can be targeted in public health interventions.

Introduction

"Diabetes is a chronic disease that occurs either when the pancreas does not produce enough insulin or when the body cannot effectively use the insulin it produces. Insulin is a hormone that regulates blood sugar. Hyperglycaemia, or raised blood sugar, is a common effect of uncontrolled diabetes and over time leads to serious damage to many of the body's systems, especially the nerves and blood vessels" [1]. Globally, 8.5% of adults (≥18 years) had diabetes in 2014 [1] and 19.3% of older adults (65-99 years) were estimated to live with diabetes in 2019 [2]. Some of the recent epicentres of diabetes include China and India [2]. Among older adults (≥50 years) in nine countries, the overall self-reported prevalence of diabetes was 7.9% and ranged from 3.8% in Ghana to 17.6% in Mexico [3]. In India in 2015-2016, the national adult prevalence of diabetes among adults was 7.1% [4], in six major cities in India in 2000 the prevalence of diabetes among adults was 12.1% [5], and among older adults (≥50 years) the self-reported prevalence of diabetes was 7.1% in 2007 in India [6].There is a lack of more recent national data on the prevalence and correlates of self-reported diabetes among older adults in India.

Factors associated with diabetes may include, as reviewed by Vonglokham et al. [7], "sociodemographic factors (age, sex, education, economic status, and residence status), health status (central obesity, overweight, hypertension, and hypercholesterolemia), and health risk behaviors (poor dietary pattern, sedentary behavior, physical inactivity and substance use)." Similar risk factors were found for diabetes in India [4, 5, 8, 9]. This study aimed to determine the prevalence and correlates of self-reported diabetes in older community-dwelling adults in India in 2017-2018.

OUR STUDY

This secondary data analysis utilized data from the cross-sectional and nationally representative Longitudinal Ageing Study in India (LASI) Wave 1, 2017-2018; "the overall household response rate is 96%, and the overall individual response rate is 87%" [11]. In a household survey, "interview, physical measurement and biomarker data were collected from individuals aged 45 and above and their spouses, regardless of age" [11]. We restricted our analysis to those 50 years and older. Specific details on the sampling approach are found elsewhere [23]. The study was approved by the "Indian Council of Medical Research (ICMR) Ethics Committee and written informed consent was obtained from the participants" [11].

Outcome variable

Self-reported diabetes was sourced from the item, "Has any health professional ever told you that you have diabetes or high blood sugar?" (Yes, No) [11].

Covariates

Sociodemographic variables consisted of years of education, age group (50-59, 60-69, 70-79, and 80 or more years), sex (male, female), marital status (currently married vs. widowed/divorced/separated/deserted/live-in relationship/never married), and residence (rural, urban). Subjective socioeconomic status was assessed with the question, "Please imagine a ten-step ladder, where at the bottom are the people who are the worst off – who have the least money, least education, and the worst jobs or no jobs, and at the top of the ladder are the people who are the best off – those who have the most money, most education, and best jobs. Please indicate the number (1-10) on the rung on the ladder where you would place yourself" [11]. Steps 1 to 3 on the socioeconomic ladder were defined as low, 4-5 as medium, and 6-10 as high socioeconomic status.

Childhood economic status was assessed with the question, "Now think about your family when you were growing up from birth to age 16. Compared to other families in your community, would you say your family during that time was pretty well off financially, about average, or poor?" [11].

Health factors variables

Anthropometry: "Height and weight of adults were measured using the Seca 803 digital scale" [11]. "Body Mass Index=BMI was calculated according to Asian criteria: underweight (<18.5 kg/m^2), normal weight (18.5-22.9 kg/m^2), overweight (23.0-24.9 kg/m^2), class I obesity (25.0-29.9 kg/m^2), and class II obesity (≥ 30.0 kg/m^2)" [12].

Waist Circumference was measured with a soft measuring tape (Gulik Tape) to the nearest 0.1 cm [11]. Central or abdominal obesity was defined using South Asian criteria for men ≥ 90 cm and for women ≥ 80 cm [13].

Vigorous physical activity. " For vigorous activity, respondents were asked about their involvement in running or jogging, swimming, going to a health centre/gym, cycling, digging with a spade or shovel, heavy lifting, chopping, farm work, fast bicycling, and cycling with loads." [11]. Participants, "who more than once a week engaged in vigorous physical activity were defined as having sufficient physical activity." [14].

Current tobacco use was assessed from 1) "Do you currently smoke any tobacco products (cigarettes, bidis, cigars, hookah, cheroot, etc.)? and 2) Do you use smokeless tobacco (such as chewing tobacco, gutka, pan masala, etc.)?" [11].

Lifetime alcohol use was assessed with the question, "Have you ever consumed any alcoholic beverages such as beer, wine, liquor, country liquor, etc.?" (Yes, No) [11].

Hypertension or raised blood pressure (BP) was defined as "systolic BP ≥140 mm Hg and/or diastolic BP ≥90 mm Hg (based on the last two averaged of three readings) or where the participant is currently on antihypertensive medication" [15]. Self-reported high-cholesterol diabetes was sourced from the question, "Has any health professional ever told you that you have high cholesterol? (Yes/No)" [11].

Data analysis

Descriptive statistics were applied to describe health status, sociodemographic information, and diabetes prevalence. Unadjusted and adjusted logistic regression was utilized to assess the predictors of self-reported diabetes; variables found significant in univariate analyses were included in the adjusted model. $P < 0.05$ was accepted as significant, missing values were excluded, and no multi-collinearity was found. Statistical analyses were conducted using STATA software version 15.0 (Stata Corporation, College Station, TX, USA), taking the complex study design into account.

FINDINGS

The sample included 52,393 older adults (50 years and older), with a median age of 62 years (14 years interquartile range), 53.3% were female and 46.7% male. Majority (70.1%) of participants were married, 69.0% were residing in rural areas, 38.2% had low subjective socioeconomic status, and 42.2% had poor childhood economic tatus. Almost half of the participants (45.4%) had hypertension, 6.4% obesity class II (≥30 kg/m^2), 48.2% central obesity, 33.0% current tobacco use, 14.9% had ever engaged in alcohol use, 62.3% did not engage in vigorous physical activity, and 2.4% had high cholesterol. The prevalence of self-reported diabetes was 13.4% diabetes, 13.2% among women and 13.8% among men (see Table 1).

Table 1. Sample and diabetes characteristics among older adults in India, 2017-2018

Variable	Sample	Diabetes self-reported
	N (%)	%
All	**52393**	**13.4**
Sociodemographic factors		
Age in years		
50-59	20916 (38.1)	12.1
60-69	18979 (36.2)	14.5
70-79	9108 (18.7)	15.5
≥80	3390 (7.0)	9.8
Sex		
Female	27815 (53.3)	13.2
Male	24578 (46.7)	13.8
Marital status		
Not married	15151 (29.9)	12.9
Married	37236 (70.1)	13.7
Education		
No schooling	25983 (53.0)	8.6
1-4 years	6138 (11.0)	14.5
5-9 years	11246 (19.5)	17.2
≥10 years	9026 (16.5)	24.0
Subjective socioeconomic status		
Low	17462 (38.2)	10.0
Medium	20070 (37.4)	13.4
High	13176 (24.4)	19.0

Variable	**Sample**	**Diabetes self-reported**
	N (%)	**%**
Childhood economic status		
Poor	20398 (42.2)	9.0
Average	27834 (49.9)	16.0
High	3911 (7.9)	20.7
Residence		
Rural	34099 (69.0)	9.0
Urban	18294 (31.0)	23.5
Health factors		
Body mass index		
Normal	17179 (37.2)	9.4
Underweight	9428 (23.0)	4.0
Overweight	6922 (13.7)	17.4
Obesity class I	9846 (19.7)	22.3
Obesity class II	3271 (6.4)	30.3
Central obesity	23760 (48.2)	20.0
Vigorous physical activity		
Never	32762 (62.3)	15.5
Once/week	4262 (8.8)	9.4
>once/week	14930 (28.9)	10.1
Current tobacco use	16403 (33.0)	8.5
Ever alcohol use	9346 (14.9)	10.8
Hypertension	22826 (45.4)	20.5
High cholesterol	1946 (2.4)	37.0

Associations with self-reported diabetes

In the adjusted logistic regression analysis, older age, higher childhood economic status, urban residence, overweight and obesity, hypertension and high cholesterol were positively associated with self-reported diabetes, while vigorous physical activity, and current tobacco use were negatively associated with diabetes. In addition, in unadjusted analysis, higher subjective socioeconomic status was positively and lifetime alcohol use was negatively associated with self-reported diabetes (see Table 2).

Table 2. Associations with self-reported diabetes among older adults in India, 2017-2018

Variable	Unadjusted Odds Ratio (95% CI)	Adjusted Odds Ratio (95% CI)
Sociodemographic factors		
Age in years		
50-59	1 (Reference)	1 (Reference)
60-69	1.23 (1.07, 1.41)***	1.41 (1.15, 1.72)***
70-79	1.33 (1.17, 1.50)***	1.61 (1.20, 2.16)***
≥80	0.79 (0.56, 1.11)	1.04 (0.74, 1.44)
Sex		
Female	1 (Reference)	---
Male	1.05 (0.91, 1.21)	
Marital status		
Not married	1 (Reference)	---
Married	1.08 (0.87, 1.34)	
Education		
No schooling	1 (Reference)	1 (Reference)
1-4 years	1.81 (1.48, 2.21)***	1.62 (1.32, 1.98)***
5-9 years	2.21 (1.84, 2.65)***	1.57 (1.39, 1.77)***
≥10 years	3.36 (2.87, 3.94)***	1.74 (1.51, 2.01)***
Subjective		
socioeconomic	1 (Reference)	1 (Reference)
status	1.39 (1.07, 1.81)*	1.01 (0.85, 1.21)
Low	2.13 (1.79, 2.52)***	1.05 (0.83, 1.32)
Medium		
High		
Childhood		
economic status	1 (Reference)	1 (Reference)
Poor	1.94 (1.59, 2.37)***	1.31 (1.18, 1.45)***
Average	2.65 (1.75, 4.00)***	1.47 (1.15, 1.87)**
High		
Residence		
Rural	1 (Reference)	1 (Reference)
Urban	3.13 (2.22, 4.42)***	1.59 (1.23, 2.06)***
Health factors		
Body mass index		
(BMI)	1 (Reference)	1 (Reference)
Normal	0.40 (0.33, 0.48)***	0.49 (0.41, 0.59)***
Underweight	2.03 (1.81, 2.28)***	1.57 (1.39, 1.77)***
Overweight	2.77 (2.29, 3.35)***	1.81 (1.56, 2.11)***
Obesity class I	4.19 (2.88, 6.09)***	2.26 (1.68, 3.04)***
Obesity class II		
Central obesity	3.43 (2.93, 4.02)***	Not included because of overlap with BMI

Variable	Unadjusted Odds Ratio (95% CI)	Adjusted Odds Ratio (95% CI)
Health factors		
Vigorous physical activity		
Never	1 (Reference)	1 (Reference)
Once/week	0.57 (0.49, 0.67)***	0.81 (0.68, 0.97)*
>once/week	0.62 (0.55, 0.69)***	0.85 (0.75, 0.96)**
Current tobacco use	0.50 (0.39, 0.65)***	0.81 (0.68, 0.94)**
Ever alcohol use	0.75 (0.58, 0.98)*	0.97 (0.86, 1.10)
Hypertension	3.38 (2.91, 3.92)***	2.34 (2.12, 2.59)***
High Cholesterol	3.98 (2.48, 6.41)***	1.84 (1.22, 2.77)**

CI=Confidence Interval; ***$p<0.001$; ** $p<0.01$; *$p<0.05$.

DISCUSSION

In this nationally representative sample of older adults (≥50 years) in India in 2017-2018, the prevalence of self-reported diabetes was 14.3%, which is higher than in the 2007 India national survey among older adults (≥50 years) (7.1%) [6], and in a study among older adults (≥50 years) in nine countries [3], but was lower than in Mexico (17.6%, ≥50 years). One of the possible reasons of the increase of self-reported diabetes among older adults in India may the related to the effect of the "National Program for Prevention and Control of Diabetes, Cardiovascular Disease, and Stroke (NPCDCS)," launched 2008, with a "special focus on risk reduction, early diagnosis and appropriate management of diabetes for the prevention of diabetes" [16, 17], led to an increased awareness of one's diabetes status.

Consistent with previous research that found an association between older age [5, 8, 18], higher education [9, 19], higher income [5, 8], higher socioeconomic status [9], urban residence [8, 18, 20, 21] and diabetes, this study found increased odds for self-reported diabetes in older adults (60-79 years), higher education, higher childhood economic status and urban residence. The decrease in the prevalence of diabetes after the age of 79 years may be related to survivor bias, "possibly reflecting deaths at earlier ages due to complications of diabetes" [8]. It is possible that older adults with higher education and urban residence increasingly adopted sedentary lifestyles, engaged in jobs requiring less physical activity and changed their dietary behaviour [22], increasing the risk for the development of diabetes [19]. Similar to a study in Laos, this study did not find significant gender differences in the prevalence of self-reported diabetes.

In line with previous findings on the positive association between abdominal obesity, generalised obesity [5, 8, 19, 23], hypertension [8, 23] and high cholesterol [24] with diabetes, this study found similar results showing major "modifiable cardiometabolic risk factors" [22, 24]. This "combination of cardiometablic risk factors calls for a multiple rather than a single risk intervention approach in this population." [7].

While some previous studies showed an association between physical inactivity [5, 19, 25], tobacco use and alcohol misuse [26], this study only found a positive association between physical inactivity and diabetes. Current tobacco use was negatively associated with diabetes and alcohol use was not associated with diabetes. Similar results were found among older adults in Ghana [21]. It is possible that persons who have been diadnosed with diabetes subsequently quit tobacco use. Physical activity may decrease the risk of weight again and obesity and thereby reducing the risk of developing diabetes [21].

Study limitations include the cross-sectional design, the assessment of some variables by self-report, including diabetes. Some variables that may affect diabetes, such as dietary behaviour, were not assessed and should be included in future studies. The different types of diabetes, such such diabetes type 1 and type 2, were not assessed, and the prevalence of diabetes may have been underestimated because of a high proportion of nondiagnosed diabetes in India [22].

CONCLUSION

One in eight older adults in India reported having been diagnosed with diabetes. Several potential risk factors for diabetes, such as older age, higher childhood economic status, urban residence, overweight and obesity, physical inactivity, hypertension and high cholesterol, were identified, which can be targeted in public health interventions.

ACKNOWLEDGMENTS

The Longitudinal Aging Study in India Project is funded by the Ministry of Health and Family Welfare, Government of India, the National Institute on Aging (R01 AG042778, R01 AG030153), and United Nations Population Fund, India.

REFERENCES

[1] World Health Organization. Factsheet diabetes, 2021. URL: https://www.who.int/news-room/fact-sheets/detail/diabetes.

[2] Sinclair A, Saeedi P, Kaundal A, Karuranga S, Malanda B, Williams R. Diabetes and global ageing among 65-99-year-old adults: Findings from the International Diabetes Federation Diabetes Atlas, 9th edition. Diabetes Res Clin Pract 2020;162:108078. doi: 10.1016/j.diabres.2020.108078.

[3] Tyrovolas S, Koyanagi A, Garin N, Olaya B, Ayuso-Mateos JL, Miret M, et al. Diabetes mellitus and its association with central obesity and disability among older adults: a global perspective. Exp Gerontol 2015;64:70-7. doi: 10.1016/j.exger.2015.02.010.

[4] Vennu V, Abdulrahman TA, Bindawas SM. The prevalence of overweight, obesity, hypertension, and diabetes in India: Analysis of the 2015-2016 National Family Health Survey. Int J Environ Res Public Health 2019;16(20):3987. doi: 10.3390/ijerph16203987.

[5] Ramachandran A, Snehalatha C, Kapur A, Vijay V, Mohan V, Das AK, et al. High prevalence of diabetes and impaired glucose tolerance in India: National Urban Diabetes Survey. Diabetologia 2001;44(9):1094-101. doi: 10.1007/s001250100627.

[6] Agrawal S, Fledderjohann J, Ghosh S. Risk factors for self-reported cataract symptoms, diagnosis, and surgery uptake among older adults in India: Findings from the WHO SAGE data. Glob Public Health 2020 Oct 22. doi: 10.1080/17441692.2020.1836246.

[7] Vonglokham M, Kounnavong S, Sychareun V, Pengpid S, Peltzer K. Prevalence and social and health determinants of pre-diabetes and diabetes among adults in Laos: a

cross-sectional national population-based survey, 2013. Trop Med Int Health 2019;24(1):65-72. doi: 10.1111/tmi.13164.

[8] Anjana RM, Pradeepa R, Deepa M, Datta M, Sudha V, Unnikrishnan R, et al. Prevalence of diabetes and prediabetes (impaired fasting glucose and/or impaired glucose tolerance) in urban and rural India: phase I results of the Indian Council of Medical Research-INdia DIABetes (ICMR-INDIAB) study. Diabetologia 2011;54(12):3022-7. doi: 10.1007/s00125-011-2291-5.

[9] Corsi DJ, Subramanian SV. Socioeconomic Gradients and Distribution of Diabetes, Hypertension, and Obesity in India. JAMA Netw Open 2019;2(4):e190411. doi: 10.1001/jamanetworkopen.2019.0411.

[10] International Institute for Population Sciences (IIPS), NPHCE, MoHFW, Harvard TH Chan School of Public Health (HSPH) and the University of Southern California (USC). Longitudinal Ageing Study in India (LASI) Wave 1, 2017-18, India Report. Mumbai: International Institute for Population Sciences, 2020.

[11] Harvard School of Public Health. Abdominal obesity measurement guidelines for different ethnic groups, 2020. URL: https://www.hsph.harvard.edu/obesity-prevention-source/waist-circumference-guidelines-for-different-ethnic-groups/.

[12] Lübs L, Peplies J, Drell C, Bammann K. Cross-sectional and longitudinal factors influencing physical activity of 65 to 75-year-olds: a pan European cohort study based on the survey of health, ageing and retirement in Europe (SHARE). BMC Geriatr 2018;18(1):94. doi: 10.1186/s12877-018-0781-8.

[13] Chobanian AV, Bakris GL, Black HR, Cushman WC, Green LA, Izzo Jr JL, et al. The seventh report of the joint national committee on prevention, detection, evaluation, and treatment of high blood pressure: the JNC 7 report. JAMA 2003;289(19):2560–71

[14] Kumar A, Goel MK, Jain RB, Khanna P, Chaudhary V. India towards diabetes control: Key issues. Australas Med J 2013;6(10):524-31. doi:10.4066/AMJ.2013.1791.

[15] Ministry of Health and Family Welfare. National Programme for Prevention and Control of Cancer, Diabetes, Cardiovascular Diseases & Stroke (NPCDCS): Operational guidelines. New Delhi: Government of India, 2010. URL: http://health.bih.nic.in/Docs/Guidelines-NPCDCS.pdf.

[16] Xu Y, Wang L, He J, Bi Y, Li M, Wang T, et al. Prevalence and control of diabetes in Chinese adults. JAMA 2013;310(9):948–59. https://doi.org/10.1001/jama.2013.168118.

[17] Gatimu SM, Milimo BW, Sebastian MS. Prevalence and determinants of diabetes among older adults in Ghana. BMC Public Health 2016;16(1):1174. doi: 10.1186/s12889-016-3845-8.

[18] Latt TS, Zaw KK, Ko K, Hlaing MM, Ohnmar M, Oo ES, et al. Measurement of diabetes, prediabetes and their associated risk factors in Myanmar 2014. Diabetes Metab Syndr Obes 2019;12:291–8. https://doi.org/10.2147/DMSO.S156270.

[19] Tarekegne FE, Padyab M, Schröders J, Stewart Williams J. Sociodemographic and behavioral characteristics associated with self-reported diagnosed diabetes mellitus in adults aged 50+ years in Ghana and South Africa: results from the WHO-SAGE wave 1. BMJ Open Diabetes Res Care 2018;6(1):e000449. doi: 10.1136/bmjdrc-2017-000449.

[20] Arokiasamy P, Salvi S, Selvamani Y. Global burden of diabetes mellitus. In: Haring R, ed. Handbook of global health. Cham: Springer, 2021:1-42. https://doi.org/10.1007/978-3-030-05325-3_28-1.

[21] Wen CP, David Cheng TY, Tsai SP, Chan HT, Hsu HL, et al. Are Asians at greater mortality risks for being overweight than Caucasians? Redefining obesity for Asians. Public Health Nutr 2009;12(4):497-506. doi: 10.1017/S1368980008002802.

[22] Animaw W, Seyoum Y. Increasing prevalence of diabetes mellitus in a developing country and its related factors. PLoS One 2017;12(11):e0187670. https://doi.org/10.1371/journal.pone.0187670 eCollection 2017.

[23] Balde NM, Camara A, Diallo AA, Kake, Dialloa AM, Diakite M, et al. Prevalence and awareness of diabetes in Guinea: findings from a WHO STEPS. J Endocr Metab Diabetes S Afr 2017;22:36–42.

[24] Pengpid S, Peltzer K. Prevalence and correlates of pre-diabetes and diabetes among a national population-based sample of adults in Zambia: Results of the first national STEPS survey in 2017. Int J Diabetes Dev Ctries 2021. https://doi.org/10.1007/s13410-020-00910-8.

[25] Barcia JM, Flores-Bellver M, Muriach M, Sancho-Pelluz J, Lopez-Malo D, Urcaneta AC, et al. Matching diabetes and alcoholism: Oxidative stress, inflammation, and neurogenesis are commonly involved. Mediators Inflamm 2015;2015:624287. doi: 10.1155/2015/624287.

In: Social and Health Issues … ISBN: 978-1-53619-937-6
Editors: S Pengpid, K Peltzer et al.

Chapter 9

ANGINA PECTORIS AMONG MIDDLE-AGED AND OLDER ADULTS IN INDIA: PREVALENCE AND CORRELATES FROM A NATIONAL CROSS-SECTIONAL SURVEY IN 2017-2018

Karl Peltzer[1,2], MA Clin Psych, PhD, Dr Habil and Supa Pengpid[1,3,*], MPH, DrPH, MBA

[1]Department of Research Administration and Development, University of Limpopo, Turfloop, South Africa

[2]Department of Psychology, College of Medical and Health Science, Asia University, Taichung, Taiwan

[3]ASEAN Institute for Health Development, Mahidol University, Salaya, Phutthamonthon, Nakhon Pathom, Thailand

[*] *Correspondence*: Professor Supa Pengpid, ASEAN Institute for Health Development, Mahidol University, 25/25 Phutthamonthon Road 4, Salaya, Phutthamonton, Nakhon Pathom 73170, Thailand. Email: supaprom@yahoo.com.

Abstract

In this chapter we estimate the prevalence and correlates of angina pectoris among middle-aged and older adults in India. The cross-sectional sample consisted of 72,262 individuals (≥45 years) from the Longitudinal Ageing Study in India (LASI) Wave 1 in 2017-2018. Angina was assessed with the World Health Organization's Rose angina questionnaire. Results indicate that the overall prevalence of angina pectoris was 8.6%, 9.2% among women and 7.7% among men. In adjusted logistic regression analysis, factors positively associated with angina were food insecurity (Adjusted Odds Ratio-AOR: 1.64, Confidence Interval-CI: 1.44-1.87), stressful events (AOR: 1.25, CI: 1.08-1.45), high discrimination experiences (AOR: 1.26, CI: 1.06-1.50), insomnia symptoms (AOR: 1.76, CI: 1.57-1.97), major depressive disorder (AOR: 1.30, CI: 1.13-1.49), hypertension (AOR: 1.24, CI: 1.13-1.37) and diabetes (AOR: 1.33, CI: 1.16-1.54). Factors negatively associated with angina were male sex (AOR: 0.96, CI: 0.77-0.95), higher education (AOR: 0.71, CI: 0.60-0.83), receipt of health insurance (AOR: 0.78, CI: 0.70-0.86), urban residence (AOR: 0.76, CI: 0.68-0.84) and edentulism (AOR: 0.75, CI: 0.63-0.89). Almost one in ten middle-aged and older adults in India had angina and several associated factors were identified.

Introduction

"Angina pectoris is the main manifestation of symptomatic myocardial ischemia and is generally associated with coronary artery disease leading to insufficient blood reaching the heart. Although stable angina is a common initial presentation of coronary disease, and it greatly affects quality of life, work capacity, and costs to society" [1]. In a large epidemiological study in 31 countries, the angina (assessed with the Rose questionnaire) prevalence was 6.7%, ranging from 0.7 to 14.4% [2]. In population-based surveys among older adults (≥50 years), the prevalence of angina was 9.9% in China, 9.5% in South Africa, 13.9% in Mexico and 18.8% in 2007 in India [3]. There is a lack of more recent national data on the prevalence and correlates of angina pectoris among middle-aged and older adults in India. It is estimated that in 2018, 27% of all deaths in India were attributed to cardiovascular diseases (CVDs) [4].

Several factors associated with angina pectoris have been identified, including female sex among 55-64 year-olds [2], higher socioeconomic status [1], higher household income in South Africa [3], lower wealth status in China, India and Russia [3], perceived stress [5], psychological distress [6], depression [7-9], anxiety [10], hypertension [7, 9], diabetes [9], edentulism [1], obesity in Russia [3], physical inactivity [1], low and moderate physical activity in China [3], smoking in India, South Africa [3] and Mexico [7]. Protective factors associated with angina pectoris may include moderate alcohol use in China [3] and adequate vegetable and fruit consumption in Ghana [3] and India [11]. This study aimed to assess the prevalence and correlates of prevalence and correlates of angina among middle-aged and older persons in India in 2017-2018.

OUR STUDY

This secondary data analysis utilized data from the cross-sectional and nationally representative Longitudinal Ageing Study in India (LASI) Wave 1, 2017-2018; "the overall household response rate is 96%, and the overall individual response rate is 87%." [12]. In a household survey, "interview, physical measurement and biomarker data were collected from individuals aged 45 and above and their spouses, regardless of age." [12]. Specific details on the sampling approach are found elsewhere [12]. The study was approved by the "Indian Council of Medical Research (ICMR) Ethics Committee and written informed consent was obtained from the participants" [12].

Measures

Angina was assessed with the "World Health Organization's Rose angina questionnaire" [13], defined on the basis of "discomfort at walking uphill or hurrying, or at an ordinary pace on level ground. Furthermore, the pain should be located at the sternum or in the left chest and arm, causing the patient to stop or slow down, and the pain should resolve within 10 minutes when the patient stops or slows down." [14].

Exposure variables

Sociodemographic variables consisted of education (none, ≥1-9 years, ≥10 years), age group (45-69, 60-69, and 70 or more years), sex (male, female), marital status (currently married vs. widowed/divorced/separated/ deserted/live-in relationship/never married), and residence status [12]. Subjective socioeconomic status was assessed with the question, "Please imagine a ten-step ladder, where at the bottom are the people who are the worst off – who have the least money, least education, and the worst jobs or no jobs, and at the top of the ladder are the people who are the best off – those who have the most money, most education, and best jobs. Please indicate the number (1-10) on the rung on the ladder where you would place yourself." [12]. Steps 1 to 3 on the socioeconomic ladder were defined as low, 4-5 as medium, and 6-10 as high socioeconomic status.

Food insecurity was sourced from four items, 1) "In the last 12 months, did you ever reduce the size of your meals or skip meals because there was not enough food at your household? (Yes/No) 2) In the last 12 months, were you hungry but didn't eat because there was not enough food at your household? (Yes/No) 3) In the past 12 months, did you ever not eat for a whole day because there was not enough food at your household? 4) Do you think that you have lost weight in the last 12 months because there was not enough food in your household?" [12]. Any positive response to the four questions was scored as one.

Poor childhood health: "Would you say your childhood health was very good, good, fair, poor or very poor on the basis of what you remember, or what you heard or perceived from your parents?" (coded poor or very poor = 1) [12].

Stressful life events included 1) ill-treatment ("Have you felt that you were ill-treated in the past year?" Yes/No), 2) victim of violent crime ("In the last 12 months, have you been the victim of a violent crime, such as assault/mugging/threat to life/others?" (Yes/No), 3) disaster exposure causing health effects ("In the last five years, has your health been severely affected by disasters such as floods, landslides, extreme cold and hot weather, cyclone/typhoons, droughts, earthquakes, tsunamis, or any other natural calamities?" (Yes/No), and 4) man-made incident causing health effects ("In the last five years, has your health been severely affected by man-made incidents such as riots, terrorism, building collapses, fires, traffic accidents or any other man-made incidents?" (Yes/No) [12]. Any yes answer was coded as "1".

Discrimination experiences were assessed with the six-item Everyday Discrimination Scale (EDS) (Short version) [15]. Response options ranged from 1 = "never" to 6 = "almost every day", and were dichotomised to 'never' = 0 and 'ever' (collapsing those reporting 'less than once a year' or greater into one category) = 1; Cronbach's alpha for the EDS in this study was 0.86.

Anthropometry: "Height and weight of adults were measured using the Seca 803 digital scale." [12]. "Body Mass Index = BMI was calculated according to Asian criteria: underweight (<18.5 kg/m^2), normal weight (18.5-22.9 kg/m^2), overweight (23.0-24.9 kg/m^2), class I obesity (25.0-29.9 kg/m^2), and class II obesity (≥30.0 kg/m^2)" [16].

Insomnia symptoms were assessed with four questions: 1) "How often do you have trouble falling asleep?" 2) "How often do you have trouble with waking up during the night?" 3) "How often do you have trouble with waking up too early and not being able to fall asleep again?" 4) "How often do you feel really rested when you wake up in the morning?" Responses options were "never, rarely (1-2 nights per week), occasionally (3-4 nights per week), and frequently five or more nights per week)" [12]. Participants who reported "frequently" with any of these four symptoms were classified as having insomnia symptoms [17].

Major depressive disorder (MDD) in the past 12 months was assessed with the Health and Retirement Study (HRS) Composite International Diagnostic Interview short form (CIDI-SF) [18], using criteria of the Diagnostic and Statistical Manual of Mental Disorders (DSM; American Psychiatric Association [19]. Study respondents were required to "endorse either anhedonia or depressed mood for most of the day for most of a 2-week period or more," and those who fulfilled this criterion "completed an additional seven symptoms: lost interest, feeling tired, change in weight, trouble with sleep, trouble concentrating, feeling down, and thoughts of death." [20]. "Those with a score ≥3 were considered to meet the criteria for having MDD in the previous 12 months; MDD symptomology scores ranged from 0 to 7." [20].

Vigorous physical activity. "For vigorous activity, respondents were asked about their involvement in running or jogging, swimming, going to a health centre/gym, cycling, digging with a spade or shovel, heavy lifting, chopping, farm work, fast bicycling, and cycling with loads." [12]. Responses were trichotomized into 1 = hardly ever/never, 2 = less than twice a week, and 3 = more than once a week [21].

Current tobacco use was assessed from 1) "Do you currently smoke any tobacco products (cigarettes, bidis, cigars, hookah, cheroot, etc.)? and 2) Do you use smokeless tobacco (such as chewing tobacco, gutka, pan masala, etc.)?" (Yes, No) [12].

Heavy episodic alcohol use was assessed with the question, "In the last 3 months, how frequently on average, have you had at least 5 or more drinks on one occasion?" [12] and defined as "one to three days per month, one to four days per week, five or more days per week, or daily."

Hypertension or raised blood pressure (BP) was defined as "systolic BP ≥140 mm Hg and/or diastolic BP ≥90 mm Hg (based on the last two averaged of three readings) or where the participant is currently on antihypertensive medication." [22].

Diabetes was sourced from the question, "Has any health professional ever told you that you have diabetes or high blood sugar?" (Yes/No)." [12].

Edentulism was assessed with the question "Have you lost some or all of your natural teeth?" and defined as "lost all natural teeth" [12].

Data analysis

Descriptive statistics were applied to describe health status, sociodemographic information, and angina. Unadjusted and adjusted logistic regression was utilized to assess the predictors of angina; variables found significant in univariate analyses were included in the adjusted model. $P < 0.05$ was accepted as significant, missing values were excluded, and no multi-collinearity was found. Statistical analyses were conducted using "STATA software version 15.0 (Stata Corporation, College Station, TX, USA)," considering the complex study approach.

FINDINGS

The sample consisted of 72,226 middle- and older aged individuals from India. Table 1 shows the detailed participant characteristics. The overall prevalence of angina was 8.6%, 9.2% among women and 7.7% among men (see Table 1).

Table 1. Sample and angina status among middle and older adults in India, 2017-2018

Variable	Sample N (%)	Angina
Sociodemographic factors		
All	**72262**	**8.6**
Age in years		
45-59	40785 (54.1)	8.0
60-69	18979 (26.8)	9.4
≥70	12498 (19.0)	9.1
Sex		
Women	41685 (58.0)	9.2
Men	30577 (42.0)	7.7
Marital status		
Not married	16852 (24.4)	8.5
Married	55401 (75.6)	8.9
Education		
≥10 years	14079 (18.5)	5.5
1-9 years	24967 (32.0)	8.9
No schooling	33213 (49.5)	9.5

Table 1. (Continued)

Variable	Sample	Angina
	N (%)	
Subjective socioeconomic status		
Low (1-3)	23625 (37.2)	9.0
Medium (4-5)	28380 (38.7)	9.3
High (6-10)	18134 (24.1)	7.1
Has health insurance	16558 (20.7)	6.9
Residence		
Rural	46539 (68.2)	9.5
Urban	25723 (31.8)	6.7
Stressors		
Food insecurity	5806 (9.7)	14.4
Poor childhood health	1068 (1.6)	12.1
Stressful events	5345 (9.0)	11.9
Discrimination experiences		
Low (0)	60008 (82.7)	8.3
Medium (1-2)	6126 (10.7)	8.8
High (3-6)	4247 (6.6)	11.8
Health status		
Body mass index (overweight/obesity)	29497 (42.5)	9.0
Insomnia symptoms	8367 (12.7)	14.3
Major depressive disorder	4352 (7.6)	13.4
Vigorous physical activity		
Hardly ever/never	43224 (58.9)	8.3
≤Once a week	6183 (9.1)	9.5
>Once a week	22210 (32.0)	8.8
Current tobacco use	21074 (30.4)	8.8
Heavy episodic alcohol use	2600 (2.9)	6.7
Hypertension	27964 (40.4)	9.8
Type 2 diabetes	8716 (11.6)	10.0
Edentulism	4599 (6.8)	7.2

Associations with angina

In adjusted logistic regression analysis, factors positively associated with angina were food insecurity (Adjusted Odds Ratio-AOR: 1.64, Confidence Interval-CI: 1.44-1.87), stressful events (AOR: 1.25, CI: 1.08-1.45), high discrimination experiences (AOR: 1.26, CI: 1.06-1.50), insomnia symptoms

Table 2. Associations with angina

Variable	Unadjusted OR (95% CI)	Adjusted OR (95% CI)
Sociodemographic factors		
Age in years		
45-59	1 (Reference)	1 (Reference)
60-69	1.18 (1.06, 1.31)**	1.05 (0.95, 1.17)
≥70	1.14 (0.99, 1.31)	1.02 (0.88, 1.19)
Sex		
Women	1 (Reference)	1 (Reference)
Men	0.82 (0.74, 0.90)***	0.96 (0.77, 0.95)**
Marital status		
Not married	1 (Reference)	---
Married	0.95 (0.85, 1.06)	
Education		
No schooling	1 (Reference)	1 (Reference)
1-9 years	0.93 (0.84, 1.03)	1.01 (0.91, 1.13)
≥10 years	0.56 (0.48, 0.64)***	0.71 (0.60, 0.83)***
Subjective socioeconomic status		
Low or medium (0-5	1 (Reference)	1 (Reference)
High (6-10)	0.76 (0.68, 0.86)***	0.87 (0.77, 0.97)*
Has health insurance	0.74 (0.67, 0.82)***	0.78 (0.70, 0.86)***
Residence		
Rural	1 (Reference)	1 (Reference)
Urban	0.69 (0.62, 0.77)***	0.76 (0.68, 0.84)***
Stressors		
Food insecurity	1.93 (1.70, 2.19)***	1.64 (1.44, 1.87)***
Poor childhood health	1.47 (1.14, 1.91)**	1.15 (0.87, 1.52)
Stressful events	1.50 (1.31, 1.71)***	1.25 (1.08, 1.45)**
Discrimination experiences		
Low (0)	1 (Reference)	1 (Reference)
Medium (1-2)	1.19 (1.02, 1.38)*	0.98 (0.84, 1.15)
High (3-5)	1.60 (1.36, 1.87)***	1.26 (1.06, 1.50)**
Health status		
Body mass index (overweight/obesity)	1.06 (0.96, 1.17)	---
Insomnia symptoms	1.97 (1.78, 2.19)***	1.76 (1.57, 1.97)***
Major depressive disorder	1.72 (1.50, 1.97)***	1.30 (1.13, 1.49)***
Vigorous physical activity		
Hardly ever/never	1 (Reference)	---
≤Once a week	1.16 (0.98, 1.37)	
>Once a week	1.06 (0.96, 1.17)	
Current tobacco use	1.05 (0.96, 1.15)	---
Heavy episodic alcohol use	0.76 (0.60, 0.96)*	0.77 (0.59, 1.01)
Hypertension	1.24 (1.12, 1.37)***	1.24 (1.13, 1.37)***
Type 2 diabetes	1.21 (1.05, 1.39)**	1.33 (1.16, 1.54)***
Edentulism	0.82 (0.70, 0.97)*	0.75 (0.63, 0.89)**

OR = Odds Ratio; CI = Confidence Interval.

(AOR: 1.76, CI: 1.57-1.97), major depressive disorder (AOR: 1.30, CI: 1.13-1.49), hypertension (AOR: 1.24, CI: 1.13-1.37) and diabetes (AOR: 1.33,

CI: 1.16-1.54). Factors negatively associated with angina were male sex (AOR: 0.96, CI: 0.77-0.95), higher education (AOR: 0.71, CI: 0.60-0.83), receipt of health insurance (AOR: 0.78, CI: 0.70-0.86), urban residence (AOR: 0.76, CI: 0.68-0.84) and edentulism (AOR: 0.75, CI: 0.63-0.89) (see Table 2).

DISCUSSION

In this national 2017-2018 India LASI survey (≥45 years), the prevalence of angina pectoris was 8.6%, which is lower than in India (18.3%, ≥50 years) in 2007 [3], China (9.9%) [3], and South Africa (9.5%) [3], but higher than in Mexico (6.4%) [7]. It is possible that the prevalence of angina pectoris declined due to various prevention efforts, e.g., "25-50% of primary health care centres reported offering CVD risk stratification and reported having CVD guidelines that are utilized in at least 50% of health facilities in 2017 in India" [4]. In addition, the study population in this study was slightly younger than in the 2007 India study, which may have also contributed to a lower angina pectoris prevalence.

Consistent with previous studies [1-3], this study found that female sex, lower education, lower subjective socioeconomic status, and not having health insurance were associated with angina. In line with former research [5, 6], different stressors (food insecurity, exposure to stressful events and discrimination experiences) increased the odds of angina. Furthermore, in agreement with previous studies [3, 6-9] major depressive disorder, insomnia symptoms, hypertension, and diabetes were associated with angina.

While other studies [1, 3] found an association between tobacco use, alcohol use, physical inactivity, overweight/obesity, and angina, we did not find a significant relationship between lifestyle factors and angina. It is possible that tobacco use and overweight/obesity do not impact on early stage cardiovascular symptoms such as angina but impact on further progressed cardiovascular disease [9]. The prevalence of heavy episodic alcohol use (2.9%) was fairly low in this study in India and may therefore not have impacted on the angina prevalence. Contrary to expectation, edentulism reduced the odds of angina, while in a previous study [1], edentulism increased the odds of angina. It is possible that angina is associated with edentulism, as this was found in a study among older adults in Mexico [23].

Study limitations

The study was limited by its cross-sectional design and the self-report of most data collected. Some variables, such as dietary behaviour, were not assessed and should be included in future studies.

CONCLUSION

Almost one in ten middle-aged and older adults in India had angina. Sociodemographic factors (older age, no education, food insecurity, rural residence, low socioeconomic status, and not having health insurance), stressors (food insecurity, exposure to stressful events, and high discrimination experiences) and health status variables (insomnia symptoms, major depressive disorder, hypertension, and diabetes) were identified for angina, which can be utilized in targeting interventions.

ACKNOWLEDGMENTS

The Longitudinal Aging Study in India Project is funded by the Ministry of Health and Family Welfare, Government of India, the National Institute on Aging (R01 AG042778, R01 AG030153), and United Nations Population Fund, India.

REFERENCES

[1] Medina-Solís CE, Pontigo-Loyola AP, Pérez-Campos E, Hernández-Cruz P, Ávila-Burgos L, Kowolik MJ, et al. Association between edentulism and angina pectoris in Mexican adults aged 35 years and older: a multivariate analysis of a population-based survey. J Periodontol 2014;85(3):406-16. doi: 10.1902/jop.2013.130186.

[2] Hemingway H, Langenberg C, Damant J, Frost C, Pyörälä K, Barrett-Connor E. Prevalence of angina in women versus men: a systematic review and meta-analysis of international variations across 31 countries. Circulation 2008;117(12):1526-36. doi: 10.1161/CIRCULATIONAHA.107.720953.

[3] Ruan Y, Guo Y, Zheng Y, Huang Z, Sun S, Kowal P, et al. Cardiovascular disease (CVD) and associated risk factors among older adults in six low-and middle-income countries: results from SAGE Wave 1. BMC Public Health 2018;18(1):778. doi: 10.1186/s12889-018-5653-9.

[4] World Health Organization. Noncommunicable diseases (NCD) country profiles, India, 2018. URL: https://www.who.int/nmh/countries/ind_en.pdf.

[5] Nielsen NR, Kristensen TS, Prescott E, Larsen KS, Schnohr P, Grønbaek M. Perceived stress and risk of ischemic heart disease: causation or bias? Epidemiology 2006;17(4):391-7.

[6] Tsai CC, Chuang SY, Hsieh IC, Ho LH, Chu PH, Jeng C. The association between psychological distress and angina pectoris: A population-based study. PLoS One 2019;14(11):e0224451. doi: 10.1371/journal.pone.0224451.

[7] Pengpid S, Peltzer K. Prevalence and correlates of angina pectoris among a nationally representative population-based sample of older adults in Mexico. Int J Disabil Hum Dev 2020;19(3):575-580.

[8] Loerbroks A, Bosch JA, Mommersteeg PM, Herr RM, Angerer P, Li J. The association of depression and angina pectoris across 47 countries: Findings from the 2002 World Health Survey. Eur J Epidemiol 2014;29(7):507-15. doi: 10.1007/s10654-014-9926-z.

[9] Quashie NT, D'Este C, Agrawal S, Naidoo N, Kowal P. Prevalence of angina and co-morbid conditions among older adults in six low- and middle-income countries: Evidence from SAGE Wave 1. Int J Cardiol 2019;285:140-6. doi: 10.1016/ j.ijcard.2019.02.068.

[10] Ketterer MW, Bekkouche NS, Goldberg AD, McMahon RP, Krantz DS. Symptoms of anxiety and depression are correlates of angina pectoris by recent history and an ischemia-positive treadmill test in patients with documented coronary artery disease in the pimi study. Cardiovasc Psychiatry Neurol 2011;2011:134040. doi: 10.1155/2011/134040.

[11] Patel S, Ram F, Patel SK, Kumar K. Association of behavioral risk factors with self-reported and symptom or measured chronic diseases among adult population (18-

69 years) in India: evidence from SAGE study. BMC Public Health 2019;19(1):560. doi: 10.1186/s12889-019-6953-4.

[12] International Institute for Population Sciences (IIPS), NPHCE, MoHFW, Harvard TH Chan School of Public Health (HSPH) and the University of Southern California (USC). Longitudinal Ageing Study in India (LASI) Wave 1, 2017-18, India Report. Mumbai: International Institute for Population Sciences, 2020.

[13] Rose GA. The diagnosis of ischaemic heart pain and intermittent claudication in field surveys. Bull World Health Organ 1962;27:645–58.

[14] Achterberg S, Soedamah-Muthu SS, Cramer MJ, Kappelle LJ, van der Graaf Y, Algra A, et al. Prognostic value of the Rose questionnaire: a validation with future coronary events in the SMART study. Eur J Prev Cardiol 2012;19(1):5-14. doi: 10.1177/1741826710391117.

[15] Sternthal MJ, Slopen N, Williams DR. Racial disparities in health: How much does stress really matter? Du Bois Rev 2011;8(1):95-113. doi: 10.1017/S1742058X11000087.

[16] Wen CP, David Cheng TY, Tsai SP, Chan HT, Hsu HL, Hsu CC, et al. Are Asians at greater mortality risk for being overweight than Caucasians? Redefining obesity for Asians. Public Health Nutr 2009; 12(4):497-506. doi: 10.1017/S1368980008002802.

[17] Cho E, Chen TY. The bidirectional relationships between effort-reward imbalance and sleep problems among older workers. Sleep Health 2020;6(3):299-305. doi: 10.1016/j.sleh.2020.01.008.

[18] Kessler RC, Andrews A, Mroczek D, Ustun B, Wittchen HU. The World Health Organization Composite International Diagnostic Interview Short-Form (CIDI-SF). Int J Methods Psychiatr Res 1998;7:171–85.

[19] American Psychiatric Association. Diagnostic and statistical manual of mental disorders (DSM-5), 5th ed. Washington, DC: American Psychiatric Publishing, 2013.

[20] Steffick D. Documentation of affective functioning measures in the Health and Retirement Study, 2000. URL: http://hrsonline. isr.umich.edu/sitedocs/userg/dr-005.pdf

[21] Lübs L, Peplies J, Drell C, Bammann K. Cross-sectional and longitudinal factors influencing physical activity of 65 to 75-year-olds: A pan European cohort study based on the survey of health, ageing and retirement in Europe (SHARE). BMC Geriatr 2018;18(1):94. doi: 10.1186/s12877-018-0781-8.

[22] Chobanian AV, Bakris GL, Black HR, Cushman WC, Green LA, Izzo Jr JL, et al. The seventh report of the joint national committee on prevention, detection, evaluation, and treatment of high blood pressure: the JNC 7 report. JAMA 2003;289(19):2560–71.

[23] Casanova-Rosado AJ, Casanova-Rosado JF, Minaya-Sánchez M, Robles-Minaya JL, Casanova-Sarmiento JA, Márquez-Corona MdL, et al. Association of edentulism with various chronic diseases in mexican elders 60+ years: Results of a population-based survey. *Healthcare* 2021;9(4):404. https://doi.org/10.3390/healthcare9040404.

In: Social and Health Issues …
Editors: S Pengpid, K Peltzer et al.
ISBN: 978-1-53619-937-6

Chapter 10

PREVALENCE AND DETERMINANTS OF STROKE AMONG OLDER ADULTS IN INDIA: RESULTS OF A NATIONAL COMMUNITY-DWELLING SURVEY IN 2017-2018

Supa Pengpid[1,2], MPH, DrPH, MBA
and Karl Peltzer[2,3,*], MA Clin Psych, PhD, Dr Habil
[1]ASEAN Institute for Health Development, Mahidol University, Salaya, Phutthamonthon, Nakhon Pathom, Thailand
[2]Department of Research Administration and Development, University of Limpopo, Turfloop, South Africa
[3]Department of Psychology, College of Medical and Health Science, Asia University, Taichung, Taiwan

* *Correspondence*: Professor Karl Peltzer, Department of Research Administration and Development, University of Limpopo, Turfloop Campus, Private Bag X1106, Sovenga 0727, South Africa. Email: kfpeltzer@gmail.com.

Abstract

In this study we aimed to estimate the prevalence and determinants of stroke among older adults in India. The cross-sectional sample consisted of 52,393 individuals (≥50 years) from the Longitudinal Ageing Study in India (LASI) Wave 1 in 2017-2018. Stroke was assessed by self-reported health care provider diagnosis of stroke. Results indicate that the overall prevalence of stroke was 2.2%, 1.6% among women and 2.9% among men. In adjusted logistic regression analysis, factors positively associated with stroke were older age (≥80 years) (Adjusted Odds Ratio-AOR: 1.66, Confidence Interval-CI: 1.12-2.48), male sex (AOR: 1.70, CI: 1.34-2.15), food insecurity (AOR: 1.47, CI: 1.09-1.98), physical inactivity (AOR: 1.81, CI: 1.47-2.24), hypertension (AOR: 2.12, CI: 1.70-2.65), and diabetes (AOR: 2.02, CI: 1.57-2.62). Factors negatively associated with stroke were high spirituality or religiosity (AOR: 0.71, CI: 0.56-0.90), moderate social network (AOR: 0.75, CI: 0.59-0.96), and underweight (AOR: 0.72, CI: 0.53-0.98). More than one in 50 older adults in India had a history of stroke and several associated factors were identified.

Introduction

Globally, "stroke is the third leading cause of disability and second leading cause of death" [1]. "One in four people over age 25 will have a stroke in their lifetime" [2]. "Metabolic risks (high systolic blood pressure (SBP), high body-mass index (BMI), high fasting plasma glucose (FPG), high total cholesterol, and low glomerular filtration rate) account for 72.1% of stroke burden" [2]. Over the past 30 years, the prevalence of stroke has declined in high-income countries [3], while middle-income countries, such as India, are confronted with a high stroke incidence [4]. In population-based surveys in six low- and middle-income countries among older adults (≥50 years), the prevalence of self-reported stroke "ranged from 2.0% in India in 2007 to 6.1% in Russia" [5], 2.6% in Ghana [6], and 3.1% in Mexico [7]. In a two sites study among older adults (≥64 years) in India the prevalence of self-reported stroke was 1.9% in urban sites and 1.1% in rural sites [8]. However, there is a lack of more recent national studies on the prevalence and determinants of stroke in older adults in India.

As previously reviewed [6], factors associated with stroke may include chronic conditions, such as diabetes, hypertension and obesity, lifestyle factors, such as alcohol use, physical inactivity, smoking, "adding salt at the table," "low green leafy vegetable consumption," and stress, and sociodemographic factors, such as age, sex, wealth status and educational level. In addition, in a US community-dwelling study among adults "having a small social network was associated with excess risk of incident stroke" [9]. In a study among adults in India, tobacco use was positively and underweight was negatively associated with stroke [10]. This study aimed to determine the prevalence and determinants of stroke in older community dwelling adults in India in 2017-2018.

OUR STUDY

This secondary data analysis utilized data from the cross-sectional and nationally representative Longitudinal Ageing Study in India (LASI) Wave 1, 2017-2018; "the overall household response rate is 96%, and the overall individual response rate is 87%" [11]. In a household survey, "interview, physical measurement and biomarker data were collected from individuals aged 45 and above and their spouses, regardless of age" [11]. We restricted our analysis on those 50 years and older. Specific details on the sampling approach are found elsewhere [11]. The study was approved by the "Indian Council of Medical Research (ICMR) Ethics Committee and written informed consent was obtained from the participants" [11].

MEASURES

Stroke was assessed with the question, "Has any health professional ever diagnosed you with stroke?" (Yes, No) [11].

Sociodemographic variables consisted of education (none, ≥1 years), age group (50-59, 60-69, 70-79, and 80 or more years), sex (male, female), marital status (currently married vs. widowed/divorced/separated/ deserted/live-in relationship/never married), and residence (rural, urban). Subjective socioeconomic status was assessed with the question, "Please imagine a ten-step ladder, where at the bottom are the people who are the worst off – who have the least money, least education, and the worst jobs or no jobs, and at the top of the ladder are the people who are the best off – those who have the most money, most education, and best jobs. Please indicate the number (1-10) on the rung on the ladder where you would place yourself." [11]. Steps 1 to 3 on the socioeconomic ladder were defined as low, 4-5 as medium, and 6-10 as high socioeconomic status.

Stressors included food insecurity, exposure to stressful events and discrimination experiences.

Food insecurity was sourced from four items, 1) "In the last 12 months, did you ever reduce the size of your meals or skip meals because there was not enough food at your household? (Yes/No), 2) In the last 12 months, were you hungry but didn't eat because there was not enough food at your household? (Yes/No), 3) In the past 12 months, did you ever not eat for a whole day because there was not enough food at your household? 4) Do you think that you have lost weight in the last 12 months because there was not enough food in your household?" [11]. Any positive response to the four questions was scored as one.

Stressful life events included 1) ill-treatment ("Have you felt that you were ill-treated in the past year?" Yes/No), 2) victim of violent crime ("In the last 12 months, have you been the victim of a violent crime, such as assault/mugging/threat to life/others?" (Yes/No), 3) disaster exposure causing health effects ("In the last five years, has your health been severely affected by disasters such as floods, landslides, extreme cold and hot weather, cyclone/typhoons, droughts, earthquakes, tsunamis, or any other natural calamities?" (Yes/No), and 4) man-made incident causing health effects ("In the last five years, has your health been severely affected by man-made incidents such as riots, terrorism, building collapses, fires, traffic accidents or any other man-made incidents?" (Yes/No) [11]. Any yes answer was coded as "1."

Discrimination experiences were assessed with the six-item Everyday Discrimination Scale (EDS) (Short version) [12]. Response options ranged from 1="never" to 6="almost every day," and were dichotomised to 'never'=0 and 'ever' (collapsing those reporting 'less than once a year' or greater into one category)=1; Cronbach's alpha for the EDS in this study was 0.86.

Social support included spirituality/religiosity, organisational religiosity and social network.

Spirituality/religiosity was measured with four items from the Daily Spiritual Experience Scale (DSES) [13], 1) "Do you think that you have a feeling of deep inner peace?" 2) "Do you think that you are spiritually touched by the beauty of creation?" 3) "Do you think that you are thankful for whatever you received in your life?" and 4) "Do you think that you are selflessly caring for others?" Responses ranged from 1=never to 5=every day in a week, and the summed scores were trichotomized to 4-7=low, 8-11=medium, and 12-20=high. Cronbach's alpha for the DSES in this study was 0.86.

Organizational religiosity was assessed with the question, "In the past year, how often have you attended religious services (at a temple/mosque/church, etc.)?" Response options ranged from 1=not at all to 6=every day, and grouped into 1: not at all (low), 2: <weekly (medium) and 3: ≥weekly (high) [11].

Social network was measured with 11 items, e.g., "Eat-out-of-house (restaurant/hotel)" [11]. Responses were coded 1= daily to at least once a month and 0=rarely/once a year or never (Cronbach's alpha 0.67).

Health status variables included body mass index, physical activity, tobacco use, alcohol use, hypertension, diabetes and angina.

Anthropometry: "Height and weight of adults were measured using the Seca 803 digital scale." [11]. "Body Mass Index=BMI was calculated according to Asian criteria: underweight (<18.5 kg/m^2), normal weight (18.5-22.9 kg/m^2), overweight (23.0-24.9 kg/m^2), class I obesity (25.0-29.9 kg/m^2), and class II obesity (≥30.0 kg/m^2)" [14].

Physical inactivity was defined as hardly ever or never vigorous and moderate activity [11].

Current tobacco use was assessed from 1) "Do you currently smoke any tobacco products (cigarettes, bidis, cigars, hookah, cheroot, etc.)? and 2) Do you use smokeless tobacco (such as chewing tobacco, gutka, pan masala, etc.)?" [11].

Heavy episodic alcohol use was assessed with the question, "In the last 3 months, how frequently on average, have you had at least 5 or more drinks on one occasion?" [11] and defined as "one to three days per month, one to four days per week, five or more days per week, or daily."

Hypertension or raised blood pressure (BP) was defined as "systolic BP ≥140 mm Hg and/or diastolic BP ≥90 mm Hg (based on the last two averaged of three readings) or where the participant is currently on antihypertensive medication." [15].

Diabetes was sourced from the question, "Has any health professional ever told you that you have diabetes or high blood sugar?" (Yes/No)." [11].

Angina was assessed with the "World Health Organization's Rose angina questionnaire" [16], defined on the basis of "discomfort at walking uphill or hurrying, or at an ordinary pace on level ground. Furthermore, the pain should be located at the sternum or in the left chest and arm, causing the patient to stop or slow down, and the pain should resolve within 10 minutes when the patient stops or slows down." [17].

Data analysis

Descriptive statistics were applied to describe health status, stressors, social support, sociodemographic information, and stroke. Unadjusted and adjusted logistic regression was utilized to assess the predictors of stroke; variables found significant in univariate analyses were included in the adjusted model. $P < 0.05$ was accepted as significant, missing values were excluded, and no multi-collinearity was found. Statistical analyses were conducted using STATA software version 15.0 (Stata Corporation, College Station, TX, USA), taking the complex study design into account.

FINDINGS

The sample consisted of 52,393 older adults from India. Table 1 shows the detailed participant characteristics. The overall prevalence of angina was 2.2%, 1.6% among women and 2.9% among men (see Table 1).

Table 1. Sample characteristics and stroke status among older adults in India, 2017-2018

Variable	Sample	Stroke
	N (%)	%
Sociodemographic factors		
All	**52393**	**2.2**
Age in years		
50-59	20916 (38.1)	1.4
60-69	18979 (36.2)	2.2
70-79	9108 (18.7)	3.4
≥80	3390 (7.0)	3.6
Sex		
Female	27815 (53.3)	1.6
Male	24578 (46.7)	2.9
Marital status		
Not married	15151 (29.9)	2.4
Married	37236 (70.1)	2.2
Education		
≥1 years	26410 (47.0)	2.5
No schooling	25983 (53.0)	2.0
Subjective socioeconomic status		
Low	17462 (38.2)	2.1
Medium	20070 (37.4)	2.1
High	13176 (24.4)	2.0
Residence		
Rural	34099 (69.0)	2.1
Urban	18294 (31.0)	2.6
Stressors		
Food insecurity	4336 (9.9)	3.5
Stressful events	3986 (9.1)	3.3
Discrimination experiences		
Low (0)	43281 (82.7)	2.0
Medium (1-2)	4483 (10.7)	2.2
High (3-6)	3151 (6.6)	3.4

Table 1. (Continued)

Variable	Sample	Stroke
	N (%)	%
Social support		
Spirituality/Religiosity		
Low	14474 (31.7)	2.7
Moderate	16896 (33.3)	1.8
High	19520 (35.0)	1.8
Organisational religiosity		
Low	13095 (27.1)	3.5
Moderate	23276 (45.6)	1.8
High	15926 (27.4)	1.6
Social network		
Low	19995 (41.3)	2.8
Moderate	15547 (29.1)	2.0
High	16100 (29.6)	1.6
Health status		
Body mass index		
Normal	17179 (37.2)	2.0
Underweight	9428 (23.0)	1.4
Overweight/Obesity	20039 (39.8)	2.1
Physical inactivity	14771 (27.3)	4.4
Current tobacco use	16403 (33.0)	2.0
Heavy episodic alcohol use	1942 (2.9)	3.7
Hypertension	22826 (45.4)	3.1
Diabetes	7423 (13.4)	4.3
Angina	4510 (8.9)	2.6

Associations with stroke

In adjusted logistic regression analysis, factors positively associated with stroke were older age (≥80 years) (Adjusted Odds Ratio-AOR: 1.66, Confidence Interval-CI: 1.12-2.48), male sex (AOR: 1.70, CI: 1.34-2.15), food insecurity (AOR: 1.47, CI: 1.09-1.98), physical inactivity (AOR: 1.81, CI: 1.47-2.24), hypertension (AOR: 2.12, CI: 1.70-2.65), and diabetes (AOR: 2.02, CI: 1.57-2.62). Factors negatively associated with stroke were high spirituality or religiosity (AOR: 0.71, CI: 0.56-0.90), moderate social network (AOR: 0.75, CI: 0.59-0.96), and underweight (AOR: 0.72, CI: 0.53-0.98) (see Table 2).

Table 2. Associations with stroke

Variable	Unadjusted OR (95% CI)	Adjusted OR (95% CI)
Sociodemographic factors		
Age in years		
50-59	1 (Reference)	1 (Reference)
60-69	1.61 (1.16, 2.23)**	1.53 (1.18, 1.98)***
70-79	2.43 (1.74, 3.41)***	1.87 (1.40, 2.50)***
≥80	2.65 (1.78, 3.95)***	1.66 (1.12, 2.48)*
Sex		
Female	1 (Reference)	1 (Reference)
Male	1.78 (1.45, 2.27)***	1.70 (1.34, 2.15)***
Marital status		
Not married	1 (Reference)	---
Married	0.91 (0.74, 1.13)	
Education		
≥1 years	1 (Reference)	---
No schooling	0.81 (0.66, 1.00)	
Subjective socioeconomic status		
Low	1 (Reference)	---
Medium	0.99 (0.77, 1.29)	
High	0.93 (0.69, 1.25)	
Residence		
Rural	1 (Reference)	---
Urban	1.27 (0.99, 1.62)	
Stressors		
Food insecurity	1.72 (1.11, 2.68)*	1.47 (1.09, 1.98)*
Stressful events	1.72 (1.03, 2.88)*	1.21 (0.88, 1.66)
Discrimination experiences		
Low (0)	1 (Reference)	---
Medium (1-2)	1.14 (0.86, 1.52)	
High (3-6)	1.78 (0.92, 3.45)	
Social support		
Spirituality/Religiosity		
Low	1 (Reference)	1 (Reference)
Moderate	0.65 (0.49, 0.85)**	0.70 (0.54, 0.91)**
High	0.65 (0.50, 0.84)***	0.71 (0.56, 0.90)**
Organisational religiosity		
Low	1 (Reference)	1 (Reference)
Moderate	0.51 (0.40, 0.65)***	0.89 (0.70, 1.14)
High	0.46 (0.35, 0.60)***	0.83 (0.62, 1.10)
Social network		
Low	1 (Reference)	1 (Reference)
Moderate	0.70 (0.51, 0.95)*	0.75 (0.59, 0.96)*
High	0.57 (0.45, 0.72)***	0.76 (0.58, 1.00)

Table 2. (Continued)

Variable	Unadjusted OR (95% CI)	Adjusted OR (95% CI)
Health status		
Body mass index		
Normal	1 (Reference)	1 (Reference)
Underweight	0.69 (0.51, 0.92)*	0.72 (0.53, 0.98)*
Overweight/Obesity	1.03 (0.83, 1.28)	0.99 (0.78, 1.25)
Physical inactivity	3.25 (2.65, 3.99)***	1.81 (1.47, 2.24)***
Current tobacco use	0.87 (0.70, 1.07)	---
Heavy episodic alcohol use	1.74 (0.50, 6.02)	---
Hypertension	2.63 (2.10, 3.30)***	2.12 (1.70, 2.65)***
Diabetes	2.31 (1.85, 2.88)***	2.02 (1.57, 2.62)***
Angina	1.21 (0.89, 1.64)	---

OR=Odds Ratio; CI=Confidence Interval.

DISCUSSION

In this national 2017-2018 India LASI survey among community-dwelling older adults (≥50 years), the prevalence of stroke was 2.2%, which seems similar to the 2007 India survey among older adults (≥50 years) (2.0%) [5], a little higher than in a previous study among older adults (≥64 years) in urban sites (1.9%) and rural sites (1.1%) in India [8], and lower than in Ghana (≥50 years) (2.6%) [6], in Mexico (≥50 years) (3.1%) [7] and in Russia (≥50 years) (6.1%) [5]. In October 2010 the Indian Ministry of Health and Family Welfare launched the "National Programme for Prevention and Control of Cancer, Diabetes, Cardiovascular Disease (CVD) and Stroke (NPCDCS)," which is to provide "preventive, promotive, curative and supportive services (core and integrated services) in cancer, diabetes, CVDs and stroke at various government health facilities" [18]. Medical Officers are expected to "give best possible initial treatment in medical emergencies like myocardial infarction and stroke, before referring to higher level of care" [18]. There is also a need to screen routinely for comorbidities of hypertension and diabetes and improve its management in reducing the stroke burden in India. Considering the poor awareness of the warning symptoms of stroke among the general public in India [4], large awareness programmes are needed with the "information that would permit the population to identify the manifestations of a cerebral-vascular event and permit the urgent transportation to a hospital" [19].

Consistent with previous research [6, 7], older age was associated with stroke. While some studies [6] did not find significant sex differences in the prevalence of stroke, this study showed that men had higher odds of stroke than women. In a review, it was found that "age-specific stroke rates are higher in men, but, because of their longer life expectancy and much higher incidence at older ages, women have more stroke events than men." [20]. Our study did not find an association between subjective socioeconomic status, level of education, marital status and stroke. In a study among older adults in Ghana, higher level of education and not married were associated with stroke, while no association was found between wealth status and stroke [6].

Consistent with previous studies [21, 22], exposure to stressors (food insecurity, and stressful events in univariate analysis) were positively associated with stroke. "Stress can increase the cerebrovascular disease risk by modulating symphaticomimetic activity, affecting the blood pressure reactivity, cerebral endothelium, coagulation or heart rhythm." [21]. Social support (high spirituality/religiosity, medium social network and in univariate analysis high organisational religiosity) was found protective against stroke, which was also found among US community-dwelling adults [9].

In line with previous investigations (hypertension and diabetes [2, 6, 22], and physical inactivity [23, 24]), having hypertension, diabetes and physical inactivity increased the odds of stroke. This result is not surprising since hypertension, diabetes and physical inactivity are major risk factors for stroke [2]. Consistent with a previous study in India [10], this study showed a negative associated between underweight and stroke. While other studies [6, 10, 22] showed an association between tobacco use and stroke, we did not find a significant association.

Study limitations

The study was limited by its cross-sectional design and the self-report of most data collected, including stroke. Some variables, such as dietary behaviour, were not assessed and should be included in future studies.

CONCLUSION

More than one in 50 older adults in India had a history of stroke. Sociodemographic factors (older age and male sex), stressors (food insecurity, and stressful events in univariate analysis), lack of social support (low spirituality/religiosity, low social network and in univariate analysis no organisational religiosity), and health status variables (not having underweight, physical inactivity, hypertension, and diabetes) were identified for stroke, which can be utilized in targeting interventions.

ACKNOWLEDGMENTS

The Longitudinal Aging Study in India Project is funded by the Ministry of Health and Family Welfare, Government of India, the National Institute on Aging (R01 AG042778, R01 AG030153), and United Nations Population Fund, India.

REFERENCES

[1] Feigin VL, Forouzanfar MH, Krishnamurthi R, Mensah GA, Connor M, Bennett DA, et al. Global and regional burden of stroke during 1990–2010: Findings from the global burden of disease study 2010. Lancet 2014;383(9913):245–54.

[2] World Stroke Organization. Global stroke fact sheet, 2020. URL: https://www.world-stroke.org/assets/downloads/WSO_Global_Stroke_Fact_Sheet.pdf.

[3] Feigin VL, Lawes CM, Bennett DA, Barker-Collo SL, Parag V. Worldwide stroke incidence and early case fatality reported in 56 population-based studies: a systematic review. Lancet Neurol 2009;8(4):355-69. doi: 10.1016/S1474-4422(09)70025-0.

[4] Banerjee TK, Das SK. Fifty years of stroke researches in India. Ann Indian Acad Neurol 2016;19(1):1-8. doi:10.4103/0972-2327.168631.

[5] Ruan Y, Guo Y, Zheng Y, Huang Z, Sun S, Kowal P, et al. Cardiovascular disease (CVD) and associated risk factors among older adults in six low-and middle-income countries: results from SAGE Wave 1. BMC Public Health 2018;18(1):778. doi: 10.1186/s12889-018-5653-9.

[6] Sanuade OA, Dodoo FN, Koram K, de-Graft Aikins A. Prevalence and correlates of stroke among older adults in Ghana: Evidence from the Study on Global AGEing and adult health (SAGE). PLoS One 2019;14(3):e0212623. doi: 10.1371/ journal.pone.0212623. eCollection 2019.

[7] Peltzer K. Pengpid S. Prevalence and correlates of stroke among a nationally representative population-based sample of older adults in Mexico. Int J Disabil Hum Dev 2020;19(3):555-60.

[8] Ferri CP, Schoenborn C, Kalra L, Acosta D, Guerra M, Huang Y, et al. Prevalence of stroke and related burden among older people living in Latin America, India and China. J Neurol Neurosurg Psychiatry 2011;82(10):1074-82. doi: 10.1136/jnnp. 2010.234153.

[9] Nagayoshi M, Everson-Rose SA, Iso H, Mosley TH Jr, Rose KM, Lutsey PL. Social network, social support, and risk of incident stroke: Atherosclerosis Risk in Communities study. Stroke 2014;45(10):2868-73. doi: 10.1161/STROKEAHA. 114.005815.

[10] Patel S, Ram F, Patel SK, Kumar K. Association of behavioral risk factors with self-reported and symptom or measured chronic diseases among adult population (18-69 years) in India: evidence from SAGE study. BMC Public Health 2019;19(1):560. doi: 10.1186/s12889-019-6953-4.

[11] International Institute for Population Sciences (IIPS), NPHCE, MoHFW, Harvard TH Chan School of Public Health (HSPH) and the University of Southern California (USC). Longitudinal Ageing Study in India (LASI) Wave 1, 2017-18, India Report. Mumbai: International Institute for Population Sciences, 2020.

[12] Sternthal MJ, Slopen N, Williams DR. Racial disparities in health: How much does stress really matter? Du Bois Rev 2011;8(1):95-113. doi: 10.1017/S1742058X 11000087.

[13] Underwood LG, Teresi JA. The Daily Spiritual Experience Scale: Development, theoretical description, reliability, exploratory factor analysis, and preliminary construct validity using health-related data. Ann Behav Med 2002;24:22-33.

[14] Wen CP, David Cheng TY, Tsai SP, Chan HT, Hsu HL, Hsu CC, et al. Are Asians at greater mortality risks for being overweight than Caucasians? Redefining obesity for Asians. Public Health Nutr 2009;12(4):497-506. doi: 10.1017/S1368980008002802.

[15] Chobanian AV, Bakris GL, Black HR, Cushman WC, Green LA, Izzo Jr JL, et al. The seventh report of the joint national committee on prevention, detection, evaluation, and treatment of high blood pressure: the JNC 7 report. JAMA 2003;289(19):2560–71.

[16] Rose GA. The diagnosis of ischaemic heart pain and intermittent claudication in field surveys. Bull World Health Organ 1962;27:645–58.

[17] Achterberg S, Soedamah-Muthu SS, Cramer MJ, Kappelle LJ, van der Graaf Y, Algra A, et al. Prognostic value of the Rose questionnaire: a validation with future coronary events in the SMART study. Eur J Prev Cardiol 2012;19(1):5-14. doi: 10.1177/1741826710391117.

[18] National Centre for Disease Control Directorate General of Health Services Ministry of Health and Family Welfare, India. National Programme for Prevention and Control of Cancer, Diabetes, Cardiovascular Diseases and Stroke, 2017. URL: http://nhsrcindia.org/sites/default/files/Module%20for%20MOs%20for%20Prevention%2CControl%20%26%20PBS%20of%20Hypertension%2CDiabetes%20%26%20Common%20Cancer.pdf.

[19] Góngora-Rivera F. Perspective on stroke in Mexico. Medicina Universitaria 2015;17(68):184-7.

[20] Reeves MJ, Bushnell CD, Howard G, Gargano JW, Duncan PW, Lynch G, et al. Sex differences in stroke: epidemiology, clinical presentation, medical care, and outcomes. Lancet Neurol 2008;7(10):915-26. doi: 10.1016/S1474-4422(08)70193-5.

[21] Kotlęga D, Gołąb-Janowska M, Masztalewicz M, Ciećwież S, Nowacki P. The emotional stress and risk of ischemic stroke. Neurol Neurochir Pol 2016;50(4):265-70. doi: 10.1016/j.pjnns.2016.03.006.

[22] O'Donnell MJ, Xavier D, Liu L, Zhang H, Chin SL, Rao-Melacini P, et al. Risk factors for ischaemic and intracerebral haemorrhagic stroke in 22 countries (the INTERSTROKE study): a case-control study. Lancet 2010;376(9735):112–23.

[23] Lee CD, Folsom AR, Blair SN. Physical activity and stroke risk: A meta-analysis. Stroke 2003;34(10):2475-81.

[24] Willey JZ, Moon YP, Sacco RL, Greenlee H, Diaz KM, Wright CB, et al. Physical inactivity is a strong risk factor for stroke in the oldest old: Findings from a multi-ethnic population (the Northern Manhattan Study). Int J Stroke 2017;12(2):197-200. doi: 10.1177/1747493016676614.

In: Social and Health Issues …
Editors: S Pengpid, K Peltzer et al.
ISBN: 978-1-53619-937-6

Chapter 11

PREVALENCE AND CORRELATES OF ARTHRITIS AMONG A NATIONALLY REPRESENTATIVE POPULATION-BASED SAMPLE OF OLDER ADULTS IN INDIA

Karl Peltzer[1,2], MA Clin Psych, PhD, Dr Habil and Supa Pengpid[1,3,*], MPH, DrPH, MBA

[1]Department of Research Administration and Development, University of Limpopo, Turfloop, South Africa

[2]Department of Psychology, College of Medical and Health Science, Asia University, Taichung, Taiwan

[3]ASEAN Institute for Health Development, Mahidol University, Salaya, Phutthamonthon, Nakhon Pathom, Thailand

* *Correspondence*: Professor Supa Pengpid, ASEAN Institute for Health Development, Mahidol University, 25/25 Phutthamonthon Road 4, Salaya, Phutthamonton, Nakhon Pathom 73170, Thailand. Email: supaprom@yahoo.com.

ABSTRACT

We here aimed to determine the prevalence and correlates of self-reported arthritis in older adults in India. The cross-sectional sample consisted of 52,393 individuals (≥50 years) from the Longitudinal Ageing Study in India (LASI) Wave 1 in 2017-2018. Results indicate that the prevalence of self-reported arthritis was 14.7%, 17.3% among women and 11.7% among men. In adjusted logistic regression analysis, older age, obesity, chronic lung disease, neurological or psychiatric problems, insomnia symptoms, hypertension, physical pain, gastrointestinal problems, periodontal disases and functional disability were positively associated with self-reported arthritis, while male sex was negatively associated with arthritis. In addition, in unadjusted analysis, physical inactivity, major depressive disorder, stroke, heart disease, angina, diabetes, high cholesterol, persistent headaches, and back pain or problems were positively, and married, high subjective socioeconomic status, current tobacco use and lifetime alcohol use were negatively associated with self-reported arthritis. One in seven older adults in India reported having been diagnosed with arthritis. Several risk factors were identified, which can be targeted in public health interventions.

INTRODUCTION

Arthritis contributes significantly to the global burden of disability [1, 2]. The global prevalence of rheumatoid arthritis was 0.24% [2], knee osteoarthritis 3.8% and hip osteoarthritis was 0.85% [1], and the global prevalence of knee osteoarthritis among persons 40 years and older was 16.0% [3]. In a six-country study among predominantly older adults in low- and middle-income settings, the prevalence of self-reported arthritis was 19.9% among women and 14.1% among men [4]. In South Africa, the prevalence of self-reported arthritis among older adults (≥50 years) was 24.7% [5], among older adults (≥50 years) in Mexico in 2014-2015 it was 9.2% [6], and in a national study among older adults (≥50 years) in India in 2007, the prevalence of self-reported arthritis was 24.5% [7]. There is a lack of more recent national data on the prevalence and correlates of arthritis among older adults in India.

Factors associated with arthritis may include sociodemographic factors, including female sex [8-12], older age [9, 11-13], lower education [10, 14], higher wealth status [9], separated, divorced or widowed [14], and rural residence [13]. Some studies found an association between physical inactivity [13-15], sedentary behaviour [16], inadequate fruit and vegetable consumption [17], alcohol use [18], obesity [5, 6, 8, 13] and arthritis. Various studies showed an association between poor mental health, such as psychological distress [5, 19, 20], mental health problems [20], depressive symptoms [6, 10, 21], sleep complaints [20] and arthritis. Furthermore, potential risk factors for arthritis include a number of physical conditions, including pain [11], functional disability [10, 11, 20], physical disability [20], hypertension [10], heart disease, stroke [12], headache [10], gastrointestinal problems [10], digestive diseases [12], bronchitis [10], chronic lung disease [12], and periodontitis [22]. This study aimed to determine the prevalence and correlates of arthritis in older community-dwelling adults in India in 2017-2018.

OUR STUDY

This secondary data analysis utilized data from the cross-sectional and nationally representative Longitudinal Ageing Study in India (LASI) Wave 1, 2017-2018; "the overall household response rate is 96%, and the overall individual response rate is 87%" [23]. In a household survey, "interview, physical measurement and biomarker data were collected from individuals aged 45 and above and their spouses, regardless of age" [23]. We restricted our analysis to those 50 years and older. Specific details on the sampling approach are found elsewhere [23]. The study was approved by the "Indian Council of Medical Research (ICMR) Ethics Committee and written informed consent was obtained from the participants" [23].

Measures

Arthritis was assessed by "self-reported healthcare professional diagnosis, Have you ever been diagnosed with arthritis or rheumatism?" (Yes, No) [23].

Sociodemographic variables consisted of education (none, ≥1 years), age group (50-59, 60-69, 70-79, and 80 or more years), sex (male, female), marital status (currently married vs. widowed/divorced/separated/ deserted/live-in relationship/never married), and residence (rural, urban). Subjective socioeconomic status was assessed with the question, "Please imagine a ten-step ladder, where at the bottom are the people who are the worst off – who have the least money, least education, and the worst jobs or no jobs, and at the top of the ladder are the people who are the best off – those who have the most money, most education, and best jobs. Please indicate the number (1-10) on the rung on the ladder where you would place yourself." [23]. Steps 1 to 3 on the socioeconomic ladder were defined as low, 4-5 as medium, and 6-10 as high socioeconomic status.

Anthropometry: "Height and weight of adults were measured using the Seca 803 digital scale" [23]. "Body Mass Index=BMI was calculated according to Asian criteria: underweight (<18.5 kg/m^2), normal weight (18.5-22.9 kg/m^2), overweight (23.0-24.9 kg/m^2), class I obesity (25.0-29.9 kg/m^2), and class II obesity (≥30.0 kg/m^2)" [24].

Physical inactivity was defined as hardly ever or never vigorous and moderate activity [23].

Current tobacco use was assessed from 1) "Do you currently smoke any tobacco products (cigarettes, bidis, cigars, hookah, cheroot, etc.)? and 2) Do you use smokeless tobacco (such as chewing tobacco, gutka, pan masala, etc.)?" [23].

Lifetime alcohol use was assessed with the question, "Have you ever consumed any alcoholic beverages such as beer, wine, liquor, country liquor etc?" (Yes, No) [23].

Chronic conditions were sourced from the question, "Has any health professional ever told you that you have…?": "1) Diabetes or high blood sugar; 2) Chronic lung disease such as asthma, chronic obstructive pulmonary disease/Chronic bronchitis or other chronic lung problems; 3) Chronic heart diseases such as Coronary heart disease (heart attack or Myocardial Infarction), congestive heart failure, or other chronic heart problems; 4) Stroke; 5) neurological or psychiatric problems, 6) Gastrointestinal problems (GERD, constipation, indigestion, piles, peptic Ulcer), and 7) High cholesterol (Yes/No)." [23].

Hypertension or raised blood pressure (BP) was defined as "systolic BP ≥140 mm Hg and/or diastolic BP ≥90 mm Hg (based on the last two averaged of three readings) or where the participant is currently on antihypertensive medication" [25].

Angina was assessed with the "World Health Organization's Rose angina questionnaire" [26], defined on the basis of "discomfort at walking uphill or hurrying, or at an ordinary pace on level ground. Furthermore, the pain should be located at the sternum or in the left chest and arm, causing the patient to stop or slow down, and the pain should resolve within 10 minutes when the patient stops or slows down." [27].

Symptom-based pain was defined as "troubled by pain and required some form of medication or treatment for relief of pain" [23].

Back pain or problem and persistent headaches were assessed based on affirmative response to the question "Have you had any of the following persistent or troublesome problems in past two years?" [23].

Functional disability was assessed with six items of Activities of Daily Living (ADL) and seven items of Instrumental Activities of Daily Living (IADL) (Yes, No) [28, 29]. Cronbach alpha was 0.87 for ADL and 0.90 for IADL in this study. Responses were trichotomized into 0, 1, and ≥2 ADL and IADL items.

Major depressive disorder in the past 12 months was assessed with the Health and Retirement Study (HRS) Composite International Diagnostic Interview short form (CIDI-SF) [30], using criteria of the Diagnostic and Statistical Manual of Mental Disorders (DSM) [31]. Study respondents were required to "endorse either anhedonia or depressed mood for most of the day for most of a 2-week period or more," and those who fulfilled this criterion "completed an additional seven symptoms: lost interest, feeling tired, change in weight, trouble with sleep, trouble concentrating, feeling down, and thoughts of death." [24]. "Those with a score ≥3 were considered to meet the criteria for having MDD in the previous 12 months; MDD symptomology scores ranged from 0 to 7" [32].

Insomnia symptoms were assessed with four questions: 1) "How often do you have trouble falling asleep?" 2) "How often do you have trouble with waking up during the night?" 3) "How often do you have trouble with waking up too early and not being able to fall asleep again?" 4) "How often did you feel unrested during the day, no matter how many hours of sleep you had?" Responses options were "never, rarely (1-2 nights per week), occasionally (3-4 nights per week), and frequently (5 or more nights per week)" [23]. Insomnia problems were coded as "frequently" for any of the four symptoms as one [33].

Periodontal disease was assessed any affirmative response to the three questions, "In the last 12 months, have you ever been diagnosed with or suffered from bleeding gums, swelling gums or ulcers lasting more than two weeks?" [23].

Data analysis

Descriptive statistics were applied to describe health status, sociodemographic information, and arthritis. Unadjusted and adjusted logistic regression was utilized to assess the predictors of arthritis; variables found significant in univariate analyses were included in the adjusted model. $P < 0.05$ was accepted as significant, missing values were excluded, and no multi-collinearity was found. Statistical analyses were conducted using STATA software version 15.0 (Stata Corporation, College Station, TX, USA), taking the complex study design into account.

FINDINGS

The sample included 52,393 older adults (50 years and older), with a median age of 62 years (14 years interquartile range), 53.3% were female and 46.7%

male. Majority (70.1%) of participants were married, 69.0% were residing in rural areas, and 38.2% had low subjective socioeconomic status. Almost half of the participants (45.4%) had hypertension, 6.4% obesity (≥30 kg/m^2), 8.9% angina, 13.4% had diabetes, 7.5% lung disease, 3.0% current tobacco use, 14.9% had ever engaged in alcohol use, and 27.3% were physical inactive. In addition, 8.0% of older adults had major depressive disorder, 13.4% insomnia symptoms, 2.2% stroke, 4.2% heart disease, 2.4% high cholesterol, 12.5% persistent headaches, 32.4% back pain or problems, 13.0% physical pain, 18.4% gastrointestinal problems, 16.0% periodontal disease and 33.8% had two or more functional disabilities. The prevalence of self-reported arthritis was 14.7%, 17.3% among women and 11.7% among men (see Table 1).

Table 1. Sample and arthritis characteristics among older adults in India, 2017-2018

Variable	Sample	Arthritis self-reported
	N (%)	%
All	**52393**	**14.7**
Age in years		
50-59	20916 (38.1)	12.4
60-69	18979 (36.2)	15.2
70-79	9108 (18.7)	18.5
≥80	3390 (7.0)	14.8
Sex		
Female	27815 (53.3)	17.3
Male	24578 (46.7)	11.7
Marital status		
Not married	15151 (29.9)	17.1
Married	37236 (70.1)	13.7
Education		
≥1 years	26410 (47.0)	15.4
No schooling	25983 (53.0)	14.4
Subjective socioeconomic status		
Low	17462 (38.2)	14.9
Medium	20070 (37.4)	14.8
High	13176 (24.4)	13.2
Residence		
Rural	34099 (69.0)	14.2
Urban	18294 (31.0)	15.9

Table 1. (Continued)

Variable	Sample	Arthritis self-reported
	N (%)	%
Body mass index (≥30 kg/m^2)	3271 (6.4)	27.1
Physical inactivity	14771 (27.3)	16.3
Current tobacco use	16403 (33.0)	13.0
Ever alcohol use	9346 (14.9)	10.7
Chronic lung disease	3297 (7.5)	24.4
Neurological or psychiatric problem	1243 (2.5)	35.1
Major depressive disorder	3263 (8.0)	18.2
Insomnia symptoms	6596 (13.4)	20.8
Stroke	1109 (2.2)	21.8
Heart disease	2154 (4.2)	26.0
Hypertension	22826 (45.4)	17.0
Angina	4510 (8.9)	19.3
Diabetes	7423 (13.4)	19.9
High cholesterol	1946 (2.4)	23.3
Persistent headaches	6492 (12.5)	19.9
Back pain/problem	18434 (32.4)	18.9
Physical pain	6050 (13.0)	26.9
Gastrointestinal problem	9803 (18.4)	18.6
Periodontal disease	7540 (16.0)	20.8
Functional disability		
0	31213 (55.5)	10.3
1	5592 (10.7)	14.7
2 or more	15318 (33.8)	22.0

Associations with self-reported arthritis

In adjusted logistic regression analysis, older age, obesity, chronic lung disease, neurological or psychiatric problems, insomnia symptoms, hypertension, physical pain, gastrointestinal problems, periodontal diseases and functional disability were positively associated with self-reported arthritis, while male sex was negatively associated with arthritis. In addition, in unadjusted analysis, physical inactivity, major depressive disorder, stroke,

Table 2. Associations with arthritis among older adults in India, 2017-2018

Variable	Unadjusted Odds Ratios (95% CI)	Adjusted Odds Ratios (95% CI)
Age in years		
50-59	1 (Reference)	1 (Reference)
60-69	1.27 (1.12, 1.44)***	1.15 (1.01, 1.32)*
70-79	1.61 (1.30, 2.00)***	1.24 (1.02, 1.50)*
≥80	1.24 (0.99, 1.54)	0.83 (0.65, 1.06)
Sex (Male)	0.67 (0.61, 0.74)***	0.77 (0.67, 0.89)***
Marital status (Married)	0.70 (0.59, 0.89)***	0.96 (0.79, 1.17)
Education (No schooling)	1.05 (0.87, 1.27)	---
Subjective socioeconomic status		
Low	1 (Reference)	1 (Reference)
Medium	0.99 (0.86, 1.15)	0.97 (0.82, 1.15)
High	0.81 (0.69, 0.96)*	0.87 (0.72, 1.05)
Residence (Urban)	1.09 (0.71, 1.67)	---
Body mass index (≥30 kg/m^2)	1.95 (1.57, 2.42)***	1.95 (1.55, 2.46)***
Physical inactivity	1.21 (1.08, 1.36)***	1.07 (0.95, 1.22)
Current tobacco use	0.82 (0.69, 0.97)*	0.98 (0.82, 1.18)
Ever alcohol use	0.67 (0.54, 0.82)***	0.90 (0.95, 1.22)
Chronic lung disease	2.15 (1.32, 3.48)**	1.25 (1.03, 1.52)*
Neurological or psychiatric problem	3.11 (2.16, 4.46)***	2.54 (1.72, 3.74)***
Major depressive disorder	1.37 (1.11, 1.69)**	0.86 (0.70, 1.05)
Insomnia symptoms	1.77 (1.55, 2.03)***	1.27 (1.12, 1.43)***
Stroke	1.86 (1.23, 2.81)**	1.25 (0.81, 1.95)
Heart disease	2.28 (1.56, 3.34)***	1.35 (0.94, 1.93)
Hypertension	1.41 (1.23, 1.62)***	1.14 (1.01, 1.28)*
Angina	1.58 (1.28, 1.96)***	0.99 (0.82, 1.20)
Diabetes	1.59 (1.18, 2.13)**	1.41 (0.95, 2.10)
High cholesterol	1.96 (1.41, 2.74)***	1.24 (0.84, 1.83)
Persistent headaches	1.57 (1.28, 1.91)***	1.05 (0.87, 1.27)
Back pain/problem	1.64 (1.49, 1.81)***	1.05 (0.92, 1.21)
Physical pain	2.64 (2.15, 3.25)***	1.98 (1.67, 2.34)***
Gastrointestinal problem	1.51 (1.26, 1.81)***	1.20 (1.05, 1.36)**
Periodontal disease	1.74 (1.35, 2.24)***	1.37 (1.05, 1.79)*
Functional disability		
0	1 (Reference)	1 (Reference)
1	1.68 (1.50, 1.88)***	1.42 (1.22, 1.66)***
2 or more	2.77 (2.39, 3.21)***	1.94 (1.64, 2.29)***

CI=Confidence Interval; ****p*<0.001; ** *p*<0.01; **p*<0.05.

heart disease, angina, diabetes, high cholesterol, persistent headaches, and back pain or problems were positively, and married, high, subjective socioeconomic status, current tobacco use and lifetime alcohol use ere negatively associated with self-reported arthritis (see Table 2).

Discussion

In this nationally representative sample of older adults in India in 2017-2018, the prevalence of self-reported arthritis was 14.7% (17.3% in women and 11.7% in men) which is lower than in the six-country study among predominantly older adults in low- and middle-income settings (19.9% among women and 14.1% among men) [4], and lower than in the 2007 India study among older adults (24.5%) [7] and among older adults in South Africa (24.7%) [5], but higher than in a national study among older adults in Mexico (9.2%) [6]. More research is needed to establish a possible decline of the prevalence of self-reported arthritis in India.

Consistent with previous research [8-12], this study showed that female sex and older age were associated with self-reported arthritis. The sex difference may be attributed to changes in estrogen levels influencing bone metabolism [10, 34]. Some research studies found an association between lower education [10, 14] and arthritis, but we did not find a significant association. Higher subjective socioeconomic status was in unadjusted analysis protective against arthritis, while in a study among older adults in Ghana higher wealth status was associated with arthritis [9]. Consistent with previous findings [14], being married was found protective against arthritis. It is possible that those who are not married or widowed are older than those who are married and therefore more likely have arthritis. Unlike in a previous investigation [13], we did not find any significant differences in the prevalence of arthritis between rural and urban older adults.

Consistent with previous research [5, 6, 8, 13], this study found an association between obesity and arthritis. Obesity may "exhibit a chronic subclinical inflammatory state" increasing the risk for rheumatoid arthritis [35]. Some studies found an association between physical inactivity and arthritis [13-15], while this study found this association in univariate analysis. "Sedentary behaviour may exacerbate already heightened inflammation in rheumatoid arthritis and hold relevance for disease-related outcomes" [16]. In unadjusted analysis, we found that current tobacco use and lifetime alcohol use was protective against arthritis. Similar results were previously found for alcohol use [18].

Furthermore, the study found associations between poor mental health (neurological or psychiatric problems, insomnia symptoms, and in unadjusted analysis major depressive disorder), which is consistent with previous results [5, 6, 10, 19-21]. The association between insomnia symptoms and arthritis may be related to overnight pain and discomfort [20]. Prothero et al. [19] showed that "psychological interventions resulted in small to moderate improvements in biopsychosocial outcomes for patients with rheumatoid arthritis in addition to those achieved by standard care."

Consistent with some previous research [10-12, 20, 22], this study found a positive association between physical pain, functional disability, chronic lung disease, hypertension, gastrointestinal problems, periodontal disease and arthritis. Previous research [10, 12] also found an association between heart disease, stroke, headache, and arthritis, while this study found these associations in univariate analysis. It is possible that across these diverse physical conditions, there is an underlying connection via pain and associated inflammatory dysfunction [10].

Study limitations include the cross-sectional design, the assessment of some variables by self-report. Some variables that may affect arthritis, such as dietary behaviour, were not assessed and should be included in future studies. Some determinants, such as physical pain, insomnia symptoms, depression, lung disease, or hypertension [10, 12], may also be consequences. Longitudinal studies are needed to determine causality.

CONCLUSION

One in seven older adults in India reported having been diagnosed with arthritis. Several potential risk factors for arthritis, such as older age, female sex, obesity, chronic lung disease, neurological or psychiatric problems, insomnia symptoms, hypertension, physical pain, gastrointestinal problems, periodontal diseases and functional disability were identified, which can be targeted in public health interventions.

ACKNOWLEDGMENTS

The Longitudinal Aging Study in India Project is funded by the Ministry of Health and Family Welfare, Government of India, the National Institute on Aging (R01 AG042778, R01 AG030153), and United Nations Population Fund, India.

REFERENCES

[1] Cross M, Smith E, Hoy D, Nolte S, Ackerman I, Fransen M, et al. The global burden of hip and knee osteoarthritis: estimates from the global burden of disease 2010 study. Ann Rheum Dis 2014;73(7):1323–30. doi:10.1136/annrheumdis-2013-204763.

[2] Cross M, Smith E, Hoy D, Carmona L, Wolfe F, Vos T, et al. The global burden of rheumatoid arthritis: estimates from the global burden of disease 2010 study. Ann Rheum Dis 2014;73(7):1316–22. doi:10.1136/annrheumdis-2013-204627.

[3] Cui A, Li H, Wang D, Zhong J, Chen Y, Lu H. Global, regional prevalence, incidence and risk factors of knee osteoarthritis in population-based studies. EClinicalMedicine 2020;29-30:100587. oi:10.1016/j.eclinm.2020.100587.

[4] Brennan-Olsen SL, Cook S, Leech MT, Bowe SJ, Kowal P, Naidoo N, et al. Prevalence of arthritis according to age, sex and socioeconomic status in six low and middle income countries: analysis of data from the World Health Organization study on global AGEing and adult health (SAGE) Wave 1. BMC Musculoskelet Disord 2017;18(1):271. doi: 10.1186/s12891-017-1624-z.

[5] Peltzer K, Phaswana-Mafuya N. Arthritis and associated factors in older adults in South Africa. Turk J Geriatr 2013;16(4):389-94.

[6] Pengpid S, Peltzer K. Prevalence and correlates of arthritis among a nationally representative population-based sample of older adults in Mexico. Int J Disabil Hum Dev 2020;19(3):603-10.

[7] Agrawal S, Fledderjohann J, Ghosh S. Risk factors for self-reported cataract symptoms, diagnosis, and surgery uptake among older adults in India: Findings from

the WHO SAGE data. Glob Public Health 2020 Oct 22:1-15. doi: 10.1080/17441692.2020.1836246.

[8] Silverwood V, Blagojevic-Bucknall M, Jinks C, Jordan JL, Protheroe J, Jordan KP. Current evidence on risk factors for knee osteoarthritis in older adults: a systematic review and meta-analysis. Osteoarthritis Cartilage 2015;23(4):507–15. doi:10.1016/j.joca.2014.11.019.

[9] Nakua EK, Otupiri E, Dzomeku VM, Owusu-Dabo E, Agyei-Baffour P, Yawson AE, et al. Gender disparities of chronic musculoskeletal disorder burden in the elderly Ghanaian population: study on global ageing and adult health (SAGE WAVE 1). BMC Musculoskelet Disord 2015;16:204. doi: 10.1186/s12891-015-0666-3.

[10] Blay SL, Fillenbaum GG, Andreoli SB, Gastal FL. Prevalence and concomitants of arthritis in the elderly in Rio Grande do Sul, Brazil. PLoS One 2012;7(9):e45418. doi: 10.1371/journal.pone.0045418.

[11] French HP, Galvin R, Horgan NF, Kenny RA. Prevalence and burden of osteoarthritis amongst older people in Ireland: findings from The Irish LongituDinal Study on Ageing (TILDA). Eur J Public Health 2016;26(1):192-8. doi: 10.1093/eurpub/ckv109.

[12] Li C, Liu T, Sun W, Wu L, Zou ZY. Prevalence and risk factors of arthritis in a middle-aged and older Chinese population: the China health and retirement longitudinal study. Rheumatology 2015;54(4):697-706. doi: 10.1093/rheumatology/keu391.

[13] Patel S, Ram F, Patel SK, Kumar K. Association of behavioral risk factors with self-reported and symptom or measured chronic diseases among adult population (18-69 years) in India: evidence from SAGE study. BMC Public Health 2019;19(1):560. doi:10.1186/s12889-019-6953-4.

[14] Arokiasamy P, Uttamacharya, Kowal P, Capistrant BD, Gildner TE, Thiele E, et al. Chronic noncommunicable diseases in 6 low- and middle-income countries: findings from wave 1 of the world health organization's Study on Global Ageing and Adult Health (SAGE). Am J Epidemiol 2017;185(6):414-28. https://doi.org/10.1093/aje/kww125.

[15] Tierney M, Fraser A, Kennedy N. Physical activity in rheumatoid arthritis: a systematic review. J Phys Act Health 2012;9(7):1036–48. doi:10.1123/jpah.9.7.1036.

[16] Fenton SAM, Veldhuijzen van Zanten JJCS, Duda JL, Metsios GS, Kitas GD. Sedentary behaviour in rheumatoid arthritis: definition, measurement and implications for health. Rheumatology 2018;57(2):213–26. doi:10.1093/rheumatology/kex053.

[17] Pattison DJ, Harrison RA, Symmons DP. The role of diet in susceptibility to rheumatoid arthritis: a systematic review. J Rheumatol 2004;31(7):1310–9.

[18] Scott IC, Tan R, Stahl D, Steer S, Lewis CM, Cope AP. The protective effect of alcohol on developing rheumatoid arthritis: A systematic review and meta-analysis. Rheumatology 2013;52(5):856–67. doi:10.1093/rheumatology/kes376.

[19] Prothero L, Barley E, Galloway J, Georgopoulou S, Sturt J. The evidence base for psychological interventions for rheumatoid arthritis: A systematic review of reviews. Int J Nurs Stud 2018;82:20–9. doi:10.1016/j.ijnurstu.2018.03.008.

[20] Machado GM, Barreto SM, Passos VM, Lima-Costa MF. Health status indicators among community-dwelling elders with arthritis: The Bambuí health and aging study. J Rheumatol 2006;33(2):342–7.

[21] Vennu V, Misra H, Misra A. Depressive symptoms and the risk of arthritis: A survival analysis using data from the osteoarthritis initiative. Indian J Psychiatry 2019;61(5):444-50. doi: 10.4103/psychiatry.IndianJPsychiatry_241_18.

[22] Dumitrescu AL. Occurrence of self-reported systemic medical conditions in patients with periodontal disease. Rom J Intern Med 2006;44(1):35-48.

[23] International Institute for Population Sciences (IIPS), NPHCE, MoHFW, Harvard TH Chan School of Public Health (HSPH) and the University of Southern California (USC). Longitudinal Ageing Study in India (LASI) Wave 1, 2017-18, India Report. Mumbai: International Institute for Population Sciences, 2020.

[24] Wen CP, David Cheng TY, Tsai SP, Chan HT, Hsu HL, Hsu CC, et al. Are Asians at greater mortality risks for being overweight than Caucasians? Redefining obesity for Asians. Public Health Nutr 2009;12(4):497-506. doi: 10.1017/S1368980008002802.

[25] Chobanian AV, Bakris GL, Black HR, Cushman WC, Green LA, Izzo Jr JL, et al. The seventh report of the joint national committee on prevention, detection, evaluation, and treatment of high blood pressure: The JNC 7 report. JAMA 2003;289(19):2560–71.

[26] Rose GA. The diagnosis of ischaemic heart pain and intermittent claudication in field surveys. Bull World Health Organ 1962;27:645–58.

[27] Achterberg S, Soedamah-Muthu SS, Cramer MJ, Kappelle LJ, van der Graaf Y, Algra A; SMART Study Group. Prognostic value of the Rose questionnaire: A validation with future coronary events in the SMART study. Eur J Prev Cardiol 2012;19(1):5-14. doi: 10.1177/1741826710391117.

[28] Katz S, Ford AB, Moskowitz RW, Jackson BA, Jaffe MW. Studies of illness in the aged. the index of adl: a standardized measure of biological and psychosocial function. JAMA 1963;185:914-9. doi: 10.1001/jama.1963.03060120024016.

[29] Lawton MP, Brody EM. Assessment of older people: self-maintaining and instrumental activities of daily living. Gerontologist 1969;9(3):179-86.

[30] Kessler RC, Andrews A, Mroczek D, Ustun B, Wittchen HU. The World Health Organization Composite International Diagnostic Interview Short-Form (CIDI-SF). Int J Methods Psychiatr Res 1998;7:171–85.

[31] American Psychiatric Association. Diagnostic and statistical manual of mental disorders (DSM-5), 5th ed. Washington, DC: American Psychiatric Publishing, 2013.

[32] Steffick D. Documentation of affective functioning measures in the Health and Retirement Study, 2000. URL: http://hrsonline. isr.umich.edu/sitedocs/userg/dr-005.pdf.

[33] Cho E, Chen TY. The bidirectional relationships between effort-reward imbalance and sleep problems among older workers. Sleep Health 2020;6(3):299-305. doi: 10.1016/j.sleh.2020.01.008.

[34] Grumbach MM. Estrogen, bone, growth and sex: a sea change in conventional wisdom. J Pediatr Endocrinol Metab 2000;13(Suppl 6):1439-55. doi: 10.1515/jpem-2000-s619.

[35] George MD, Baker JF. The obesity epidemic and consequences for rheumatoid arthritis care. Curr Rheumatol Rep 2016;18(1):6. doi:10.1007/s11926-015-0550-z.

In: Social and Health Issues …
Editors: S Pengpid, K Peltzer et al.
ISBN: 978-1-53619-937-6

Chapter 12

PREVALENCE AND CORRELATES OF BACK PAIN OR PROBLEMS AMONG A NATIONALLY REPRESENTATIVE POPULATION-BASED SAMPLE OF OLDER ADULTS IN INDIA IN 2017-2018

Supa Pengpid*[1,2], *MPH, DrPH, MBA
and Karl Peltzer*[2,3,*], *MA Clin Psych, PhD, Dr Habil
[1]ASEAN Institute for Health Development, Mahidol University, Salaya, Phutthamonthon, Nakhon Pathom, Thailand
[2]Department of Research Administration and Development, University of Limpopo, Turfloop, South Africa
[3]Department of Psychology, College of Medical and Health Science, Asia University, Taichung, Taiwan

* *Correspondence*: Professor Karl Peltzer, Department of Research Administration and Development, University of Limpopo, Turfloop Campus, Private Bag X1106, Sovenga 0727, South Africa. Email: kfpeltzer@gmail.com.

ABSTRACT

In this study we aimed to determine the prevalence and correlates of self-reported back pain or problem in older adults in India. The cross-sectional sample consisted of 52,393 individuals (≥50 years) from the Longitudinal Ageing Study in India (LASI) Wave 1 in 2017-2018. Results indicate that the prevalence of past 2-years back pain or problem was 32.4%, 36.8% among women and 27.1% among men. In adjusted logistic regression analysis, older age, married, food insecurity, experiencing 3-6 types of discrimination, exposure to stressful life events, and major depressive disorder were positively associated with 2-year back pain or problem, while male sex, higher education and underweight were negatively associated with 2-year back pain or problem. In addition, in unadjusted analysis, higher subjective socioeconomic status, overweight and lifetime alcohol use were negatively associated with 2-year back pain or problem. Almost two in five older adults in India reported 2-year back pain or problem. Several risk factors were identified, which can be targeted in public health interventions.

INTRODUCTION

"Back problems are a range of conditions related to the bones, joints, connective tissue, muscles and nerves of the back, and include pain in the neck, lower, middle and upper back, pain, tingling, numbness or weakness in the legs starting from the lower back, narrowing of the spine canal through which the spinal cord passes, degeneration of the disc and spinal joints, pressure on the spinal nerve attached to the spinal cord" [1]. "Low back pain is the leading worldwide cause of years lost to disability" [2], with a "global point prevalence of 9.4%" and a growing trend in low- and middle-income countries because of ageing [3]. In a six-country study among older adults (≥50 years) in low- and middle-income settings, the prevalence of the past month (any day) back pain ranged from 22.0% in China to 55.7% in Russia, and 31.9% in 2007 in India [4]. In an adult community survey in the Northern states of India, the past year prevalence of low back pain was 48% [5]. There is a lack of more recent national data on the prevalence and correlates of back pain among older adults in India.

Risk factors for back pain, as reviewed previously [6], include "sociodemographic factors (female sex, lower education, lower wealth, marital status and rural residence), stress, anxiety, depression, heavy physical load, smoking, alcohol consumption, hypertension, physical inactivity and obesity." This study aimed to determine the prevalence and correlates of self-reported pack pain or problems in older community-dwelling adults in India in 2017-2018.

OUR STUDY

This secondary data analysis utilized data from the cross-sectional and nationally representative Longitudinal Ageing Study in India (LASI) Wave 1, 2017-2018; "the overall household response rate is 96%, and the overall individual response rate is 87%" [7]. In a household survey, "interview, physical measurement and biomarker data were collected from individuals aged 45 and above and their spouses, regardless of age" [7]. We restricted our analysis to those 50 years and older. Specific details on the sampling approach are found elsewhere [7]. The study was approved by the "Indian Council of Medical Research (ICMR) Ethics Committee and written informed consent was obtained from the participants" [7].

Measures

"Have you had any of the following persistent or troublesome problems in past two years?" back pain or problems (Yes, No) [7].

Covariates

Sociodemographic variables consisted of number of years of education, age group (50-59, 60-69, 70-79, and 80 or more years), sex (male, female), marital status (currently married vs. widowed/divorced/separated/

deserted/live-in relationship/never married), and residence status (urban, rural). Subjective socioeconomic status was assessed with the question, "Please imagine a ten-step ladder, where at the bottom are the people who are the worst off – who have the least money, least education, and the worst jobs or no jobs, and at the top of the ladder are the people who are the best off – those who have the most money, most education, and best jobs. Please indicate the number (1-10) on the rung on the ladder where you would place yourself." [7]. Steps 1 to 3 on the socioeconomic ladder were defined as low, 4-5 as medium, and 6-10 as high socioeconomic status.

Sociopsychological factors

Food insecurity was assessed with four questions, 1) "In the last 12 months, did you ever reduce the size of your meals or skip meals because there was not enough food at your household? (Yes/No), 2) In the last 12 months, were you hungry but didn't eat because there was not enough food at your household? (Yes/No), 3) In the past 12 months, did you ever not eat for a whole day because there was not enough food in your household? and 4) Do you think that you have lost weight in the last 12 months because there was not enough food in your household?" [7]. Any positive response to the four questions was scored as one.

Life event stressors assessed included 1) ill-treatment ("Have you felt that you were ill-treated in the past year?" Yes/No), 2) victim of violent crime ("In the last 12 months, have you been the victim of a violent crime, such as assault/mugging/ threat to life/others?" (Yes/No), 3) disaster exposure causing health effects ("In the last five years, has your health been severely affected by disasters such as floods, landslides, extreme cold and hot weather, cyclone/typhoons, droughts, earthquakes, tsunamis, or any other natural calamities?" (Yes/No), and 4) man-made incident causing health effects ("In the last five years, has your health been severely affected by man-made incidents such as riots, terrorism, building collapses, fires, traffic accidents or any other man-made incidents?" (Yes/No) [7]. Any affirmative response was coded with 1 and none=0.

Discrimination experiences were assessed with the six-item Everyday Discrimination Scale (EDS) (Short version) [8]. Response options ranged from 1 = "never" to 6 = "almost every day", and were dichotomised to 'never' = 0 and 'ever' (collapsing those reporting 'less than once a year' or greater into one category) = 1). Total responses were trichotomized into 0, 1-2, and 3-6 discrimination experiences. Cronbach's alpha for the EDS in this study was 0.86.

Major depressive disorder in the past 12 months was assessed with the Health and Retirement Study (HRS) Composite International Diagnostic Interview short form (CIDI-SF) [9], using criteria of the Diagnostic and Statistical Manual of Mental Disorders (DSM) [10]. Study respondents were required to "endorse either anhedonia or depressed mood for most of the day for most of a 2-week period or more," and those who fulfilled this criterion "completed an additional seven symptoms: lost interest, feeling tired, change in weight, trouble with sleep, trouble concentrating, feeling down, and thoughts of death." [11]. "Those with a score ≥3 were considered to meet the criteria for having MDD in the previous 12 months; MDD symptomology scores ranged from 0 to 7" [11].

Health factors

Anthropometry: "Height and weight of adults were measured using the Seca 803 digital scale" [7]. "Body Mass Index = BMI was calculated according to Asian criteria: underweight (<18.5 kg/m^2), normal weight (18.5-22.9 kg/m^2), overweight (23.0-24.9 kg/m^2), class I obesity (25.0-29.9 kg/m^2), and class II obesity (≥30.0 kg/m^2)" [12].

Vigorous physical activity. " For vigorous activity, respondents were asked about their involvement in running or jogging, swimming, going to a health centre/gym, cycling, digging with a spade or shovel, heavy lifting, chopping, farm work, fast bicycling, and cycling with loads" [7]. Responses were trichotomized into 1 = hardly ever/never, 2 = less than twice a week, and 3 = more than once a week [13].

Current tobacco use was assessed from 1) "Do you currently smoke any tobacco products (cigarettes, bidis, cigars, hookah, cheroot, etc.)? and 2) Do you use smokeless tobacco (such as chewing tobacco, gutka, pan masala, etc.)?" (Yes/No) [7].

Lifetime alcohol use was assessed with the question, "Have you ever consumed any alcoholic beverages such as beer, wine, liquor, country liquor, etc?" (Yes, No) [7].

Hypertension or raised blood pressure (BP) was defined as "systolic BP ≥140 mm Hg and/or diastolic BP ≥90 mm Hg (based on the last two averaged of three readings) or where the participant is currently on antihypertensive medication" [14].

Data analysis

Descriptive statistics were applied to describe health status, sociodemographic information, and back pain prevalence. Unadjusted and adjusted logistic regression was utilized to assess the predictors of self-reported back pain or problem; variables found significant in univariate analyses were included in the adjusted model. $P < 0.05$ was accepted as significant, missing values were excluded, and no multi-collinearity was found. Statistical analyses were conducted using STATA software version 15.0 (Stata Corporation, College Station, TX, USA), taking the complex study design into account.

FINDINGS

The sample included 52,393 older adults (50 years and older), with a median age of 62 years (14 years interquartile range), 53.3% were female and 46.7% male. Majority (70.1%) of participants were married, 69.0% were residing in rural areas, and 53.9% had no schooling. Almost half of the participants (45.4%) had hypertension, 6.4% obesity class II (≥30 kg/m^2), 33.0% had current tobacco use, 14.9% had ever engaged in alcohol use, and 62.3% did not engage in vigorous physical activity. One in ten older adults (9.9%) had food insecurity, 17.3% had discrimination experiences, 9.1% had been exposed to stressful events, and 8.0% had a major depressive disorder. The prevalence of past 2-years back pain or problem was 32.4%, 36.8% among women and 27.1% among men (see Table 1).

Table 1. Sample and back pain or problem characteristics among older adults in India, 2017-2018

Variable	Sample	Back pain or problem
	N (%)	%
All	**52393**	**32.4**
Sociodemographic factors		
Age in years		
50-59	20916 (38.1)	29.6
60-69	18979 (36.2)	32.7
70-79	9108 (18.7)	35.7
≥80	3390 (7.0)	36.4
Sex		
Female	27815 (53.3)	36.8
Male	24578 (46.7)	27.2
Marital status		
Not married	15151 (29.9)	34.2
Married	37236 (70.1)	31.6
Education		
No schooling	25983 (53.0)	36.3
1-4 years	6138 (11.0)	32.4
5-9 years	11246 (19.5)	27.3
≥10 years	9026 (16.5)	25.4
Subjective socioeconomic status		
Low	17462 (38.2)	34.5
Medium	20070 (37.4)	32.3
High	13176 (24.4)	28.6
Residence		
Rural	34099 (69.0)	32.9
Urban	18294 (31.0)	31.2
Sociopsychological factors		
Food insecurity	4336 (9.9)	44.0
Discrimination experiences		
0	43281 (82.7)	31.0
1-2	4483 (10.7)	36.7
3-6	3151 (6.6)	41.0
Stressful life events	3986 (9.1)	41.2
Major depressive disorder	3263 (8.0)	47.5

Table 1. (Continued)

Variable	Sample	Back pain or problem
	N (%)	%
Health factors		
Body mass index		
Normal	17179 (37.2)	32.3
Underweight	9428 (23.0)	32.5
Overweight	6922 (13.7)	30.1
Obesity class I	9846 (19.7)	31.8
Obesity class II	3271 (6.4)	39.4
Vigorous physical activity		
Never	32762 (62.3)	32.5
Once/week	4262 (8.8)	34.7
>once/week	14930 (28.9)	31.5
Current tobacco use	16403 (33.0)	31.3
Ever alcohol use	9346 (14.9)	28.8
Hypertension	22826 (45.4)	33.3

Associations with back pain or problems

In adjusted logistic regression analysis, older age, married, food insecurity, experiencing 3-6 types of discrimination, exposure to stressful life events, and major depressive disorder were positively associated with 2-year back pain or problem, while male sex, higher education and underweight were negatively associated with 2-year back pain or problem. In addition, in unadjusted analysis, higher subjective socioeconomic status, overweight and lifetime alcohol use were negatively associated with 2-year back pain or problem (see Table 2).

Table 2. Associations with back pain or problems among older adults in India

Variable	Unadjusted Odds Ratio (95% CI)	Adjusted Odds Ratio (95% CI)
Sociodemographic factors		
Age in years		
50-59	1 (Reference)	1 (Reference)
60-69	1.15 (1.05, 1.26)**	1.25 (1.15, 1.36)***
70-79	1.32 (1.21, 1.43)***	1.45 (1.28, 1.64)***
≥80	1.36 (1.17, 1.57)***	1.58 (1.28, 1.94)***

Variable	**Unadjusted Odds Ratio (95% CI)**	**Adjusted Odds Ratio (95% CI)**
Sex		
Female	1 (Reference)	1 (Reference)
Male	0.64 (0.59, 0.70)***	0.63 (0.58, 0.70)***
Marital status		
Not married	1 (Reference)	1 (Reference)
Married	0.89 (0.81, 0.98)*	1.19 (1.04, 1.37)*
Education		
No schooling	1 (Reference)	1 (Reference)
1-4 years	0.84 (0.75, 0.95)**	0.94 (0.83, 1.07)
5-9 years	0.66 (0.55, 0.79)***	0.77 (0.62, 0.96)*
≥10 years	0.60 (0.48, 0.74)***	0.69 (0.58, 0.83)***
Subjective socioeconomic status		
Low	1 (Reference)	1 (Reference)
Medium	0.91 (0.76, 1.08)	1.03 (0.88, 1.31)
High	0.76 (0.64, 0.90)**	0.91 (0.76, 1.08)
Residence		
Rural	1 (Reference)	---
Urban	0.93 (0.65, 1.32)	
Sociopsychological factors		
Food insecurity	1.74 (1.42, 2.14)***	1.54 (1.27, 1.87)***
Discrimination experiences		
0	1 (Reference)	1 (Reference)
1-2	1.31 (1.17, 1.47)***	1.08 (0.88, 1.31)
3-6	1.61 (1.32, 1.96)***	1.32 (1.08, 1.61)**
Stressful life events	1.59 (1.36, 1.85)***	1.38 (1.15, 1.66)***
Major depressive disorder	2.00 (1.70, 2.35)***	1.64 (1.37, 1.96)***
Health factors		
Body mass index		
Normal	1 (Reference)	1 (Reference)
Underweight	1.01 (0.93, 1.10)	0.91 (0.84, 0.99)*
Overweight	0.91 (0.83, 0.99)*	0.98 (0.88, 1.08)
Obesity class I	0.98 (0.83, 1.15)	1.11 (1.00, 1.23)
Obesity class II	1.36 (0.88, 2.11)	1.43 (0.92, 2.24)
Vigorous physical activity		
Never	1 (Reference)	---
Once/week	1.12 (0.97, 1.29)	
>once/week	1.00 (0.85, 1.17)	
Current tobacco use	0.93 (0.81, 1.06)	---
Ever alcohol use	0.82 (0.71, 0.95)*	1.07 (0.93, 1.25)
Hypertension	1.06 (0.93, 1.21)	---

CI = Confidence Interval; ***$p < 0.001$; ** $p < 0.01$; *$p < 0.05$.

DISCUSSION

In this nationally representative sample of older adults in India in 2017-2018, the past 2-year back pain or problem prevalence was 32.4%, which was similar to the 2007 national survey among older adults in India (31.9% past month back pain) [4], higher than in China (22.0% past month back pain) [4], and lower than in Mexico (35.6% past month) [6], in Russia (55.7% past month) [4], and Northern states in India (48% past year) [5]. Connelly et al. [15] propose "behaviour and exercise therapy and lifestyle change, in addition to pharmacological interventions for the treatment and management for back pain."

Consistent with previous research [4, 5, 16, 17, 18], this study found that female sex and lower education was associated with back pain. "Multiple biological and psychosocial mechanisms" may contribute to the sex differences in the prevalence of back pain [4]. Less educated older adults in India may be more frequently involved in more strenuous physical labour activities than higher educated older adults, which may make them more vulnerable to back pain [4].

Consistent with previous research, this study found an association between stress factors (food insecurity, stressful events [18-20], and discrimination experiences [21, 22]) and back pain. Possible mechanisms relate to stressors that are uncontrollable and unpredictable and thus detrimental to health, initiating a process of physiological responses, such as increased cortisol secretion, blood pressure, and chronic pain [22, 23]. Furthermore, major depressive disorder was found associated with back pain or problems in this study. In a systematic review of prospective studies, back pain was found to be a risk factor for depressive symptoms and in the review of cross-sectional studies back pain was associated with depressive symptoms [24]. In another systematic review investigating the "effect of depression on the course of acute and subacute low back pain" found that "depression might have an adverse effect on the prognosis of low back pain" [25]. Therefore, the direction of the relationship between major depressive disorder and back pain may need to be further investigated in a longitudinal study in India.

In a previous review [26], overweight and obesity were associated with chronic low back pain, but in this study underweight was negatively and in unadjusted analysis only overweight was also negatively associated with back pain. Contrary to previous studies [6, 27, 28], physical inactivity was not significantly associated with back pain or problems in this study. In a meta-analysis, Shiri et al. [29] found that "smokers have a higher prevalence and incidence of low back pain than never smokers," while this study did not find an association with current tobacco users. In a systematic review, Ferreira et al. [30] showed that "alcohol consumption appears to be associated with complex and chronic lower back pain only and in people with alcohol dependence," while in this study lifetime alcohol use was protective against back pain in unadjusted analysis.

Study limitations include the cross-sectional design, the assessment of some variables, such as back pain by self-report. Some determinants, such as depression or substance use, may also be consequences. Longitudinal studies are needed to determine causality. Furthermore, the study did not assess some variables, such as sedentary behaviour, which could have impacted on back pain, and future studies should include scales that measure back pain.

Conclusion

Almost two in five older adults in India reported past 2-year back pain or problem. Several risk factors, such as female sex, older age, married, lower education, food insecurity, experiencing 3-6 types of discrimination, exposure to stressful life events, and major depressive disorder were were identified for past 2-year back pain or problem, which can be targeted in public health interventions.

ACKNOWLEDGMENTS

The Longitudinal Aging Study in India Project is funded by the Ministry of Health and Family Welfare, Government of India, the National Institute on Aging (R01 AG042778, R01 AG030153), and United Nations Population Fund, India.

REFERENCES

[1] Australian Institute of Health and Welfare. Musculoskeletal fact sheet: back problems. Arthritis series no. 21. Cat. no. PHE 185. Canberra: AIHW, 2015. URL: https://www.aihw.gov.au/getmedia/72d28f53-cf36-40b9-b122-8415de81b1f7/back-problems-factsheet-phe185.pdf.aspx?inline=true.

[2] Buchbinder R, van Tulder M, Öberg B, Costa LM, Woolf A, Schoene M, et al. Low back pain: a call for action. Lancet 2018;391(10137):2384-8. doi: 10.1016/S0140-6736(18)30488-4.

[3] Hoy D, March L, Brooks P, Blyth F, Woolf A, Bain C, et al. The global burden of low back pain: estimates from the Global Burden of Disease 2010 study. Ann Rheum Dis 2014;73(6):968–74.

[4] Stewart Williams J, Ng N, Peltzer K, Yawson A, Biritwum R, Maximova T, et al. Risk factors and disability associated with low back pain in older adults in low- and middle-income countries. Results from the WHO Study on Global AGEing and Adult Health (SAGE). PLoS One 2015;10(6):e0127880. doi: 10.1371/journal.pone.0127880. eCollection 2015.

[5] Bansal D, Asrar MM, Ghai B, Pushpendra D. Prevalence and impact of low back pain in a community-based population in Northern India. Pain Physician 2020;23(4):E389-98.

[6] Peltzer K, Pengpid S. Prevalence and correlates of back pain among a nationally representative population-based sample of older adults in Mexico. Int J Disabil Hum Dev 2020;19(3):595-602.

[7] International Institute for Population Sciences (IIPS), NPHCE, MoHFW, Harvard TH Chan School of Public Health (HSPH) and the University of Southern California (USC). Longitudinal Ageing Study in India (LASI) Wave 1, 2017-18, India Report. Mumbai: International Institute for Population Sciences, 2020.

[8] Sternthal MJ, Slopen N, Williams DR. Racial disparities in health: How much does stress really matter? Du Bois Rev 2011;8(1):95-113. doi: 10.1017/S1742058X1 000087.

[9] Kessler RC, Andrews A, Mroczek D, Ustun B, Wittchen HU. The World Health Organization Composite International Diagnostic Interview Short-Form (CIDI-SF). Int J Methods Psychiatr Res 1998;7:171–85.

[10] American Psychiatric Association. Diagnostic and statistical manual of mental disorders (DSM-5), (5th ed. Washington, DC: American Psychiatric Publishing, 2013.

[11] Steffick D. Documentation of affective functioning measures in the Health and Retirement Study, 2000. URL: http://hrsonline. isr.umich.edu/sitedocs/userg/dr-005.pdf.

[12] Wen CP, David Cheng TY, Tsai SP, Chan HT, Hsu HL, Hsu CC, et al. Are Asians at greater mortality risks for being overweight than Caucasians? Redefining obesity for Asians. Public Health Nutr 2009;12(4):497-506. doi: 10.1017/S1368980008002302.

[13] Lübs L, Peplies J, Drell C, Bammann K. Cross-sectional and longitudinal factors influencing physical activity of 65 to 75-year-olds: a pan European cohort study based on the survey of health, ageing and retirement in Europe (SHARE). BMC Geriatr 2018;18(1):94. doi: 10.1186/s12877-018-0781-8.

[14] Chobanian AV, Bakris GL, Black HR, Cushman WC, Green LA, Izzo Jr JL, et al. The seventh report of the joint national committee on prevention, detection, evaluation, and treatment of high blood pressure: the JNC 7 report. JAMA 2003;289(19):2560–71.

[15] Connelly LB, Woolf A, Brooks P. Cost-effectiveness of interventions for musculoskeletal conditions. In: Jamison DT, Breman BJ, Measham AR, Alleyne G, Claeson M, et al, eds. Disease control priorities in developing countries, 2nd ed. Washington, DC: World Bank, 2006.

[16] Jesus-Moraleida FR, Ferreira PH, Ferreira ML, Silva JP, Maher CG, Enthoven WTM, et al. Back complaints in the elders in Brazil and the Netherlands: A cross-sectional comparison. Age Ageing 2017;46(3):476-81. doi: 10.1093/ageing/afw230.

[17] Peláez-Ballestas I, Alvarez-Nemegyei J, Loyola-Sánchez A, Escudero ML. Prevalence and factors associated with musculoskeletal disorders and rheumatic diseases in indigenous Maya-Yucateco people: a cross-sectional community-based study. Clin Rheumatol 2016;35(Suppl 1):15-23. doi: 10.1007/s10067-015-3085-9.

[18] Hoy D, Brooks P, Blyth F, Buchbinder R. The epidemiology of low back pain. Best Pract Res Clin Rheumatol 2010;24(6):769-81. doi: 10.1016/j.berh.2010.10.002.

[19] Buscemi V, Chang WJ, Liston MB, McAuley JH, Schabrun SM. The role of perceived stress and life stressors in the development of chronic musculoskeletal pain disorders: A systematic review. J Pain 2019;20(10):1127-39. doi: 10.1016/j.jpain.2019.02.008..

[20] Manek NJ, MacGregor AJ. Epidemiology of back disorders: prevalence, risk factors, and prognosis. Curr Opin Rheumatol 2005;17(2):134-40.

[21] Mouzon DM, Taylor RJ, Woodward A, Chatters LM. Everyday racial discrimination, everyday non-racial discrimination, and physical health among African Americans. J Ethn Cult Divers Soc Work 2017;26(1-2):68-80. doi: 10.1080/15313204. 2016.1187103.

[22] Gee GC, Spencer MS, Chen J, Takeuchi D. A nationwide study of discrimination and chronic health conditions among Asian Americans. Am J Public Health 2007;97(7):1275-82. doi: 10.2105/AJPH.2006.091827.

[23] Pascoe EA, Smart Richman L. Perceived discrimination and health: a meta-analytic review. Psychol Bull 2009;135(4):531-54. doi: 10.1037/a0016059.

[24] Amiri S, Behnezhad S, Azad E. Back pain and depressive symptoms: A systematic review and meta-analysis. Int J Psychiatry Med 2020:91217420913001. doi: 10.1177/0091217420913001.

[25] Pinheiro MB, Ferreira ML, Refshauge K, Maher CG, Ordoñana JR, Andrade TB, et al. Symptoms of depression as a prognostic factor for low back pain: a systematic review. Spine J 2016;16(1):105-16. doi: 10.1016/j.spinee.2015.10.037.

[26] Shiri R, Karppinen J, Leino-Arjas P, Solovieva S, Viikari-Juntura E. The association between obesity and low back pain: A meta-analysis. Am J Epidemiol 2010;171(2):135-54. doi: 10.1093/aje/kwp356.

[27] Øverås CK, Villumsen M, Axén I, Cabrita M, Leboeuf-Yde C, Hartvigsen J, et al. Association between objectively measured physical behaviour and neck- and/or low back pain: A systematic review. Eur J Pain 2020 Febr 24. doi: 10.1002/ejp.1551.

[28] De Carvalho DE, de Luca K, Funabashi M, Breen A, Wong AYL, Johansson MS, et al. Association of exposures to seated postures with immediate increases in back pain: A systematic review of studies with objectively measured sitting time. J Manipulative Physiol Ther 2020;pii: S0161-4754(19)30432-4. doi: 10.1016/j.jmpt.2019.10.001.

[29] Shiri R, Karppinen J, Leino-Arjas P, Solovieva S, Viikari-Juntura E. The association between smoking and low back pain: A meta-analysis. Am J Med 2010;123(1):87.e7-35. doi: 10.1016/j.amjmed.2009.05.028.

[30] Ferreira PH, Pinheiro MB, Machado GC, Ferreira ML. Is alcohol intake associated with low back pain? A systematic review of observational studies. Man Ther 2013;18(3):183-90. doi: 10.1016/j.math.2012.10.007.

In: Social and Health Issues … ISBN: 978-1-53619-937-6
Editors: S Pengpid, K Peltzer et al.

Chapter 13

PREVALENCE AND CORRELATES OF ORAL HEALTH PROBLEMS AMONG A NATIONALLY REPRESENTATIVE SAMPLE OF OLDER ADULTS IN INDIA, 2017-2018

Karl Peltzer[1,2], MA Clin Psych, PhD, Dr Habil and Supa Pengpid[1,3,*], MPH, DrPH, MBA

[1]Department of Research Administration and Development, University of Limpopo, Turfloop, South Africa
[2]Department of Psychology, College of Medical and Health Science, Asia University, Taichung, Taiwan
[3]ASEAN Institute for Health Development, Mahidol University, Salaya, Phutthamonthon, Nakhon Pathom, Thailand

[*] *Correspondence*: Professor Supa Pengpid, ASEAN Institute for Health Development, Mahidol University, 25/25 Phutthamonthon Road 4, Salaya, Phutthamonton, Nakhon Pathom 73170, Thailand. Email: supaprom@yahoo.com.

ABSTRACT

In this chapter we determine the prevalence and correlates of self-reported oral health problems in older adults in India. The cross-sectional sample consisted of 52,393 individuals (≥50 years) from the Longitudinal Ageing Study in India (LASI) Wave 1 in 2017-2018. Oral health problems were assessed by self-report. Results indicate that the prevalence of past 12-month 1 and 2-7 oral health problems were 19.7% and 30.1%, respectively. In adjusted multinomial logistic regression analysis, older age (60-69 years), diabetes, angina and poor or fair self-rated health status were positively associated with 2-7 oral health problems in the past 12 months, while male sex, and higher education (≥10 years) were negatively associated with 2-7 oral health problems in the past 12 months. In addition, lifetime alcohol use was associated with one oral health problem in the past 12 months. One in two older adults in India had at least one oral health problem in the past 12 months. Several risk factors were identified, which can be targeted in public health interventions.

INTRODUCTION

Oral health is defined by the World Health Organization (WHO) as "a state of being free from mouth and facial pain, oral and throat cancer, oral infection and sores, periodontal (gum) disease, tooth decay, tooth loss, and other diseases and disorders that limit an individual's capacity for biting, chewing, smiling, speaking, and psychosocial well-being" [1]. Globally, oral health has deteriorated over the last 25 years "due to demographic changes, including population growth and aging" [2]. "Oral diseases are highly prevalent in the globe, posing a very serious public health challenge to policy makers" [2]. Globally, poor oral health among older adults is seen by high levels of oral health problems, including "loss of teeth, edentulism, periodontitis, coronal and root caries, oral mucosal lesions, utilization of non-functional dental prostheses, xerostomia, and chewing problems" [3, 4]. In a study among adults in China, Russian Federation and in India in 2007, the prevalence of past 12-month oral health problems was 9.3% in China, 35.4% in Russia, and 10.2% in India, and among those 60 years and older in India 23.1% [5]. In a study among older adults (≥50 years) in Mexico, the past 12-month prevalence of oral health problems was 17.8% [6]. There is a lack of recent national population-based data on self-reported oral health problems among older adults in India.

As reviewed previously [5], factors associated with oral health problems include "age, education, socioeconomic status, sex, residence status, body mass index, smoking, alcohol use, diabetes, hypertension, and coronary heart disease." This study aimed to determine the prevalence and correlates of self-reported oral health problems in older community-dwelling adults in India in 2017-2018.

OUR STUDY

This secondary data analysis utilized data from the cross-sectional and nationally representative Longitudinal Ageing Study in India (LASI) Wave 1, 2017-2018; "the overall household response rate is 96%, and the overall individual response rate is 87%" [7]. In a household survey, "interview, physical measurement and biomarker data were collected from individuals aged 45 and above and their spouses, regardless of age" [7]. We restricted our analysis to persons 50 years and older. Specific details on the sampling approach are found elsewhere [7]. The study was approved by the "Indian Council of Medical Research (ICMR) Ethics Committee and written informed consent was obtained from the participants" [7].

Measures

Oral health problems were assessed with seven questions, "In the last 12 months, have you ever been diagnosed with or suffered from any of the following oral problem(s)? 1) Painful teeth, 2) Ulcers lasting more than two weeks, 3) Bleeding gums, 4) Swelling gums, 5) Loose teeth, 6) Dental cavity/dental caries and 7) Soreness or cracks in the corner of the mouth." (Yes, No, multiple responses were possible) [7]. Oral health problems were summed and trichotomized into 0 = none, 1 = 1 and 2 = 2-7 oral health problems.

Covariates

Sociodemographic variables consisted of number of years of education, age group (50-59, 60-69, 70-79, and 80 or more years), sex (male, female), marital status (currently married vs. widowed/divorced/separated/deserted/ live-in relationship/never married), and residence (rural, urban). Subjective socioeconomic status was assessed with the question, "Please imagine a ten-step ladder, where at the bottom are the people who are the worst off – who have the least money, least education, and the worst jobs or no jobs, and at the top of the ladder are the people who are the best off – those who have the most money, most education, and best jobs. Please indicate the number (1-10) on the rung on the ladder where you would place yourself." [7]. Steps 1 to 3 on the socioeconomic ladder were defined as low, 4-5 as medium, and 6-10 as high socioeconomic status.

Health factor variables included body mass index, substance use, hypertension, diabetes, angina, and self-rated health status.

Anthropometry: "Height and weight of adults were measured using the Seca 803 digital scale." [7]. "Body Mass Index = BMI was calculated according to Asian criteria: underweight (<18.5 kg/m^2), normal weight (18.5-22.9 kg/m^2), overweight (23.0-24.9 kg/m^2), class I obesity (25.0-29.9 kg/m^2), and class II obesity (≥30.0 kg/m^2)" [8].

Vigorous physical activity. "For vigorous activity, respondents were asked about their involvement in running or jogging, swimming, going to a health centre/gym, cycling, digging with a spade or shovel, heavy lifting, chopping, farm work, fast bicycling, and cycling with loads" [7]. Responses were trichotomized into 1 = hardly ever/never, 2 = less than twice a week, and 3 = more than once a week [9].

Current tobacco use was assessed from 1) "Do you currently smoke any tobacco products (cigarettes, bidis, cigars, hookah, cheroot, etc.)? and 2) Do you use smokeless tobacco (such as chewing tobacco, gutka, pan masala, etc.)?" (Yes, No) [7].

Lifetime alcohol use was assessed with the question, "Have you ever consumed any alcoholic beverages such as beer, wine, liquor, country liquor, etc?" (Yes, No) [7].

Hypertension or raised blood pressure (BP) was defined as "systolic BP ≥140 mm Hg and/or diastolic BP ≥90 mm Hg (based on the last two averaged of three readings) or where the participant is currently on antihypertensive medication" [10].

Diabetes was sourced from the question, "Has any health professional ever told you that you have diabetes or high blood sugar?" (Yes/No)" [7].

Angina was assessed with the "World Health Organization's Rose angina questionnaire" [11], defined based on "discomfort at walking uphill or hurrying, or at an ordinary pace on level ground. Furthermore, the pain should be located at the sternum or in the left chest and arm, causing the patient to stop or slow down, and the pain should resolve within 10 minutes when the patient stops or slows down" [12].

Self-rated health status was sourced from the question, "In general, would you say your health is excellent, very good, good, fair, or poor?" Responses were coded as "1 = poor, 2 = fair, 3 = good, 4 = very good and 5 = excellent" [7].

Data analysis

Descriptive statistics were applied to describe health status, sociodemographic information, and oral health problems prevalence. Adjusted multinominal logistic regression was utilized to assess the predictors of 1 and 2-7 oral health problems in the past 12 months, with no oral health problems in the past 12 months as the reference category. $P < 0.05$ was accepted as significant, missing values were excluded, and no multi-collinearity was found. Statistical analyses were conducted using STATA software version 15.0 (Stata Corporation, College Station, TX, USA), taking the complex study design into account.

FINDINGS

The sample included 52,393 older adults (50 years and older), with a median age of 62 years (14 years interquartile range), 53.3% were female, and 46.7% male, 69.0% were residing in rural areas, and 53.9% had no schooling. Almost half of the participants (45.4%) had hypertension, 13.4% diabetes, 8.9% angina, 43.3% poor or fair self-rated health status, 6.4% obesity class II (≥30 kg/m^2), 33.0% had current tobacco use, 14.9% had ever engaged in alcohol use, and 62.3% did not engage in vigorous physical activity. The prevalence of past 12-month 1 and 2-7 oral health problems were 19.7% and 30.1%, respectively (see Table 1).

Table 1. Sample and oral health problems characteristics among older adults in India, 2017-2018

Variable	Sample	Number of oral health problems		
		0	1	2-7
	N (%)	%	%	%
All	**52393**	**50.2**	**19.7**	**30.1**
Sociodemographic factors				
Age in years				
50-59	20916 (38.1)	52.6	18.7	28.7
60-69	18979 (36.2)	47.6	20.0	32.4
70-79	9108 (18.7)	49.0	20.6	30.4
≥80	3390 (7.0)	54.1	21.2	24.7
Sex				
Female	27815 (53.3)	47.9	20.4	31.8
Male	24578 (46.7)	52.9	18.9	28.2
Education				
No schooling	25983 (53.0)	48.9	19.9	31.2
1-4 years	6138 (11.0)	48.8	20.4	30.8
5-9 years	11246 (19.5)	49.9	20.1	30.0
≥10 years	9026 (16.5)	55.8	18.1	26.0
Subjective socioeconomic status				
Low	17462 (38.2)	48.0	20.3	31.7
Medium	20070 (37.4)	49.2	20.1	30.4
High	13176 (24.4)	54.6	18.7	26.7

Variable	Sample	Number of oral health problems		
		0	1	2-7
	N (%)	%	%	%
Residence				
Rural	34099 (69.0)	50.3	19.8	29.9
Urban	18294 (31.0)	49.9	19.6	30.5
Health factors				
Body mass index				
Normal	17179 (37.2)	50.0	19.8	30.2
Underweight	9428 (23.0)	51.0	19.0	30.0
Overweight	6922 (13.7)	48.9	19.9	31.2
Obesity class I	9846 (19.7)	48.3	21.0	30.7
Obesity class II	3271 (6.4)	45.9	20.9	33.2
Vigorous physical activity				
Never	32762 (62.3)	50.0	20.0	30.0
Once/week	4262 (8.8)	48.4	20.4	31.2
>once/week	14930 (28.9)	51.1	19.0	29.9
Current tobacco use	16403 (33.0)	50.4	19.2	30.4
Ever alcohol use	9346 (14.9)	49.5	20.9	29.6
Hypertension	22826 (45.4)	48.0	21.1	30.9
Diabetes	7423 (13.4)	44.4	21.0	34.5
Angina	4510 (8.9)	42.0	18.7	39.3
Self-rated health (poor or fair)	21248 (43.3)	45.0	20.6	34.4

Associations with oral health problems

In adjusted multinomial logistic regression analysis, older age (60-69 years), diabetes, angina, and poor or fair self-rated health status were positively associated with 2-7 oral health problems in the past 12 months, while male sex, and higher education (≥10 years) were negatively associated with 2-7 oral health problems in the past 12 months. In addition, lifetime alcohol use was associated with one oral health problem in the past 12 months (see Table 2).

Table 2. Associations with past 12-month 1 and 2-7 oral health problems in older adults in India

Variable	1 oral health problem	2-7 oral health problems
	ARRR (95% CI)	ARRR (95% CI)
Sociodemographic factors		
Age in years		
50-59	1 (Reference)	1 (Reference)
60-69	1.12 (0.99, 1.25)	1.20 (1.11, 1.30)***
70-79	1.16 (0.94, 1.42)	1.09 (0.96, 1.22)
≥80	1.11 (0.87, 1.40)	0.85 (0.69, 1.04)
Sex		
Female	1 (Reference)	1 (Reference)
Male	0.81 (0.69, 0.95)**	0.75 (0.66, 0.85)***
Education		
No schooling	1 (Reference)	1 (Reference)
1-4 years	1.03 (0.92, 1.14)	1.02 (0.92, 1.13)
5-9 years	1.03 (0.90, 1.19)	1.00 (0.89, 1.11)
≥10 years	0.86 (0.74, 0.99)*	0.81 (0.69, 0.95)**
Subjective socioeconomic status		
Low	1 (Reference)	1 (Reference)
Medium	1.01 (0.95, 1.11)	1.01 (0.84, 1.21)
High	0.87 (0.72, 1.05)	0.87 (0.76, 1.01)
Residence		
Rural	1 (Reference)	1 (Reference)
Urban	1.04 (0.70, 1.55)	1.04 (0.70, 1.55)
Health factors		
Body mass index		
Normal	1 (Reference)	1 (Reference)
Underweight	0.90 (0.79, 1.02)	0.94 (0.82, 1.06)
Overweight	1.03 (0.95, 1.11)	1.10 (0.98, 1.23)
Obesity class I	1.10 (0.94, 1.29)	1.11 (0.96, 1.26)
Obesity class II	1.12 (0.94, 1.34)	1.16 (0.80, 1.72)
Vigorous physical activity		
Never	1 (Reference)	1 (Reference)
Once/week	1.11 (0.93, 1.33)	1.02 (0.88, 1.18)
>once/week	1.02 (0.84, 1.24)	1.10 (0.86, 1.40)
Ever alcohol use	1.22 (1.04, 1.35)*	1.19 (0.99, 1.43)
Hypertension	1.10 (0.97, 1.25)	1.00 (0.92, 1.09)
Diabetes	1.16 (0.95, 1.42)	1.26 (1.13, 1.41)***
Angina	1.02 (0.82, 1.27)	1.42 (1.18, 1.69)***
Self-rated health (poor or fair)	1.21 (1.10, 1.34)***	1.48 (1.32, 1.66)***

ARRR = Adjusted Relative Risk Ratio; CI = Confidence Interval; ***$p < 0.001$; ** $p < 0.01$; *$p < 0.05$.

DISCUSSION

In this nationally representative sample of older adults in India in 2017-2018, the prevalence of self-rated oral health problems was at least one 49.2%, 19.7% one and 30.1% 2-7 oral health problems, which is higher than in previous studies among older adults in India in 2007 (23.1%, ≥60 years) [5] and in Mexico (17.8%, ≥50 years) [6]. One possible reason for these differences may be attributed to differences in the measurement tools used to assess oral health problems. While some of the reported studies [5, 6] used one item to assess oral health problems ("having any problems with your mouth and/or teeth, including problems with swallowing") in the past 12 months, this study used seven items on different oral health problems in the past 12 months. In a study on oral health problems among adults in Kuwait, 13 different oral health problems in the past six months were assessed, with the result that only 9.4% reported not having any oral health problems, and 41.8% had three or more oral health problems [13]. Nevertheless, the found prevalence of oral health problems among older adults in India is high and needs urgent attention through the national oral health programme [14].

Consistent with previous studies [15, 16], this study showed that poor general self-rated health status was associated with a higher prevalence of oral health problems. Contrary to a study that found beneficial effects of physical activity on oral health [17], this study did not find a significant association between physical activity and oral health problems. Previous research [13, 18] showed that cigarette smoking increased the risk for oral health problems, such as missing teeth, decayed teeth and periodontal disease, while this study did not find a significant association. Alcohol use was found associated with oral health problems in Russia and China, but not in India [5]. We also did not find a significant association between lifetime alcohol use and multiple oral health problems, but found an inverse relationship with a single oral health problem in this study.

In line with some previous research [5, 19, 20], this study found that female sex, diabetes, and angina increased the odds of oral health problems. The female gender bias may be attributed to genetic, hormonal, and cultural influences, such as "(a) the relative value of sons and daughters, (b) frequent fasting among Hindu women, and (c) the belief that dietary restrictions result in easier childbirth" [19]. Older adults belonging to a cardiovascular risk group ("hypertension, diabetes, dyslipidemia, previous myocardial infarction, or angina") were found to have a higher prevalence of periodontal disease than those not belonging to the cardiovascular risk group [20].

Furthermore, we found that higher education was protective against oral health problems. It is possible that those with higher education are more aware of and practice oral hygiene and dental care utilization, thereby reducing oral health problems. Like a previous study among older adults in Mexico [6], we did not find significant differences in the prevalence of oral health problems in terms of age, residence status, body mass index and hypertension.

Study limitations include the cross-sectional design, the assessment of some variables, including oral health status, by self-report, and that certain relevant variables, such as certain dietary behaviours (e.g., sugar and soft drink intake) oral health risk behaviour (inadequate tooth brushing, low oral hygiene behaviours, dental attendance), were not assessed.

CONCLUSION

One in two older adults in India had at least one oral health problem in the past 12 months, and several associated factors were identified, such as female sex, older age (60-69 years), lower education, diabetes, angina and poor or fair self-rated health status, that could assist in programmes promoting oral health in older adults in India.

ACKNOWLEDGMENTS

The Longitudinal Aging Study in India Project is funded by the Ministry of Health and Family Welfare, Government of India, the National Institute on

Aging (R01 AG042778, R01 AG030153), and United Nations Population Fund, India.

REFERENCES

[1] Petersen PE, WHO Oral Health Programme. The World Oral Health Report 2003: Continuous improvement of oral health in the 21st century–the approach of the WHO Global Oral Health Programme. Geneva: World Health Organization, 2003.

[2] Kassebaum NJ, Smith AGC, Bernabé E, Fleming TD, Reynolds AE, Vos T, et al. Global, regional, and national prevalence, incidence, and Disability-Adjusted Life Years for oral conditions for 195 countries, 1990-2015: A systematic analysis for the global burden of diseases, injuries, and risk factors. J Dent Res 2017;96(4):380-7. doi: 10.1177/0022034517693566.

[3] Petersen PE, Ueda H. WHO Oral Health Programme and WHO Centre for Health Developmentin ageing societie Oral health .s: Iand general ntegration of oral health health. Report of a meeting convened at the WHO Centre for Health Development in Kobe,Japan 2005 Jun 3-1. URL: https://apps.who.int/iris/handle/10665/43531.

[4] Castrejón-Pérez RC, Borges-Yáñez SA, Gutiérrez-Robledo LM, Avila-Funes JA. Oral health conditions and frailty in Mexican community-dwelling elderly: A cross sectional analysis. BMC Public Health 2012;12:773. doi: 10.1186/1471-2458-12-773.

[5] Bawankule R, Singh A, Kumar K, Pedgaonkar S. Oral problems and associated risk indicators in adults in the Russian Federation, India, and China. BMC Oral Health 2019;19(1):114. doi: 10.1186/s12903-019-0811-8.

[6] Pengpid S, Peltzer K. Prevalence and correlates of oral health problems among a nationally representative sample of older adults in Mexico. Int J Disabil Hum Dev 2020;19(3):535-42.

[7] International Institute for Population Sciences (IIPS), NPHCE, MoHFW, Harvard TH Chan School of Public Health (HSPH) and the University of Southern California (USC). Longitudinal Ageing Study in India (LASI) Wave 1, 2017-18, India Report. Mumbai: International Institute for Population Sciences, 2020.

[8] Wen CP, David Cheng TY, Tsai SP, Chan HT, Hsu HL, Hsu CC, et al. Are Asians at greater mortality risks for being overweight than Caucasians? Redefining obesity for Asians. Public Health Nutr 2009;12(4):497-506. doi: 10.1017/S1368980008002802.

[9] Lübs L, Peplies J, Drell C, Bammann K. Cross-sectional and longitudinal factors influencing physical activity of 65 to 75-year-olds: a pan European cohort study based on the survey of health, ageing and retirement in Europe (SHARE). BMC Geriatr 2018;18(1):94. doi: 10.1186/s12877-018-0781-8.

[10] Chobanian AV, Bakris GL, Black HR, Cushman WC, Green LA, Izzo Jr JL, et al. The seventh report of the joint national committee on prevention, detection, evaluation,

and treatment of high blood pressure: the JNC 7 report. JAMA 2003;289(19):2560–71.

[11] Rose GA. The diagnosis of ischaemic heart pain and intermittent claudication in field surveys. Bull World Health Organ 1962;27:645–58.

[12] Achterberg S, Soedamah-Muthu SS, Cramer MJ, Kappelle LJ, van der Graaf Y, Algra A; SMART Study Group. Prognostic value of the Rose questionnaire: a validation with future coronary events in the SMART study. Eur J Prev Cardiol 2012;19(1):5-14. doi: 10.1177/1741826710391117.

[13] Al-Shammari KF, Al-Ansari JM, Al-Khabbaz AK, Dashti A, Honkala EJ. Self-reported oral hygiene habits and oral health problems of Kuwaiti adults. Med Princ Pract 2007;16(1):15-21. doi: 10.1159/000096134.

[14] Ministry of Health and Family Welfare, Government of India. National Oral Health Programme, 2020. URL: https://www.nhp.gov.in/national-oral-health-programme_pg.

[15] Brennan DS, Singh KA.General health and oral health self-ratings, and impact of oral problems among older adults. Eur J Oral Sci 2011;119(6):469-73. doi: 10.1111/j.1600-0722.2011.00873.x.

[16] Cárdenas-Bahena Á, Velázquez-Olmedo LB, Falcón-Flores JA, García-Zámano IE, Montes-Salmerón RE, Reza-Bravo GG, et al. Self-perception of oral health in older adults from Mexico City. Rev Med Inst Mex Seguro Soc 2018;56(Suppl 1):S54-63.

[17] Anderson AP, Park YM, Shrestha D, Zhang J, Liu J, Merchant AT. Cross-sectional association of physical activity and periodontal antibodies. J Periodontol 2018;89(12):1400-1406. doi: 10.1002/JPER.17-0709.

[18] Ide R, Mizoue T, Ueno K, Fujino Y, Yoshimura T. Relationship between cigarette smoking and oral health status. Sangyo Eiseigaku Zasshi 2002;44(1):6-11.

[19] Lukacs JR. Gender differences in oral health in South Asia: metadata imply multifactorial biological and cultural causes. Am J Hum Biol 2011;23(3):398-411. doi: 10.1002/ajhb.21164.

[20] Lee SK, Hwang SY. Oral health in adults with coronary artery disease and its risk factors: a comparative study using the Korea National Health and Nutrition Examination Survey data. BMC Cardiovasc Disord 2021;21(1):71. doi: 10.1186/s12872-021-01878-x.

In: Social and Health Issues … ISBN: 978-1-53619-937-6
Editors: S Pengpid, K Peltzer et al.

Chapter 14

PREVALENCE AND CORRELATES OF SELF-REPORTED CATARACT AMONG A NATIONALLY REPRESENTATIVE COMMUNITY-DWELLING SAMPLE OF OLDER ADULTS IN INDIA, 2017-2018

Supa Pengpid[1,2], MPH, DrPH, MBA and Karl Peltzer[2,3,*], MA Clin Psych, PhD, Dr Habil

[1]ASEAN Institute for Health Development, Mahidol University, Salaya, Phutthamonthon, Nakhon Pathom, Thailand

[2]Department of Research Administration and Development, University of Limpopo, Turfloop, South Africa

[3]Department of Psychology, College of Medical and Health Science, Asia University, Taichung, Taiwan

[*] *Correspondence*: Professor Karl Peltzer, Department of Research Administration and Development, University of Limpopo, Turfloop Campus, Private Bag X1106, Sovenga 0727, South Africa. Email: kfpeltzer@gmail.com.

Abstract

This chapter aimed to determine the prevalence and correlates of cataract in older adults in India. The cross-sectional sample consisted of 52,393 individuals (≥50 years) from the Longitudinal Ageing Study in India (LASI) Wave 1 in 2017-2018. Self-reported cataract diagnosis was used to assess the cataract prevalence. Results indicate that the prevalence of self-reported cataract was 16.9%, 15.2% among men and 18.4% among women. In adjusted logistic regression analysis, older age, medium subjective socioeconomic status, urban residence, poor or fair self-rated health status, hypertension and diabetes were positively associated with self-reported cataract, while male sex and married were negatively associated with self-reported cataract. In addition, in unadjusted analysis, underweight, physical inactivity, angina, arthritis, lung disease, and poor self-rated vision was positively and ever tobacco and ever alcohol use were negatively associated with self-reported cataract. More than one in six older adults reported having been diagnosed with cataract in India. Several risk factors were identified, which can be targeted in public health interventions.

Introduction

"Age-related cataracts constitute approximately 50% of the 285 million visually-impaired people globally" [1]. "Cataracts are the major cause of blindness and visual impairment in developing countries and contribute to more than 90% of the total disability adjusted life years"[2]. Based on a systematic review the global age-standardized prevalence of any cataract was 17.2% [3]. In a population-based survey among older adults (≥50 years) in six low and middle-income countries [4], the prevalence of self-reported cataract diagnosis was 4.4%, in Ghana 5.4% [5], in South Africa 4.4% [6], in Mexico 12.2% [7], and in Taiwan (40 years and older) 11.8% [8]. Among older adults (≥50 years) in India in 2007, 15.5% self-reported diagnosed cataracts in the last five years [9]. There is a lack of more recent national population-based data on the prevalence and correlates of cataract among older adults in India. As previously reviewed [6], factors associated with cataract may include "older age, lower income, lower education, urban residency, female sex, diabetes, hypertension, obesity, alcohol use, smoking and poor well-being." This study aimed to determine the prevalence and correlates of cataract in older adults in a national community-dwelling sample in India in 2017-2018.

OUR STUDY

This secondary data analysis utilized data from the cross-sectional and nationally representative Longitudinal Ageing Study in India (LASI) Wave 1, 2017-2018; "the overall household response rate is 96%, and the overall individual response rate is 87%" [10]. In a household survey, "interview, physical measurement and biomarker data were collected from individuals aged 45 and above and their spouses, regardless of age" [10]. We restricted our analysis to those 50 years and older. Specific details on the sampling approach are found elsewhere [10]. The study was approved by the "Indian Council of Medical Research (ICMR) Ethics Committee and written informed consent was obtained from the participants" [10].

Measures

Cataract was based on an affirmative response to the question. "Were you diagnosed with cataract in one or both eyes?" [10].

Sociodemographic variables consisted of education (none, ≥1 years), age group (50-59, 60-69, 70-79, and 80 or more years), sex (male, female), marital status (currently married vs. widowed/divorced/separated/deserted/ live-in relationship/never married), and residence (rural, urban). Subjective socioeconomic status was assessed with the question, "Please imagine a ten-step ladder, where at the bottom are the people who are the worst off – who have the least money, least education, and the worst jobs or no jobs, and at the top of the ladder are the people who are the best off – those who have the most money, most education, and best jobs. Please indicate the number [1-10] on the rung on the ladder where you would place yourself" [10]. Steps

1 to 3 on the socioeconomic ladder were defined as low, 4-5 as medium, and 6-10 as high socioeconomic status.

Self-rated health status was sourced from the question, "In general, would you say your health is excellent, very good, good, fair, or poor?" Responses were coded as "1 = poor, 2 = fair, 3 = good, 4 = very good and 5 = excellent" [10].

Anthropometry: "Height and weight of adults were measured using the Seca 803 digital scale." [10]. "Body Mass Index = BMI was calculated according to Asian criteria: underweight (<18.5 kg/m^2), normal weight (18.5-22.9 kg/m^2), overweight (23.0-24.9 kg/m^2), class I obesity (25.0-29.9 kg/m^2), and class II obesity (≥30.0 kg/m^2)" [11].

Physical inactivity was defined as hardly ever or never vigorous and moderate activity [10].

Lifetime tobacco use was assessed from 1) "Have you ever smoked any tobacco products (cigarettes, bidis, cigars, hookah, cheroot, etc.)? and 2) Did you ever use smokeless tobacco (such as chewing tobacco, gutka, pan masala, etc.)?" (Yes, No) [10].

Lifetime alcohol use was assessed with the question, "Have you ever consumed any alcoholic beverages such as beer, wine, liquor, country liquor, etc?" (Yes, No) [10].

Hypertension or raised blood pressure (BP) was defined as "systolic BP ≥140 mm Hg and/or diastolic BP ≥90 mm Hg (based on the last two averaged of three readings) or where the participant is currently on antihypertensive medication" [12].

Arthritis, diabetes, and chronic lung disease were assessed by self-reported health care provider diagnosis [10].

Angina was assessed with the "World Health Organization's Rose angina questionnaire" [13], defined based on "discomfort at walking uphill or hurrying, or at an ordinary pace on level ground. Furthermore, the pain should be located at the sternum or in the left chest and arm, causing the patient to stop or slow down, and the pain should resolve within 10 minutes when the patient stops or slows dow." [14].

Vision was assessed with two questions, 1) "How good is your eyesight for seeing things at a distance, like recognizing a person across the street (or

20 meters away), whether or not you wear glasses, contacts, or corrective lenses?" and 2) "How good is your eyesight for seeing things up close, like reading an ordinary newspaper print whether or not you wear glasses, contacts, or corrective lenses?" [7]. Response options ranged from 1 = very good to 5 = very poor, and poor near or far vision was defined as "poor or very poor" [10].

Data analysis

Descriptive statistics were applied to describe health status, sociodemographic information, and cataract prevalence. Unadjusted and adjusted logistic regression was utilized to assess the predictors of self-reported cataract; variables found significant in univariate analyses were included in the adjusted model. $P < 0.05$ was accepted as significant, missing values were excluded, and no multi-collinearity was found. Statistical analyses were conducted using STATA software version 15.0 (Stata Corporation, College Station, TX, USA), taking the complex study design into account.

FINDINGS

The sample included 52,393 older adults (50 years and older), with a median age of 62 years (14 years interquartile range), 53.3% were female and 46.7% male. Majority (70.1%) of participants were married, 53.0% had no formal schooling, 69.0% were residing in rural areas, 27.3% were physically inactive, and 43.3% rated their health status as fair or poor. Almost half of the participants (45.4%) had hypertension, 8.9% angina, 13.4% had diabetes, 17.6% arthritis, 7.5% lung disease, 24.4% poor self-rated vision, 39.8% overweight/obesity, 38.4% had ever used tobacco and 14.9% had ever engaged in alcohol use. The prevalence of self-reported cataract was 16.9%, 12.2% among men and 18.4% among women (see Table 1).

Table 1. Sample and cataract characteristics among older adults in India, 2017-2018

Variable	Sample	Cataract
	N (%)	N (%)
Sociodemographic factors		
All	**52393**	**16.9**
Age in years		
50-59	20916 (38.1)	6.7
60-69	18979 (36.2)	18.5
70-79	9108 (18.7)	28.7
≥80	3390 (7.0)	33.5
Sex		
Female	27815 (53.3)	18.4
Male	24578 (46.7)	15.2
Marital status		
Not married	15151 (29.9)	23.8
Married	37236 (70.1)	14.0
Education		
≥1 years	26410 (47.0)	16.9
No schooling	25983 (53.0)	16.9
Subjective socioeconomic status		
Low	17462 (38.2)	15.9
Medium	20070 (37.4)	17.1
High	13176 (24.4)	18.0
Residence		
Rural	34099 (69.0)	15.3
Urban	18294 (31.0)	20.5
Health factors		
Self-rated health status (poor)	21248 (43.3)	20.7
Body mass index		
Normal	17179 (37.2)	16.0
Underweight	9428 (23.0)	17.7
Overweight/Obesity	20039 (39.8)	17.0
Physical inactivity	14771 (27.3)	21.4
Ever tobacco use	19600 (38.4)	13.9
Ever alcohol use	9346 (14.9)	12.3
Hypertension	22826 (45.4)	20.3
Diabetes	7423 (13.4)	23.2
Angina	4510 (8.9)	19.4
Arthritis	8329 (17.6)	20.4
Lung disease	3297 (7.5)	22.9
Poor self-rated vision	12650 (24.4)	20.6

Table 2. Associations with cataract in older adults in India

Variable	Unadjusted Odds Ratios (95% CI)	Adjusted Odds Ratios (95% CI)
Sociodemographic factors		
Age in years		
50-59	1 (Reference)	1 (Reference)
60-69	3.18 (2.80, 3.61)***	3.09 (2.71, 3.52)***
70-79	5.66 (4.92, 6.50)***	5.22 (4.44, 6.13)***
≥80	7.07 (5.94, 8.41)***	6.53 (5.30, 8.04)***
Sex		
Female	1 (Reference)	1 (Reference)
Male	0.79 (0.73, 0.86)***	0.81 (0.73, 0.90)***
Marital status		
Not married	1 (Reference)	1 (Reference)
Married	0.52 (0.48, 0.57)***	0.82 (0.73, 0.93)***
Education		
≥1 years	1 (Reference)	---
No schooling	1.00 (0.92, 1.09)	
Subjective socioeconomic status		
Low	1 (Reference)	1 (Reference)
Medium	1.09 (0.99, 1.21)	1.12 (1.00, 1.26)*
High	1.16 (1.03, 1.31)*	1.14 (0.98, 1.31)
Residence		
Rural	1 (Reference)	1 (Reference)
Urban	1.43 (1.29, 1.59)***	1.52 (1.36, 1.70)***
Health factors		
Self-rated health status (poor)	1.61 (1.47, 1.75)***	1.31 (1.17, 1.31)***
Body mass index		
Normal	1 (Reference)	1 (Reference)
Underweight	1.13 (1.01, 1.26)*	1.04 (0.93, 1.17)
Overweight/Obesity	1.07 (0.97, 1.19)	1.02 (0.91, 1.14)
Physical inactivity	1.52 (1.39, 1.66)***	1.08 (0.97, 1.20)
Ever tobacco use	0.86 (0.79, 0.94)***	0.99 (0.89, 1.10)
Ever alcohol use	0.79 (0.70, 0.89)***	0.98 (0.85, 1.12)
Hypertension	1.56 (1.43, 1.71)***	1.20 (1.08, 1.32)***
Diabetes	1.60 (1.40, 1.83)***	1.30 (1.09, 1.55)**
Angina	1.21 (1.05, 1.39)**	1.10 (0.94, 1.29)
Arthritis	1.33 (1.19, 1.48)***	1.02 (0.88, 1.19)
Lung disease	1.51 (1.26, 1.83)***	1.24 (0.94, 1.63)
Poor self-rated vision	1.38 (1.27, 1.51)***	1.07 (0.96, 1.19)

CI = Confidence Interval; $***p < 0.001$; $**p < 0.01$; $*p < 0.05$.

Associations with cataract prevalence

In adjusted logistic regression analysis, older age, medium subjective socioeconomic status, urban residence, poor or fair self-rated health status, hypertension and diabetes were positively associated with self-reported cataract, while male sex and married were negatively associated with self-reported cataract. In addition, in unadjusted analysis, underweight, physical inactivity, angina, arthritis, lung disease, and poor self-rated vision were positively and ever tobacco and ever alcohol use were negatively associated with self-reported cataract (see Table 2).

Discussion

In this national 2017-2018 India LASI survey among community-dwelling older adults (≥50 years), the prevalence of self-reported cataract was 16.9%, which seems similar to the 2007 India survey (≥50 years, 15.5% self-reported diagnosed cataracts in the last five years) [9], but probably higher than among older adults (50 years and older) in six low- and middle-income countries (4.4% in the last 5 years) [4], in Ghana (5.4%) [5], in South Africa (4.4%) [6], in Mexico (12.2%) [7], and in Taiwan (40 years and older) (11.8%) [8].

In line with previous results [3, 5, 6, 9], this study found a strong association between increasing age and cataract prevalence. Age related cataract is expected to increase with an ageing population in middle income countries like India [15]. Consistent with previous research [5, 6, 16], female sex and urban residency were associated with higher cataract prevalence in this study. While some studies [5, 6] found an association between lower socioeconomic status and cataract, this study did not find significant differences in terms of educational level but found that medium subjective socioeconomic status was associated with higher odds of cataract. It is possible that with higher economic status, older Indians have better access to cataract (screening) services. Consistent with previous research in India [9], not married was associated with cataract in this study. It is possible that compared to non-married older adults, married older adults may have better access to health care and eye care services [5].

Consistent with studies in Ghana [5], Bangladesh [17] and Mexico [7], this study showed that poorer perceived health status was associated with cataract. Some previous research [7, 8, 18] showed an association between low physical activity, sedentary behaviour, and cataract prevalence, while in this study physical inactivity was associated with cataract in unadjusted analysis. Some research suggests that "maintaining low levels of systemic oxidative stress by being physically active on a regular basis may contribute to the prevention of age-related cataracts in the general population" [18].

Having diabetes and/or hypertension increased the odds of cataract in this study. Several previous studies have highlighted the link between diabetes and cataract [4-7]. Because of the strong link between diabetes and cataract, Pizzol et al. [4] suggest "the introduction of health policies for the prevention, early diagnosis, and treatment of diabetes, as well as its complications such as vision diseases." Similar to studies in Ghana [5], South Africa [6], the previous India study [9], and in a systematic review on the relationship between alcohol use and cataract [15], we did not find a significant association between lifetime alcohol use, lifetime tobacco use and cataract. Likewise, we did not find a significant association between overweight/obesity and cataract, as found previously in South Africa [6] and in South Korea [16]. Unlike previous results, this study did not find an association between arthritis [9, 16], lung disease (asthma) [16], angina [16], poor vision [9], and cataract. Study limitations include the cross-sectional design, the assessment of some variables, including cataract, by self-report, and future studies should include an objective eye examination.

CONCLUSION

More than one in six older adults reported having been diagnosed with cataract in India. Several potential risk factors, such as older age, higher subjective socioeconomic status, urban residence, poor or fair self-rated health status, hypertension, female sex, and not married were identified, which can be targeted in public health interventions.

ACKNOWLEDGMENT

This paper uses data from WHO's Study on Global Ageing and Adult Health (SAGE). SAGE is supported by the US National Institute on Aging through Interagency Agreements OGHA 04034785; YA1323-08-CN-0020; Y1-AG-1005-0) and through research grants R01-AG034479 and R21-AG034263.

REFERENCES

[1] Pascolini D, Mariotti SP. Global estimates of visual impairment: 2010. Br J Ophthalmol 2012;96:614–8.

[2] Rao GN, Khanna R, Payal A. The global burden of cataract. Curr Opin Ophthalmol 2011;22(1):4-9. doi: 10.1097/ICU.0b013e3283414fc8.

[3] Hashemi H, Pakzad R, Yekta A, Aghamirsalim M, Pakbin M, Ramin S, et al. Global and regional prevalence of age-related cataract: a comprehensive systematic review and meta-analysis. Eye 2020;34:1357-70. doi: 10.1038/s41433-020-0806-3.

[4] Pizzol D, Veronese N, Quaglio G, Di Gennaro F, Deganello D, Stubbs B, et al. The association between diabetes and cataract among 42,469 community-dwelling adults in six low- and middle-income countries. Diabetes Res Clin Pract 2019;147:102-10. doi: 10.1016/j.diabres.2018.12.001.

[5] Yawson AE, Ackuaku-Dogbe EM, Seneadza NA, Mensah G, Minicuci N, Naidoo N, et al. Self-reported cataracts in older adults in Ghana: sociodemographic and health related factors. BMC Public Health 2014;14:949. doi: 10.1186/1471-2458-14-949.

[6] Phaswana-Mafuya N, Peltzer K, Crampin A, Ahame E, Sokhela Z. Prevalence of self-reported diagnosed cataract and associated risk factors among elderly South Africans. Int J Environ Res Public Health 2017;14(12). pii: E1523. doi: 10.3390/ijerph14121523.

[7] Pengpid S, Peltzer K. Prevalence and correlates of cataract among a nationally representative population-based sample of older adults in Mexico. Int J Disabil Hum Dev 2020;19(3):561-6.

[8] Shih YH, Chang HY, Lu MI, Hurng BS. Time trend of prevalence of self-reported cataract and its association with prolonged sitting in Taiwan from 2001 and 2013. BMC Ophthalmol 2014;14:128. doi: 10.1186/1471-2415-14-128.

[9] Agrawal S, Fledderjohann J, Ghosh S. Risk factors for self-reported cataract symptoms, diagnosis, and surgery uptake among older adults in India: Findings from the WHO SAGE data. Glob Public Health 2020 Oct 22:1-15. doi: 10.1080/17441692.2020.1836246.

[10] International Institute for Population Sciences (IIPS), NPHCE, MoHFW Harvard TH Chan School of Public Health (HSPH) and the University of Southern California (USC). Longitudinal Ageing Study in India (LASI) Wave 1, 2017-18, India Report. Mumbai: International Institute for Population Sciences, 2020.

[11] Wen CP, David Cheng TY, Tsai SP, Chan HT, Hsu HL, Hsu CC, et al. Are Asians at greater mortality risks for being overweight than Caucasians? Redefining obesity for Asians. Public Health Nutr 2009;12(4):497-506. doi: 10.1017/S1368980008002802.

[12] Chobanian AV, Bakris GL, Black HR, Cushman WC, Green LA, Izzo Jr JL, et al. The seventh report of the joint national committee on prevention, detection, evaluation, and treatment of high blood pressure: the JNC 7 report. JAMA 2003;289(19):2560–71.

[13] Rose GA. The diagnosis of ischaemic heart pain and intermittent claudication in field surveys. Bull World Health Organ 1962;27:645–58.

[14] Achterberg S, Soedamah-Muthu SS, Cramer MJ, Kappelle LJ, van der Graaf Y, Algra A, et al. Prognostic value of the Rose questionnaire: a validation with future coronary events in the SMART study. Eur J Prev Cardiol 2012;19(1):5-14. doi: 10.1177/1741826710391117.

[15] Wang W, Zhang X. Alcohol intake and the risk of age-related cataracts: A meta-analysis of prospective cohort studies. PLoS One 2014;9:e107820.

[16] Rim TH, Kim DW, Kim SE, Kim SS. Factors associated with cataract in Korea: A Community Health survey 2008–2012. Yonsei Med J 2015;56:1663–70.

[17] Polack S, Kuper H, Wadud Z, Fletcher A, Foster A. Quality of life and visual impairment from cataract in Satkhira district, Bangladesh. Br J Ophthalmol 2008;92(8):1026-30. doi: 10.1136/bjo.2007.134791.

[18] Zheng Selin J, Orsini N, Ejdervik Lindblad B, Wolk A. Long-term physical activity and risk of age-related cataract: a population-based prospective study of male and female cohorts. Ophthalmology 2015;122(2):274-80. doi: 10.1016/j.ophtha.2014.08.023.

In: Social and Health Issues … ISBN: 978-1-53619-937-6
Editors: S Pengpid, K Peltzer et al.

Chapter 15

SOCIAL AND HEALTH DETERMINANTS OF EDENTULISM AMONG OLDER ADULTS IN INDIA

Karl Peltzer*[1,2]*, MA Clin Psych, PhD, Dr Habil and Supa Pengpid*[1,3,*]*, MPH, DrPH, MBA
[1]Department of Research Administration and Development, University of Limpopo, Turfloop, South Africa
[2]Department of Psychology, College of Medical and Health Science, Asia University, Taichung, Taiwan
[3]ASEAN Institute for Health Development, Mahidol University, Salaya, Phutthamonthon, Nakhon Pathom, Thailand

ABSTRACT

In this chapter we estimate the associations between social and health indicators with edentulism among older adults in India. The sample

* *Correspondence*: Professor Supa Pengpid, ASEAN Institute for Health Development, Mahidol University, 25/25 Phutthamonthon Road 4, Salaya, Phutthamonton, Nakhon Pathom 73170, Thailand. Email: supaprom@yahoo.com.

included 52,393 and older adults (≥50 years) from a cross-sectional national community-dwelling survey in India in 2017-2018. Results indicate that the prevalence of edentulism was 8.4%, 8.2% among women and 8.5% among men. In the adjusted logistic regression analysis, older age (≥70 years) (Adjusted Odds Ratio-AOR: 5.77, 95% Confidence Interval-CI: 4.86-6.84), belonging to the Sikh religion (AOR: 2.67, 95% CI: 2.16-3.30), and having difficulties with two or more Activities of Daily Living (ADL)/Instrumental Activities of Daily Living (IADL) (AOR: 1.18, 95% CI: 1.02-1.36) were positively and belonging to other religions or no religion (AOR: 0.45, 95% CI: 0.26-0.79) and having overweight or obesity (AOR: 0.79, 95% CI: 0.68-0.92) were negatively associated with edentulism. In addition, in unadjusted analysis, having no education and poor or fair self-rated health status were positively, and receipt of health insurance, attendance of religious services and having a medium social network were negatively associated with edentulism. Almost one in ten older adults in India have edentulism, and several associated factors were identified that can be targeted in interventions.

Introduction

"Edentulism (=having lost all of one's natural teeth) is a significant public health problem globally because of its high prevalence (> 10% in individuals 50 years and older) and related disability" [1-3]. In a study among older adults (≥50 years) in six low- and middle-income countries, the overall prevalence of edentulism was 11.7%, ranging from 3.0% in Ghana to 21.7% in Mexico, and 16.3% in India in 2007 [2]. There is a lack of more recent national data on the prevalence and correlates of edentulism among older adults in India.

As previously reviewed [3], factors associated with edentulism include "increasing age, female gender, no or lower education, lower economic status, rural residence, smoking, having chronic diseases, diabetes, arthritis, asthma, depression, reduced physical function, functional disability, poor self-rated health and lack of social capital." In a local study in India "complete edentulousness of both the arches was highest in the middle socio-economic group and was the lowest in the low socio-economic group. Less than 50% of edentulous elderly and only 10% of partially edentulous elderly were wearing dentures" [4]. This study aimed to determine the prevalence and correlates of edentulism in older adults in a national community dwelling survey in 2017-2018 in India.

Our Study

This cross-sectional study was conducted in a nationally representative sample of community-dwelling older adults in India in 2017-2018; "the overall household response rate was 96%, and the overall individual response rate was 87%" [5]. In a household survey, "interview, physical measurement and biomarker data were collected from individuals aged 45 and above and their spouses, regardless of age" [5]. We restricted in this analysis the sample to those who were 50 years and older. Specific details on the sampling approach are found elsewhere [5]. The study was approved by the "Indian Council of Medical Research (ICMR) Ethics Committee and written informed consent was obtained from the participants" [5].

Measures

Edentulism was defined as "lost all natural teeth," following the question, "Have you lost some or all of your natural teeth?" [5].

Social and demographic variables

Sociodemographic variables consisted of education (none and ≥1 years), age, sex (male, female), receipt of health insurance, religion, urban and rural residence [5]. Subjective socioeconomic status was assessed with the question, "Please imagine a ten-step ladder, where at the bottom are the people who are the worst off – who have the least money, least education, and the worst jobs or no jobs, and at the top of the ladder are the people who are the best off – those who have the most money, most education, and best jobs. Please indicate the number (1-10) on the rung on the ladder where you would place yourself" [5]. Steps 1 to 3 on the socioeconomic ladder were defined as low, 4-5 as medium, and 6-10 as high.

Organizational religiosity was assessed with the question, "In the past year, how often have you attended religious services (at a temple/mosque/church, etc.)?" Response options were grouped into 1 (low)=not at all, 2 (medium)=1-3 times a month or 1 or more times a year, and 3(high)=once a week or more than once a week or every day [5].

Social network was measured with 11 items, e.g., "Eat-out-of-house (restaurant/hotel)" [5]. Responses were coded 1= daily to at least once a month and 0=rarely/once a year or never (Cronbach's alpha 0.67).

Health indicators

Self-rated health status was sourced from the question, "In general, would you say your health is excellent, very good, good, fair, or poor?" Responses were coded as "1=poor, 2=fair, 3=good, 4=very good and 5=excellent" [5].

Arthritis, diabetes, and chronic lung disease were assessed by self-reported health care provider diagnosis [5].

Major depressive disorder in the past 12 months was assessed with the Health and Retirement Study (HRS) Composite International Diagnostic Interview short form (CIDI-SF) [6], using criteria of the Diagnostic and Statistical Manual of Mental Disorders (DSM) [7]. Study respondents were required to "endorse either anhedonia or depressed mood for most of the day for most of a 2-week period or more," and those who fulfilled this criterion "completed an additional seven symptoms: lost interest, feeling tired, change in weight, trouble with sleep, trouble concentrating, feeling down, and thoughts of death" [8]. "Those with a score ≥3 were considered to meet the criteria for having MDD in the previous 12 months; MDD symptomology scores ranged from 0 to 7." [8].

Current tobacco use included, 1) "Do you currently smoke any tobacco products (cigarettes, bidis, cigars, hookah, cheroot, etc.)? and/or 2) Do you use smokeless tobacco (such as chewing tobacco, gutka, pan masala, etc.)?" (Yes, No) [5].

Functional disability was assessed with 6 items of "Activities of Daily Living (ADL)" and 7 items of "Instrumental Activities of Daily Living (IADL)" [9, 10]; Cronbach alpha for the 13 items was 0.89 in this study. Responses were "Yes/No," summed and were trichotomized into 0,1, or ≥2 ADL/IADL items.

Anthropometry: "Height and weight of adults were measured using the Seca 803 digital scale." [5]. "BMI was calculated according to Asian criteria: underweight (<18.5 kg/m^2), normal weight (18.5-22.9 kg/m^2), overweight (23.0-24.9 kg/m^2), class I obesity (25.0-29.9 kg/m^2), and class II obesity (≥30.0 kg/m^2)" [11].

Data analysis

Considering the clustered study design, data analyses were conducted with "STATA software version 15.0 (Stata Corporation, College Station, TX, USA)." Unadjusted and adjusted logistic regression analyses were used to calculate associations between social, demographic, and health indicators with edentulism. Variables significant in the univariate analysis were subsequently included in the multivariable model. *P*-values of below 0.05 were accepted as significant and missing values were excluded from the analysis.

FINDINGS

The sample included 52,393 older adults (50 years and older), 53.3% were female and 46.7% male. More than half of participants (53.0%) had no formal education, 24.4% had high subjective socioeconomic status, 19.6% had health insurance, and 69.0% were residing in rural areas. More than one-third of participants (34.9%) had high intrinsic religiosity, 14.0% attended at least weekly religious services, and 30.6% had a high social network. Furthermore, health indictor characteristics are shown in Table 1. The prevalence of edentulism was 8.4%, 8.2% among women and 8.5% among men (see Table 1).

Table 1. Sample characteristics among older adults (≥50 years) in India, 2017-2018 (N=52,393)

Variable	Variable specification	Sample	Edentulism
		%	%
Social and demographic factors			
All			**8.4**
Age in years	50-59	38.1	3.7
	60-69	36.2	6.9
	70 or more	25.7	17.3
Sex	Female	53.3	8.2
	Male	46.7	8.5
Education	Some	47.0	7.4
	None	53.0	9.2
Subjective socioeconomic status	Low	38.2	8.8
	Medium	37.4	7.5
	High	24.4	8.3
Has health insurance	No	80.4	8.7
	Yes	19.6	6.7
Residence	Rural	69.0	8.3
	Urban	31.0	8.4
Organised religiosity (Attendance of religious services)	Not at all	27.1	9.8
	≥ monthly	45.6	7.0
	≥1/week or every day	27.4	8.0
Social network	Low	41.3	9.5
	Medium	29.1	7.4
	High	29.6	7.6
Religion	Hindu	82.4	8.3
	Muslim	11.3	8.4
	Christian	2.8	6.2
	Sikh	1.8	18.2
	Other	1.7	4.9
Health indicators			
Self-rated health status	Fair or poor	43.3	9.4
Arthritis	Yes	17.6	7.9
Diabetes	Yes	13.4	9.3
Major depressive disorder	Yes	8.0	12.0
Chronic lung disease	Yes	7.5	9.6
Current tobacco use	Yes	33.0	8.2
ADL/IADL	0	55.5	6.5
	1	10.7	7.6
	2 or more	33.8	11.7
Body mass index (BMI)	Normal	37.2	8.4
	Underweight	23.0	10.5
	Overweight/obesity	39.8	6.0

Associations with edentulism

Table 2. Associations with edentulism estimated by logistic regression

Variable	Variable specification	Crude Odds Ratio (95% CI)	Adjusted Odds Ratio (95% CI)
Social and demographic factors			
Age in years	50-59	1 (Reference)	1 (Reference)
	60-69	1.90 (1.34, 2.68)***	2.28 (1,96, 2.66)***
	70 or more	5.38 (3.80, 7.62)***	5.77 (4.86, 6.84)***
Sex	Female	1 (Reference)	---
	Male	1.04 (0.89, 1.21)	
Education	Some	1 (Reference)	1 (Reference)
	None	1.27 (1.10, 1.47)***	0.92 (0.81, 1.05)
Subjective socioeconomic status	Low	1 (Reference)	---
	Medium	0.85 (0.70, 1.02)	
	High	0.94 (0.76, 1.16)	
Has health insurance	No	1 (Reference)	1 (Reference)
	Yes	0.74 (0.62, 0.89)***	0.91 (0.76, 1.09)
Residence	Rural	1 (Reference)	---
	Urban	1.00 (0.81, 1.25)	
Organised religiosity (Attendance of religious services)	Not at all	1 (Reference)	1 (Reference)
	≥ monthly	0.77 (0.67, 0.87)***	0.92 (0.78, 1.06)
	≥1/week or every day	0.79 (0.62, 1.02)	0.92 (0.78, 1.09)
Social network	Low	1 (Reference)	1 (Reference)
	Medium	0.76 (0.67, 0.86)***	0.90 (0.78, 1.03)
	High	0.78 (0.61, 1.00)	0.90 (0.76, 1.06)
Religion	Hindu	1 (Reference)	1 (Reference)
	Muslim	(0.60, 1.70)	0.89 (0.76, 1.01)
	Christian	0.73 (0.52, 1.03)	0.67 (0.45, 1.01)
	Sikh	2.47 (2.06, 2.97)***	2.67 (2.16, 3.30)***
	Other	0.57 (0.37, 0.89)*	0.45 (0.26, 0.79)**
Health indicators			
Self-rated health status	Fair or poor	1.31 (1.12, 1.53)***	1.04 (0.91, 1.18)
Arthritis	Yes	0.93 (0.80,1.08)	---
Diabetes	Yes	1.15 (0.77, 1.70)	---
Major depressive disorder	Yes	1.60 (0.96, 2.66)	---
Chronic lung disease	Yes	1.18 (0.95, 1.47)	---
Current tobacco use	Yes	0.97 (0.85, 1.11)	---
ADL/IADL	0	1 (Reference)	1 (Reference)
	1	1.19 (1.01, 1.40)*	1.08 (0.90, 1.29)
	2 or more	1.92 (1.64, 2.26)***	1.18 (1.02, 1.36)*
Body mass index (BMI)	Normal	1 (Reference)	1 (Reference)
	Underweight	1.29 (1.13, 1.47)***	1.11 (0.96, 1.27)
	Overweight/obesity	0.70 (0.61, 0.82)***	0.79 (0.68, 0.92)**

CI=Confidence Interval; ***$p<0.001$; ** $p<0.01$; *$p<0.05$.

In the adjusted logistic regression analysis, older age (≥70 years) (Adjusted Odds Ratio-AOR: 5.77, 95% Confidence Interval-CI: 4.86-6.84), belonging to the Sikh religion (AOR: 2.67, 95% CI: 2.16-3.30), and having difficulties with two or more ADL/IADL (AOR: 1.18, 95% CI: 1.02-1.36) were positively and belonging to other religions or no religion (AOR: 0.45, 95% CI: 0.26-0.79) and having overweight or obesity (AOR: 0.79, 95% CI: 0.68-0.92) were negatively associated with edentulism. In addition, in unadjusted analysis, having no education, and poor or fair self-rated health status were positively, and receipt of health insurance, attendance or religious services and having a medium social network were negatively associated with edentulism (see Table 2).

DISCUSSION

In this nationally representative sample of older adults in India in 2017-2018, the prevalence of edentulism was 8.4%, which is lower than in a previous study in India in 2007 (16.3%), the six middle-income countries study (11.7%), but higher than in Ghana (3.0%) [2]. The reduction of edentulism in India from 2007 to 2017-2018 may be attributed to increased comprehensive oral health care through the primary health care system in India [12].

Consistent with previous investigations [2, 13, 14], that increasing age, and in unadjusted analysis lower education and not having health insurance were associated with edentulism. Unlike some previous research [2, 13, 14], we did not observe significant sex differences in the prevalence of edentulism. Further, lower education and not having health insurance may translate to lower oral health knowledge and less access to oral health care [3]. Consistent with some previous studies [15, 16], this study found in univariate analysis a negative association between social network, attendance of religious services and edentulism. Older adults who belong to social networks may be more likely to perform health promotion behaviours and may have better health, including better self-rated oral health [2, 17, 18].

Compared to Hindus, Sikhs had a 2.7 times higher odds of edentulism in this study. This result needs further research investigation.

In agreement with previous studies [2, 3], functional disability (ADL/IADL difficulty) was found positively associated with edentulism. People with a functional disability may have more difficulty in performing proper oral hygiene and less likely access dental care services [2, 19]. Some previous research [19, 20] found a relationship between poor self-rated health status and edentulism, while this study only found this in unadjusted analysis.

Unlike in some previous investigations (arthritis [2], chronic lung disease, asthma [2], diabetes [21], depression [22]), this study did not find an association between arthritis, diabetes, chronic lung disease, major depressive disorder and edentulism. Likewise, contrary to some previous research [2, 23], this study did not find an association between tobacco use and edentulism. It is possible that no significant relationship between tobacco use and edentulism was found because of the very high prevalence of current tobacco use (33.0%).

Study limitations include the cross-sectional design, the assessment of some variables, including edentulism, by self-report, and that certain relevant variables, such as certain dietary behaviours (e.g., sugar and soft drink intake as well as fruit and vegetable consumption), and knowledge on oral health, were not assessed.

CONCLUSION

Almost one in ten older adults in India have edentulism, and several associated factors were identified, such as older age, belonging to the Sikh religion, and having difficulties with two or more ADL/IADL that could assist in programmes promoting oral health.

Acknowledgments

The Longitudinal Aging Study in India Project is funded by the Ministry of Health and Family Welfare, Government of India, the National Institute on Aging (R01 AG042778, R01 AG030153), and United Nations Population Fund, India.

References

[1] Tyrovolas S, Koyanagi A, Panagiotakos DB, Haro JM, Kassebaum NJ, Chrepa V, et al. Population prevalence of edentulism and its association with depression and self-rated health. Sci Rep 2016;6:37083. https://doi.org/10. 1038/srep37083.

[2] Peltzer K, Hewlett S, Yawson AE, Moynihan P, Preet R, Wu F, et al. Prevalence of loss of all teeth (edentulism) and associated factors in older adults in China, Ghana, India, Mexico, Russia and South Africa. Int J Environ Res Public Health 2014;11(11):11308–24. https://doi.org/10.3390/ijerph111111308.

[3] Pengpid S, Peltzer K.The prevalence of edentulism and their related factors in Indonesia, 2014/15. BMC Oral Health 2018;18(1):118. doi: 10.1186/s12903-018-0582-7.

[4] Bijjargi S, Chowdhary R. Geriatric dentistry: is rethinking still required? A community-based survey in Indian population. Gerodontology 2013;30(4):247-53. doi: 10.1111/j.1741-2358.2012.00667.x.

[5] International Institute for Population Sciences (IIPS), NPHCE, MoHFW, Harvard TH Chan School of Public Health (HSPH) and the University of Southern California (USC). Longitudinal Ageing Study in India (LASI) Wave 1, 2017-18, India Report. Mumbai: International Institute for Population Sciences, 2020.

[6] Kessler RC, Andrews A, Mroczek D, Ustun B, Wittchen HU. The World Health Organization Composite International Diagnostic Interview Short-Form (CIDI-SF). Int J Methods Psychiatr Res 1998;7:171–85.

[7] American Psychiatric Association. Diagnostic and statistical manual of mental disorders (DSM-5), 5th ed. Washington, DC: American Psychiatric Publishing, 2013.

[8] Steffick D. Documentation of affective functioning measures in the Health and Retirement Study, 2000. URL: http://hrsonline. isr.umich.edu/sitedocs/userg/dr-005.pdf.

[9] Katz S, Ford AB, Moskowitz RW, Jackson BA, Jaffe MW. Studies of illness in the aged. the index of adl: a standardized measure of biological and psychosocial function. JAMA 1963;185:914-9. doi: 10.1001/jama.1963.03060120024016.

[10] Lawton MP, Brody EM. Assessment of older people: self-maintaining and instrumental activities of daily living. Gerontologist 1969;9(3):179-86.

[11] Wen CP, David Cheng TY, Tsai SP, Chan HT, Hsu HL, Hsu CC, et al. Are Asians at greater mortality risks for being overweight than Caucasians? Redefining obesity for Asians. Public Health Nutr 2009;12(4):497-506. doi: 10.1017/S1368980008002802.

[12] Ministry of Health and Family Welfare, Government of India. National Oral Health Programme, 2019. URL: https://www.nhp.gov.in/national-oral-health-programme_pg.

[13] Pengpid S, Peltzer K. Prevalence and correlates of edentulism in a national sample of older adults in Mexico. Int J Disabil Hum Dev 2020;19(3):589-94.

[14] Ren C, McGrath C, Yang Y. Edentulism and associated factors among community-dwelling middle-aged and elderly adults in China. Gerodontology 2017;34(2):195–207. https://doi.org/10.1111/ger.12249.

[15] Kim EK, Jung YS, Kim KH, Kim KR, Kwon GH, Choi YH, et al. Social capital and oral health: the association of social capital with edentulism and chewing ability in the rural elderly. Arch Gerontol Geriatr 2018;74:100–5. https://doi.org/10.1016/j.archger.2017.10.002.

[16] Hanson BS, Liedberg B, Owall B. Social network, social support and dental status in elderly Swedish men. Community Dent Oral Epidemiol 1994;22:331–7.

[17] Tsakos G, Sabbah W, Chandola T, Newton T, Kawachi I, Aida J, et al. Social relationships and oral health among adults aged 60 years or older. Psychosom Med 2013;75(2):178-86. doi: 10.1097/PSY.0b013e31827d221b.

[18] Hanson BS, Liedberg B, Owall B. Social network, social support and dental status in elderly Swedish men. Community Dent Oral Epidemiol 1994;22(5 Pt 1):331-7. doi: 10.1111/j.1600-0528.1994.tb02063.x.

[19] Olofsson H, Ulander EL, Gustafson Y, Hörnsten C. Association between socioeconomic and health factors and edentulism in people aged 65 and older - a population-based survey. Scand J Public Health 2018;46(7):690-8. https://doi.org/10.1177/1403494817717406.

[20] Felton DA. Edentulism and comorbid factors. J Prosthodont 2009;18(2):88-96. doi: 10.1111/j.1532-849X.2009.00437.x.

[21] Saman DM, Lemieux A, Arevalo O, Lutfiyya MN. A population-based study of edentulism in the US: does depression and rural residency matter after controlling for potential confounders? BMC Public Health 2014;14:65. doi: 10.1186/1471-2458-14-65.

[22] Medina-Solís CE, Pérez-Núñez R, Maupomé G, Casanova-Rosado JF. Edentulism among Mexican adults aged 35 years and older and associated factors. Am J Public Health 2006;96(9):1578-81.

In: Social and Health Issues … ISBN: 978-1-53619-937-6
Editors: S Pengpid, K Peltzer et al.

Chapter 16

ASSOCIATIONS BETWEEN EDENTULISM AND HEALTH INDICATORS AMONG OLDER ADULTS IN INDIA

Supa Pengpid[1,2], MPH, DrPH, MBA
and Karl Peltzer[2,3,*], MA Clin Psych, PhD, Dr Habil
[1]ASEAN Institute for Health Development, Mahidol University, Salaya, Phutthamonthon, Nakhon Pathom, Thailand,
[2]Department of Research Administration and Development, University of Limpopo, Turfloop, South Africa
[3]Department of Psychology, College of Medical and Health Science, Asia University, Taichung, Taiwan

ABSTRACT

In this chapter we aimed to estimate the associations between edentulism and health indicators among older adults in a national population survey in

* *Correspondence:* Professor Karl Peltzer, Department of Research Administration and Development, University of Limpopo, Turfloop Campus, Private Bag X1106, Sovenga 0727, South Africa. Email: kfpeltzer@gmail.com.

India. The sample included 52,393 older adults (≥50 years) from a cross-sectional national community-dwelling survey in India in 2017-2018. Results indicate that the prevalence of edentulism was 8.4%. In the adjusted logistic regression analysis, edentulism was positively associated with having difficulties with one or more Activities of Daily Living (ADL) (Adjusted Odds Ratio-AOR: 1.55, 95% Confidence Interval-CI: 1.14-2.10), having difficulties with one or more Instrumental Activities of Daily Living (IADL) (AOR: 1.28, 95% CI: 1.01-1.62) and body underweight (AOR: 1.27, 95% CI: 1.12-1.44). Furthermore, edentulism was negatively associated with cognitive functioning (AOR: 0.60, 95% CI: 0.47-0.77), angina (AOR: 0.81, 95% CI: 0.68-0.97), and general overweight or obesity (AOR: 0.75, 95% CI: 0.66-0.87). In addition, in unadjusted analysis, edentulism was associated with poor or fair self-rated health status and low life satisfaction. Edentulism was positively associated with having difficulty with one or more ADL, having difficulties with one or more IADL and body underweight, and negatively associated with cognitive functioning, angina, and overweight or obesity.

INTRODUCTION

"Edentulism (=having lost all of one's natural teeth) is a significant public health problem globally because of its high prevalence (>10% in individuals 50 years and older)" [1, 2] and related deleterious consequences for oral and general health, including impaired masticatory function, unhealthy diet, social disability, poor oral health quality of life, greater risk for different systemic diseases and an increase in mortality rate" [3]. There is a lack of studies investigating the associations between edentulism and various health indicators among older adults in India.

As previously reviewed [1, 3, 4], edentulism has been associated with underweight, poor nutrition, overweight/obesity, insufficient fruit and vegetable consumption, poor cognitive functioning, depression, poor health status, arthritis, asthma, angina, hypertension, strokes, diabetes, and functional disability. This study aimed to determine the associations between edentulism and various health indicators in older adults in a national community-dwelling survey in 2017-2018 in India.

OUR STUDY

This cross-sectional study was conducted in a nationally representative sample of community-dwelling older adults in India in 2017-2018; "the overall household response rate was 96%, and the overall individual response rate was 87%" [5]. In a household survey, "interview, physical measurement and biomarker data were collected from individuals aged 45 and above and their spouses, regardless of age" [5]. We restricted in this analysis the sample to those who were 50 years and older. Specific details on the sampling approach are found elsewhere [5]. The study was approved by the "Indian Council of Medical Research (ICMR) Ethics Committee and written informed consent was obtained from the participants" [5].

Measures

Cognitive functioning was included "memory (immediate and delayed word recall), orientation (time and place), and arithmetic function (serial 7)", with a summative score ranging from 0-32, with higher scores indicating better cognitive functioning [6].

Self-rated health status was sourced from the question, "In general, would you say your health is excellent, very good, good, fair, or poor?" Responses were coded as "1 = poor, 2 = fair, 3 = good, 4 = very good and 5 = excellent" [5].

Life satisfaction was assessed with the item, "Please, think about your life as a whole. How satisfied are you with it? Are you completely satisfied, very satisfied, somewhat satisfied, not very satisfied, or not at all satisfied?" [5]. Responses were grouped into 1 (low) = not very satisfied or not at all satisfied, and 0 = somewhat satisfied or very satisfied or completely satisfied.

Hypertension or raised blood pressure (BP) was defined as "systolic BP ≥140 mm Hg and/or diastolic BP ≥ 90 mm Hg (based on the last two averaged of three readings) or where the participant is currently on antihypertensive medication" [7].

Angina was assessed with the "World Health Organization's Rose angina questionnaire" [8], defined on the basis of "discomfort at walking uphill or hurrying, or at an ordinary pace on level ground. Furthermore, the pain should be located at the sternum or in the left chest and arm, causing the patient to stop or slow down, and the pain should resolve within 10 minutes when the patient stops or slows down." [9].

Other *chronic conditions* were sourced from the question, "Has any health professional ever told you that you have…?": 1) "Diabetes or high blood sugar; 2) Chronic lung disease such as asthma, chronic obstructive pulmonary disease/Chronic bronchitis or other chronic lung problems; 3) Chronic heart diseases such as Coronary heart disease (heart attack or Myocardial Infarction), congestive heart failure, or other chronic heart problems; 4) Stroke; and 5) Arthritis or rheumatism, Osteoporosis or other bone/joint diseases" (Yes/No) [5].

Major depressive disorder in the past 12 months was assessed with the Health and Retirement Study (HRS) Composite International Diagnostic Interview short form (CIDI-SF) [10], using criteria of the Diagnostic and Statistical Manual of Mental Disorders (DSM) [11]. Study respondents were required to "endorse either anhedonia or depressed mood for most of the day for most of a 2-week period or more," and those who fulfilled this criterion "completed an additional seven symptoms: lost interest, feeling tired, change in weight, trouble with sleep, trouble concentrating, feeling down, and thoughts of death." [12]. "Those with a score ≥3 were considered to meet the criteria for having MDD in the previous 12 months; MDD symptomology scores ranged from 0 to ." [12].

Functional disability was assessed with 6 items of "Activities of Daily Living (ADL)" (Cronbach alpha 0.86) and 7 items of "Instrumental Activities of Daily Living (IADL)" (Cronbach alpha 0.87) [13, 14]. Responses were "Yes/No" and dichotomized into 0 and ≥1 ADL and IADL items, respectively.

Anthropometry: "Height and weight of adults were measured using the Seca 803 digital scale." [5]. "BMI was calculated according to Asian criteria: underweight (<18.5 kg/m^2), normal weight (18.5-22.9 kg/m^2), overweight

(23.0-24.9 kg/m^2), class I obesity (25.0-29.9 kg/m^2), and class II obesity (≥30.0 kg/m^2)" [15].

Independent variable

Edentulism was defined as "lost all natural teeth", following the question, "Have you lost some or all of your natural teeth?" [5].

Covariates consisted of education (none and ≥1 years), age, sex (male, female), receipt of health insurance, marital status, subjective socioeconomic status, and urban and rural residence [5].

Social network was measured with 11 items, e.g., "Eat-out-of-house (restaurant/hotel)" [5]. Responses were coded 1 = daily to at least once a month and 0 = rarely/once a year or never (Cronbach's alpha 0.67).

Data analysis

Considering the clustered study design, data analyses were conducted with "STATA software version 15.0 (Stata Corporation, College Station, TX, USA)." Unadjusted and adjusted logistic regression analyses were used to calculate associations between edentulism and health indicators. Multivariable regression models were adjusted for age group, sex, education, marital status, subjective socioeconomic status, area of residence, health insurance, and social network. *P*-values of below 0.05 were accepted as significant and missing values were excluded from the analysis.

FINDINGS

The sample included 52,393 older adults (50 years and older), 53.3% were female and 46.7% male. More than half of participants (53.0%) had no formal education, 24.4% had high subjective socioeconomic status, 70.1% were married, 19.6% had a health insurance, and 69.0% were residing in rural areas. Almost one in three of the participants (30.6%) had a high social network. Furthermore, health indictor characteristics are shown in Table 1.

Table 1. Sample characteristics among older adults (≥50 years) in India, 2017-2018 (N = 52,393)

Variable	Variable specification	Sample
		% or M (SD)
Social and demographic factors		
Age in years	50-59	38.1
	60-69	36.2
	70 or more	25.7
Sex	Female	53.3
	Male	46.7
Education	Some	47.0
	None	53.0
Subjective socioeconomic status	Low	38.2
	Medium	37.4
	High	24.4
Marital status	Not married	29.9
	Married	70.1
Has health insurance	No	80.4
	Yes	19.6
Residence	Rural	69.0
	Urban	31.0
Social network	Low	41.3
	Medium	29.1
	High	29.6
Health indicators		
Cognitive functioning	Scale	18.1 (5.0)
Self-rated health status	Fair or poor	43.3
Low life satisfaction	Yes	12.0
Hypertension	Yes	45.4
Stroke	Yes	2.2
Angina	Yes	8.9
Heart disease	Yes	4.2
Diabetes	Yes	13.4
Arthritis	Yes	17.6
Major depressive disorder	Yes	8.0
Chronic lung disease	Yes	7.5
Difficulty with one or more Activities of Daily Living (ADL)	Yes	19.1
Difficulty with one or more Instrumental Activities of Daily Living (IADL)	Yes	44.5
Body mass index (BMI) underweight	Yes	23.0
BMI overweight or obesity	Yes	39.8
Edentulism	Yes	8.4

Associations between edentulism and health indicators

In the adjusted logistic regression analysis, edentulism was positively associated with having difficulties with one or more ADL (Adjusted Odds Ratio-AOR: 1.55, 95% Confidence Interval-CI: 1.14-2.10), having difficulties with one or more IADL (AOR: 1.28, 95% CI: 1.01-1.62) and body underweight (AOR: 1.27, 95% CI: 1.12-1.44). Furthermore, edentulism was negatively associated with cognitive functioning (AOR: 0.60, 95% CI: 0.47-0.77), angina (AOR: 0.81, 95% CI: 0.68-0.97), and body overweight or obesity (AOR: 0.75, 95% CI: 0.66-0.87). In addition, in unadjusted analysis, edentulism was associated with poor or fair self-rated health status and low life satisfaction (see Table 2).

Table 2. Associations between edentulism and health indicators

Outcome variables		**Model 1: unadjusted Odds Ratio or exp (Coef.) (95% CI)**	**Model 2: adjusted Odds Ratio exp (Coef.) (95% CI)[a]**
Cognition	Scale	0.26 (0.20, 0.34)***	0.60 (0.47, 0.77)***
Fair or poor self-rated health status	No	1 Reference	1 Reference
	Yes	1.31 (1.12, 1.53)***	1.08 (0.95, 1.24)
Low life satisfaction	No	1 Reference	1 Reference
	Yes	1.56 (1.09, 2.22)*	1.43 (0.96, 2.11)
Hypertension	No	1 Reference	---
	Yes	0.97 (0.87, 1.09)	
Stroke	No	1 Reference	---
	Yes	1.18 (0.88, 1.58)	
Angina	No	1 Reference	1 Reference
	Yes	0.81 (0.68, 0.96)*	0.81 (0.68, 0.97)*
Heart disease	No	1 Reference	---
	Yes	1.24 (0.89, 1.74)	
Diabetes	No	1 Reference	---
	Yes	1.15 (0.77, 1.70)	
Arthritis	No	1 Reference	---
	Yes	0.93 (0.80, 1.08)	
Major depressive disorder	No	1 Reference	---
	Yes	1.60 (0.96, 2.66)	
Chronic lung disease	No	1 Reference	---
	Yes	1.18 (0.95, 1.47)	
Current smoking tobacco	No	1 Reference	1 Reference
	Yes	1.23 (1.05, 1.43)**	1.33 (1.06, 1.67)*

Table 2. (Continued)

Outcome variables		Model 1: unadjusted Odds Ratio or exp (Coef.) (95% CI)	Model 2: adjusted Odds Ratio exp (Coef.) (95% CI)[a]
Current smokeless tobacco use	No	1 Reference	1 Reference
	Yes	0.82 (0.71, 0.95)**	0.81 (0.69, 0.95)*
Difficulty with one or more Activities of Daily Living (ADL)	No	1 Reference	1 Reference
	Yes	2.12 (1.72, 2.62)***	1.55 (1.14, 2.10)**
Difficulty with one or more Instrumental Activities of Daily Living (IADL)	No	1 Reference	1 Reference
	Yes	1.72 (1.48, 1.99)***	1.28 (1.01, 1.62)*
Body mass index (BMI) underweight	No	1 Reference	1 Reference
	Yes	1.52 (1.35, 1.72)***	1.27 (1.12, 1.44)***
BMI overweight or obesity	No	1 Reference	1 Reference
	Yes	0.63 (0.55, 0.73)***	0.75 (0.66, 0.87)***

[a] Adjusted for age group, sex, education, marital status, subjective socioeconomic status, area of residence, health insurance and social network; CI = Confidence Interval; ***$p < 0.001$; ** $p < 0.01$; *$p < 0.05$.

Discussion

In this nationally representative sample of older adults in India in 2017-2018, edentulism was found to be positively associated with having difficulty with one or more ADL, having difficulties with one or more IADLs and body underweight. These findings are in agreement with previous research, in terms of underweight [4, 16-18], and functional disability [3, 19, 20]. Edentulism negatively influences nutritional intake, thereby causing malnutrition and underweight [4].

Consistent with previous research [4, 21, 22], this study found a negative association between edentulism and cognitive functioning. In a longitudinal study, Okamoto et al. [21] found that "the completely edentulous patient experienced a greater decline in cognitive function when compared to the dentate cohort."

Some studies [4, 16, 17] found a positive association between edentulism and overweight or obesity, while this study showed an inverse association between edentulism and overweight or obesity. It is possible that edentulous participants change their diet that is low in saturated fat and high in fiber, reducing the risk of obesity [3].

Furthermore, several studies showed a positive association between edentulism and a number of chronic conditions, such as hypertension [3, 23, 24], angina [25], stroke [26, 27], diabetes [4, 28], arthritis [4] and chronic lung disease, such as asthma [4], and depression [1], while in our no significant associations were found for hypertension, stroke, heart disease, diabetes, chronic lung disease, major depressive disorder and for angina a negative association was found. It appears that the dietary pattern of edentulous older adults in India does not put them at a higher risk for heart diseases and diabetes [3].

Study limitations include the cross-sectional design, the assessment of some variables, including edentulism, by self-report, and that certain relevant variables, such as certain dietary behaviours, were not assessed and should be included in future research.

CONCLUSION

The study found among this national study of older adults in India that edentulism was positively associated with having difficulties with one or more ADL, having difficulties with one or more IADL and body underweight and negatively associated with cognitive functioning, angina, and overweight or obesity.

ACKNOWLEDGMENTS

The Longitudinal Aging Study in India Project is funded by the Ministry of Health and Family Welfare, Government of India, the National Institute on Aging (R01 AG042778, R01 AG030153), and United Nations Population Fund, India.

REFERENCES

[1] Tyrovolas S, Koyanagi A, Panagiotakos DB, Haro JM, Kassebaum NJ, Chrepa V, et al. Population prevalence of edentulism and its association with depression and self-rated health. Sci Rep 2016;6:37083. https://doi.org/10. 1038/srep37083.

[2] Emami E, de Souza RF, Kabawat M, Feine JS. The impact of edentulism on oral and general health. Int J Dent 2013;2013:498305. doi: 10.1155/2013/498305.

[3] Pengpid S, Peltzer K. The prevalence of edentulism and their related factors in Indonesia, 2014/15. BMC Oral Health 2018;18(1):118. doi: 10.1186/s12903-018-0582-7.

[4] Felton DA. Complete edentulism and comorbid diseases: an update. J Prosthodont 2016;25(1):5–20. https://doi.org/10.1111/jopr.12350.

[5] International Institute for Population Sciences (IIPS), NPHCE, MoHFW, Harvard TH Chan School of Public Health (HSPH) and the University of Southern California (USC). Longitudinal Ageing Study in India (LASI) Wave 1, 2017-18, India Report. Mumbai: International Institute for Population Sciences, 2020.

[6] Lee J, Smith JP. Regional disparities in adult height, educational attainment and gender difference in late- life cognition: Findings from the Longitudinal Aging Study in India (LASI). J Econ Ageing 2014;4:26-34. doi: 10.1016/j.jeoa.2014. 02.002.

[7] Chobanian AV, Bakris GL, Black HR, Cushman WC, Green LA, Izzo Jr JL, et al. The seventh report of the joint national committee on prevention, detection, evaluation, and treatment of high blood pressure: the JNC 7 report. JAMA 2003;289(19):2560–71.

[8] Rose GA. The diagnosis of ischaemic heart pain and intermittent claudication in field surveys. Bull World Health Organ 1962;27:645–58.

[9] Achterberg S, Soedamah-Muthu SS, Cramer MJ, Kappelle LJ, van der Graaf Y, Algra A, et al. Prognostic value of the Rose questionnaire: a validation with future coronary events in the SMART study. Eur J Prev Cardiol 2012;19(1):5-14. doi: 10.1177/1741826710391117.

[10] Kessler RC, Andrews A, Mroczek D, Ustun B, Wittchen HU. The World Health Organization Composite International Diagnostic Interview Short-Form (CIDI-SF). Int J Methods Psychiatr Res 1998;7:171–85.

[11] American Psychiatric Association. Diagnostic and statistical manual of mental disorders (DSM-5), 5th ed. Washington, DC: American Psychiatric Publishing, 2013.

[12] Steffick D. Documentation of affective functioning measures in the Health and Retirement Study, 2000. URL: http://hrsonline. isr.umich.edu/sitedocs/userg/dr-005.pdf.

[13] Katz S, Ford AB, Moskowitz RW, Jackson BA, Jaffe MW. Studies of illness in the aged. the index of adl: a standardized measure of biological and psychosocial function. JAMA 1963;185:914-9. doi: 10.1001/jama.1963.03060120024016.

[14] Lawton MP, Brody EM. Assessment of older people: self-maintaining and instrumental activities of daily living. Gerontologist 1969;9(3):179-86.

[15] Wen CP, David Cheng TY, Tsai SP, Chan HT, Hsu HL, Hsu CC, et al. Are Asians at greater mortality risks for being overweight than Caucasians? Redefining obesity for Asians. Public Health Nutr 2009;12(4):497-506. doi: 10.1017/S1368980008002802.

[16] Toniazzo MP, Amorim PS, Muniz FW, Weidlich P. Relationship of nutritional status and oral health in elderly: Systematic review with meta-analysis. Clin Nutr 2018; 37(3):824-30. https://doi.org/10.1016/j.clnu.2017.03.014.

[17] Tôrres LH, da Silva DD, Neri AL, Hilgert JB, Hugo FN, Sousa ML. Association between underweight and overweight/obesity with oral health among independently living Brazilian elderly. Nutrition 2013;29(1):152–7. https://doi. org/10.1016/j.nut.2012.05.011.

[18] Zelig R, Goldstein S, Touger-Decker R, Firestone E, Golden A, Johnson Z, et al. tooth loss and nutritional status in older adults: A systematic review and meta-analysis. JDR Clin Trans Res 2020:2380084420981016. doi: 10.1177/2380084420981016.

[19] Starr JM, Hall R. Predictors and correlates of edentulism in healthy older people. Curr Opin Clin Nutr Metab Care 2010;13(1):19–23. https://doi.org/10.1097/MCO.0b013e328333aa37.

[20] Yu YH, Lai YL, Cheung WS, Kuo HK. Oral health status and self-reported functional dependence in community-dwelling older adults. J Am Geriatr Soc 2011;59(3):519–23. https://doi.org/10.1111/j.1532-5415.2010.03311.x

[21] Okamoto N, Morikawa M, Tomioka K, Yanagi M, Amano N, Kurumatani N. Association between tooth loss and the development of mild memory impairment in the elderly: the Fujiwara-kyo Study. J Alzheimers Dis 2015;44(3):777-86.

[22] Ruan Y, Guo YF, Yu M, Liu F, Zhu YL, Sun SY, et al. Association between edentulism and cognition among people aged 50 and over. Zhonghua Liu Xing Bing Xue Za Zhi 2019;40(10):1234-9. [Chinese]. doi: 10.3760/cma.j.issn.0254-6450.2019.10.012.

[23] Ayo-Yusuf OA, Ayo-Yusuf IJ. Association of tooth loss with hypertension. S Afr Med J 2008;98:381–5.

[24] Peres MA, Tsakos G, Barbato PR, Silva DA, Peres KG. Tooth loss is associated with increased blood pressure in adults: A multidisciplinary populationbased study. J Clin Periodontol 2012;39(9):824–33. https://doi.org/10.1111/j. 1600-051X.2012.01916.x.

[25] Medina-Solís CE, Pontigo-Loyola AP, Pérez-Campos E, Hernández-Cruz P, ÁvilaBurgos L, Kowolik MJ, et al. Association between edentulism and angina pectoris in Mexican adults 35 years of age and older: a multivariate analysis of a population-based survey. J Periodontol 2014;85:406–16.

[26] Del Brutto OH, Mera RM, Zambrano M, Del Brutto VJ. Severe edentulism is a major risk factor influencing stroke incidence in rural Ecuador (The Atahualpa Project). Int J Stroke 2017;12(2):201–4. https://doi.org/10.1177/

[27] Fagundes NCF, Couto RSD, Brandão APT, Lima LAO, Bittencourt LO, Souza-Rodrigues RD, et al. Association between tooth loss and stroke: A systematic review. J Stroke Cerebrovasc Dis 2020;29(8):104873. doi: 10.1016/j.jstrokecerebrovasdis.2020.104873.

[28] Emami E, de Souza RF, Kabawat M, Feine JS. The impact of edentulism on oral and general health. Int J Dent 2013;2013:498305. https://doi.org/10. 1155/2013/498305.

In: Social and Health Issues … ISBN: 978-1-53619-937-6
Editors: S Pengpid, K Peltzer et al.

Chapter 17

SELF-REPORTED HEARING LOSS AND INSTRUMENTAL ACTIVITIES OF DAILY LIVING AMONG COMMUNITY-DWELLING OLDER ADULTS IN INDIA: RESULTS OF A NATIONAL SURVEY IN 2017-2018

Karl Peltzer[1,2], MA Clin Psych, PhD, Dr Habil and Supa Pengpid[1,3,*], MPH, DrPH, MBA

[1]Department of Research Administration and Development, University of Limpopo, Turfloop, South Africa

[2]Department of Psychology, College of Medical and Health Science, Asia University, Taichung, Taiwan

[3]ASEAN Institute for Health Development, Mahidol University, Salaya, Phutthamonthon, Nakhon Pathom, Thailand

---

* *Correspondence*: Professor Supa Pengpid, ASEAN Institute for Health Development, Mahidol University, 25/25 Phutthamonthon Road 4, Salaya, Phutthamonton, Nakhon Pathom 73170, Thailand. Email: supaprom@yahoo.com.

Abstract

In this chapter we assess the association between hearing loss and seven Instrumental Activities of Daily Living (IADL) among older adults in India. The cross-sectional sample consisted of 31,477 individuals (≥60 years) from the Longitudinal Ageing Study in India (LASI) Wave 1 in 2017-2018. Results indicate that the prevalence of no hearing loss was 90.1%, hearing loss and no hearing aid 9.5%, and hearing loss plus hearing aid 0.4%. Among those with hearing loss only 4.3% reported using hearing aids. In the adjusted logistic regression analysis, compared to persons with no hearing loss, people with hearing loss and no hearing aid had a higher odds of IADL 1 (preparing hot meals) (Adjusted Odds Ratio-AOR: 1.47, Confidence Interval-CI: 1.11-193), IADL 3 (telephone calls) (AOR: 1.23, CI: 1.01-1.46), IADL 5 (house or garden work) (AOR: 1.56, CI: 1.19-2.03), IADL 6 (managing money) (AOR: 1.59, CI: 1.17-2.14), and IADL 7 (getting around) (AOR: 1.56, CI: 1.17-2.09). Compared to persons with no hearing loss, people with hearing loss and with hearing aid did not significantly differ on all of the seven IADLs. One in ten older adults in India reported hearing loss. We found a positive association between hearing loss without hearing aid and difficulty with five IADLs, and the associations were not significant in those with hearing loss and with hearing aid.

Introduction

"Globally, 5.5% of the population experience moderate or higher levels of hearing loss. The global prevalence of moderate or higher grades of hearing loss increases with age, rising from 12.7% at the age of 60 years to over 58% at 90 years. Notable is that over 58% of moderate or higher grade hearing loss is experienced by adults above the age of 60 years" [1]. In a national study among older adults (≥60 years) in Columbia, the prevalence of self-reported hearing loss was 23.4% [2], and in a local study in Puna, India, the prevalence of self-reported hearing loss was 63.1% among older adult (≥60 years) urban slum and village dwellers [3].

Some studies [2, 4, 5] found that self-reported hearing loss increased difficulty with Instrumental Activities of Daily Living (IADL). Compared to Activities of Daily Living (ADLs), IADLs are "more complex to perform and may be more vulnerable to hearing loss" [2]. There is a lack of national studies investigating self-reported hearing loss and difficulties with IADLs in Southeast Asia, such as in India.

Hearing loss is an "important issue in geriatric medicine because it is associated with numerous health issues, including accelerated cognitive decline, depression, increased risk of dementia, poorer balance, falls, hospitalization, early mortality and social implications, such as reduced communication function, social isolation, and financial decline" [5]. "Health care for persons with hearing loss and people within their communication circles requires education and counselling (e.g., increasing knowledge, changing attitudes, and reducing stigma), behaviour change (e.g., adapting communication strategies), and environmental modifications (e.g., reducing noise)" [6]. This study aimed to assess the association between hearing loss and seven Instrumental Activities of Daily Living (IADL) among older adults in India.

OUR STUDY

This secondary data analysis utilized data from the cross-sectional and nationally representative Longitudinal Ageing Study in India (LASI) Wave 1, 2017-2018; "the overall household response rate is 96%, and the overall individual response rate is 87%" [7]. In a household survey, "interview, physical measurement and biomarker data were collected from individuals aged 45 and above and their spouses, regardless of age" [7]. In this analysis, we restricted our sample to participants 60 years and older. Specific details on the sampling approach are found elsewhere [7]. The study was approved by the "Indian Council of Medical Research (ICMR) Ethics Committee and written informed consent was obtained from the participants" [7].

Table 1. Sample characteristics of older adults (≥60 years) by hearing status in India, 2017-2018

Variable	Sample	No hearing loss	Hearing loss	Hearing loss and hearing aid
	N (%)	%	%	%
Sociodemographic factors				
All	31477	90.1	9.5	0.4
Age in years				
60-69	18979 (58.5)	92.6	7.1	0.3
70-79	9108 (30.2)	87.7	11.9	0.5
80 or more	3390 (11.3)	83.4	15.7	0.9
Sex				
Female	16371 (52.5)	90.2	9.5	0.3
Male	15106 (47.5)	89.9	9.5	0.6
Education				
≥1 years	14583 (43.5)	89.9	9.4	0.7
No schooling	16894 (56.5)	90.2	9.5	0.2
Food insecurity				
No	28355 (89.5)	90.3	9.3	0.4
Yes	2747 (10.5)	88.3	11.1	0.6
Residence				
Rural	20730 (70.5)	90.4	9.2	0.3
Urban	10747 (29.5)	89.3	10.1	0.7
Has health insurance	6573 (18.2)	90.8	8.7	0.5
Health status				
Major depressive disorder	2029 (8.2)	88.8	10.9	0.2
Diabetes	4862 (14.3)	87.1	12.5	0.5
Lung disease	2371 (8.5)	80.6	18.4	1.0
Angina	2805 (9.2)	87.9	11.7	0.4
Stroke	842 (2.7)	87.5	12.2	0.2
Arthritis	5586 (19.7)	85.1	14.3	0.6
Poor distant vision	6479 (21.2)	85.8	13.9	0.3
Poor near vision	6424 (20.7)	86.5	13.0	0.5
Low cognitive functioning	4545 (18.5)	6.3	13.5	0.2

ADL = Activities of Daily Living; IADL = Instrumental Activities of Daily Living.

Measures

Hearing loss was assessed with the question, "Have you ever been diagnosed with any hearing or ear-related problem or condition?" (Yes, No)

[7]. Similar self-report measures have been used previously [2, 4]. In addition, participants were asked if they had been "using a hearing aid to assist them in the activities of daily living" (Yes, No). Respondents were grouped into 1) "those without hearing loss, 2) those with hearing loss and non-use of hearing aid, and 3) those with hearing loss and use of hearing aid" [2].

Independent variables

IADL was assessed with 7 items [8], which are shown in Table 2. Responses were "Yes/No." Cronbach alpha for the IADL measure 0.88.

Table 2. Proportion of difficulty with Instrumental Activities of Daily Living (IADL) by hearing loss (N = 31,477)

Instrumental Activities of Daily Living (IADL) items	Difficulty	No hearing loss	Hearing loss without hearing aid	Hearing loss with hearing aid
		%	%	%
Preparing a hot meal	Yes	83.9	15.5	0.5
	No	91.5	8.1	0.4
Shopping for groceries	Yes	85.5	14.0	0.5
	No	91.5	8.1	0.4
Making telephone calls	Yes	86.8	12.7	0.4
	No	91.4	8.2	0.4
Taking medications	Yes	86.4	13.2	0.5
	No	90.8	8.8	0.4
Doing work around the house or garden	Yes	84.3	15.2	0.5
	No	92.2	7.4	0.4
Managing money	Yes	85.2	14.4	0.4
	No	92.0	7.6	0.4
Getting around	Yes	85.5	14.1	0.4
	No	92.0	7.5	0.4

Confounding variables

We included education (none and ≥1 years), age, sex, residence (rural, urban), and receipt of health insurance. *Food insecurity* was sourced from four items: 1) "In the last 12 months, did you ever reduce the size of your meals or skip meals because there was not enough food at your household? (Yes/No); 2) In the last 12 months, were you hungry but didn't eat because there was not enough food at your household? (Yes/No); 3) In the past 12 months, did you ever not eat for a whole day because there was not enough food at your household?; 4) Do you think that you have lost weight in the last 12 months because there was not enough food in your household?" [7]. Any positive response to the four questions was scored as one.

Health status variables

Chronic conditions were sourced from the question, "Has any health professional ever told you that you have…?": 1) "Diabetes or high blood sugar; 2) Chronic lung disease such as asthma, chronic obstructive pulmonary disease/Chronic bronchitis or other chronic lung problems; 3) Stroke; and 4) Arthritis or rheumatism, Osteoporosis or other bone/joint diseases" (Yes, No) [7].

Angina was assessed with the "World Health Organization's Rose angina questionnaire" [9], defined on the basis of "discomfort at walking uphill or hurrying, or at an ordinary pace on level ground. Furthermore, the pain should be located at the sternum or in the left chest and arm, causing the patient to stop or slow down, and the pain should resolve within 10 minutes when the patient stops or slows down" [10].

Major depressive disorder (MDD) in the past 12 months was assessed with the Health and Retirement Study (HRS) Composite International Diagnostic Interview short form (CIDI-SF) [11], using criteria of the Diagnostic and Statistical Manual of Mental Disorders (DSM; American Psychiatric Association [12]. Study respondents were required to "endorse either anhedonia or depressed mood for most of the day for most of a 2-week period or more," and those who fulfilled this criterion "completed an additional seven symptoms: lost interest, feeling tired, change in weight, trouble with sleep, trouble concentrating, feeling down, and thoughts of death." [19]. "Those with scores ≥3 were considered to meet the criteria for having MDD in the previous 12 months; MDD symptomology scores ranged from 0 to 7" [13].

Vision was assessed with two questions, 1) "How good is your eyesight for seeing things at a distance, like recognizing a person across the street (or 20 meters away), whether or not you wear glasses, contacts, or corrective lenses?", and 2) "How good is your eyesight for seeing things up close, like reading an ordinary newspaper print whether or not you wear glasses, contacts, or corrective lenses?" [7]. Response options ranged from 1 = very good to 5 = very poor and poor near or far vision as defined as "poor or very poor."

Cognitive ability was assessed with tests for word recall (both immediate and delayed), orientation in time and place, and serial 7s [14]. Total scores ranged from 0-32; low cognitive functioning was defined as having 0-11 scores.

Data analysis

Descriptive statistics were applied to describe health status, sociodemographic information, IADL and hearing status. Unadjusted and adjusted logistic regression was utilized to assess the predictors (hearing loss without hearing aid, hearing loss with hearing aid, and no hearing loss as reference category) of each IADL difficulty, separately. Models were adjusted for age, sex, education, food insecurity, residence status, health insurance status, major depressive disorder, diabetes, lung disease, angina, stroke, arthritis, poor vision and low cognitive functioning. These factors were previously established as confounding factors [2, 4]. $P < 0.05$ was accepted as significant, missing values were excluded, and no multi-collinearity was found. Statistical analyses were conducted using STATA software version 15.0 (Stata Corporation, College Station, TX, USA), taking the complex study design into account.

Table 3. Logistic regression between hearing status and difficulties with Instrumental Activities of Daily Living (IADL)

Variable	CrOR (95% CI)	AOR (95% CI)
Preparing a hot meal (IADL 1)		
Hearing status		
1	1 (Reference)	1 (Reference)
2	2.08 (1,71, 2.54)***	1.47 (1.11, 1.93)**
3	1.52 (0.88, 2.62)	1.02 (0.49, 2.12)
Shopping for groceries (IADL 2)		
Hearing status		
1	1 (Reference)	1 (Reference)
2	1.85 (1.53, 2.25)***	1.24 (0.94, 1.62)
3	1.49 (0.88, 2.51)	1.26 (0.58, 2.77)
Making telephone calls (IADL 3)		
Hearing status		
1	1 (Reference)	1 (Reference)
2	1.64 (1.36, 1.98)***	1.23 (1.01, 1.46)*
3	1.13 (0.69, 1.85)	1.33 (0.66, 2.67)
Taking medications (IADL 4)		
Hearing status		
1	1 (Reference)	1 (Reference)
2	1.57 (1.30, 1.90)***	1.07 (0.84, 1.36)
3	1.22 (0.66, 2.24)	1.19 (0.46, 3.06)
Doing work around the house or garden (IADL 5)		
Hearing status		
1	1 (Reference)	1 (Reference)
2	2.24 (1.76, 2.85)***	1.56 (1.19, 2.03)***
3	1.51 (0.02, 2.48)	1.10 (0.55, 2.19)
Managing money (IADL 6)		
Hearing status		
1	1 (Reference)	1 (Reference)
2	2.05 (1.61, 2.60)***	1.59 (1.17, 2.14)**
3	0.99 (0.59, 1.66)	0.79 (0.35, 1.77)
Getting around (IADL 7)		
Hearing status		
1	1 (Reference)	1 (Reference)
2	2.01 (1.60, 2.53)***	1.56 (1.17, 2.09)**
3	1.10 (0.66, 1.82)	1.45 (0.72, 2.96)

1 = No hearing loss; 2 = Hearing loss with no hearing aid; 3 = Hearing loss with hearing aid;
CrOR = Crude Odds Ratio; CI = Confidence Interval; AOR = Adjusted Odd Ratio;
***p < 0.001; **p < 0.01; *p < 0.05.

Discussion

In this nationally representative sample of older adults (≥60 years) in India in 2017-2018, the prevalence of self-reported hearing loss (9.9%) was lower than in national studies among older adults ≥60 years in Columbia (21.3%) [2], and among older adults (≥60 years) in an urban slum area and a village in Puna, India (63.1%) [3]. Among those participants with hearing loss only 4.3% reported the use of hearing aids, which is lower than in the Columbia study (8.1%) [2].

Furthermore, the study found an independent association between hearing loss and difficulties in IADLs, such as preparing hot meals, making telephone calls, doing house or garden work, managing money, and getting around. These results are consistent with previous research [2, 4, 5]. In addition, compared to persons with no hearing loss, people with a hearing loss and with hearing aid did not significantly differ on all of the seven IADLs, which was also found in the study among older adults in Columbia [2]. Although age-related hearing loss can currently not be cured [6], we have shown that the use of hearing aids may reduce the negative impact on IADLs.

Possible reasons for the relationship between hearing loss and difficulties with IADLs may include that communication problems because of hearing loss may reduce participation in various activities, which in turn may further reduce IADLs, and hearing loss may make moving more difficult due to a disturbed perception of the environment [4]. It is also possible that hearing loss leads to a decline in cognitive functioning, which may, in turn reduce the capability of performing IADLs [4, 15].

Study limitations

The study was limited by its cross-sectional design and the self-report of most data collected. Self-report may lead to biased responses and possibly underreporting of assessed conditions. Since this study only included community-dwelling older adults, persons under institutional care were excluded, the prevalence of hearing loss and functional disability may have been underestimated.

CONCLUSION

One in ten older adults in India reported hearing loss. We found a positive association between hearing loss without hearing aid and difficulties with five IADLs, and the associations were not significant in persons with hearing loss and with hearing aid, supporting the importance of treating hearing loss among older adults in India.

ACKNOWLEDGMENTS

The Longitudinal Aging Study in India Project is funded by the Ministry of Health and Family Welfare, Government of India, the National Institute on Aging (R01 AG042778, R01 AG030153), and United Nations Population Fund, India.

REFERENCES

[1] World Health Organization. World report on hearing. Geneva: World Health Organization, 2021.

[2] Borda MG, Reyes-Ortiz CA, Heredia RA, Castellanos-Perilla N, Ayala Copete AM, Soennesyn H, et al. Association between self-reported hearing impairment, use of a hearing aid and performance of instrumental activities of daily living. Arch Gerontol Geriatr 2019;83:101-105. doi: 10.1016/j.archger.2019.04.001.

[3] Thakur R, Banerjee A, Nikumb V. Health problems among the elderly: a cross-sectional study. Ann Med Health Sci Res 2013;3(1):19-25. doi: 10.4103/2141-9248.109466.

[4] Mikkola TM, Polku H, Portegijs E, Rantakokko M, Rantanen T, Viljanen A. self-reported hearing status is associated with lower limb physical performance, perceived mobility, and activities of daily living in older community-dwelling men and women. J Am Geriatr Soc 2015;63(6):1164-9. doi: 10.1111/jgs.13381.

[5] Yamada M, Nishiwaki Y, Michikawa T, Takebayashi T. Self-reported hearing loss in older adults is associated with future decline in instrumental activities of daily living but not in social participation. J Am Geriatr Soc 2012;60(7):1304-9. doi: 10.1111/j.1532-5415.2012.04039.x.

[6] Davis A, McMahon CM, Pichora-Fuller KM, Russ S, Lin F, Olusanya BO, et al. Aging and hearing health: The life-course approach. Gerontologist 2016;56(Suppl 2):S256-67. doi: 10.1093/geront/gnw033.

[7] International Institute for Population Sciences (IIPS), NPHCE, MoHFW, Harvard TH Chan School of Public Health (HSPH) and the University of Southern California (USC). Longitudinal Ageing Study in India (LASI) Wave 1, 2017-18, India Report. Mumbai: International Institute for Population Sciences, 2020.

[8] Lawton MP, Brody EM. Assessment of older people: self-maintaining and instrumental activities of daily living. Gerontologist 1969;9(3):179-86.

[9] Rose GA. The diagnosis of ischaemic heart pain and intermittent claudication in field surveys. Bull World Health Organ 1962;27:645–58.

[10] Achterberg S, Soedamah-Muthu SS, Cramer MJ, Kappelle LJ, van der Graaf Y, Algra A, et al. Prognostic value of the Rose questionnaire: a validation with future coronary events in the SMART study. Eur J Prev Cardiol 2012;19(1):5-14. doi: 10.1177/1741826710391117.

[11] Kessler RC, Andrews A, Mroczek D, Ustun B, Wittchen HU. The World Health Organization Composite International Diagnostic Interview Short-Form (CIDI-SF). Int J Methods Psychiatr Res 1998;7:171–85.

[12] American Psychiatric Association. Diagnostic and statistical manual of mental disorders (DSM-5), 5th ed. Washington, DC: American Psychiatric Publishing, 2013.

[13] Steffick D. Documentation of affective functioning measures in the Health and Retirement Study, 2000. URL: http://hrsonline. isr.umich.edu/sitedocs/userg/dr-005.pdf

[14] Lee J, Smith JP. Regional disparities in adult height, educational attainment and gender difference in late- life cognition: Findings from the Longitudinal Aging Study in India (LASI). J Econ Ageing 2014;4:26-34. doi: 10.1016/j.jeoa.2014.02.002.

[15] Buchman AS, Boyle PA, Leurgans SE, Barnes LL, Bennett DA. Cognitive function is associated with the development of mobility impairments in community-dwelling elders. Am J Geriatr Psychiatry 2011;19(6):571-80. doi: 10.1097/JGP.0b013e3181ef7a2e.

In: Social and Health Issues … ISBN: 978-1-53619-937-6
Editors: S Pengpid, K Peltzer et al.

Chapter 18

PREVALENCE AND DETERMINANTS OF SMOKING TOBACCO AND SMOKELESS TOBACCO USE AMONG A NATIONALLY REPRESENTATIVE POPULATION-BASED SAMPLE OF OLDER ADULTS IN INDIA

Supa Pengpid[1,2], MPH, DrPH, MBA
and Karl Peltzer[2,3,*], MA Clin Psych, PhD, Dr Habil
[1]ASEAN Institute for Health Development, Mahidol University, Salaya, Phutthamonthon, Nakhon Pathom, Thailand
[2]Department of Research Administration and Development, University of Limpopo, Turfloop, South Africa
[3]Department of Psychology, College of Medical and Health Science, Asia University, Taichung, Taiwan

* *Correspondence*: Professor Karl Peltzer, Department of Research Administration and Development, University of Limpopo, Turfloop Campus, Private Bag X1106, Sovenga 0727, South Africa. Email: kfpeltzer@gmail.com.

Abstract

This chapter aimed to determine the prevalence and correlates of smoking tobacco and smokeless tobacco use in older adults in India. The cross-sectional sample consisted of 52,393 individuals (≥50 years) from the Longitudinal Ageing Study in India (LASI) Wave 1 in 2017-2018. Results indicate that the prevalence of current tobacco use was 33.0%, 13.7% current smoking tobacco, and 21.0% current smokeless tobacco use. In adjusted logistic regression analysis, male sex, exposure to stressful life events, underweight, vigorous physical activity, lifetime alcohol use and major depressive disorder were positively associated with current tobacco use, while older age (≥80 years), married, higher subjective socioeconomic status, urban residence, spirituality or religiosity, overweight/obesity, hypertension, diabetes, and lung disease were negatively associated with current tobacco use. While current smoking tobacco decreased with age, current smokeless tobacco use did not significantly decrease with age. Having multiple types of discrimination experiences increased the odds of current smoking tobacco but decreased the odds of current smokeless tobacco use. Higher social support (spirituality/religiosity and social engagement) decreased the odds of current smokeless tobacco use. Low or fair self-rated health status was positively associated with current smoking tobacco. One thirds of older adults in India reported current tobacco use. Several risk factors were identified, which can be targeted in public health interventions.

Introduction

"Tobacco kills more than 8 million people each year; 80% of the world's 1.1 billion smokers live in low- and middle-income countries" [1]. "Smoking is known to cause various illnesses, including cancer, heart disease, stroke, lung diseases, diabetes, and chronic obstructive pulmonary disease (COPD)" [2]. Older adults seem to continue tobacco use to a high extent and may be more unaware of its harmful effects [3-5]. In a systematic review on tobacco use among the elderly, the "overall prevalence of tobacco use was 13% in both genders (22% male and 8% female" [3]. In a study among older adults (≥50 years) in six low- and middle-income countries, the prevalence of current tobacco use ranged from 10.2% in Ghana to 49.4% in India in 2007 [6]. In a study among older adults (≥60 years) in seven states in India in

2011, the prevalence of current tobacco use was 27.8%, with 9.2% smoking tobacco only and 16.9% smokeless tobacco use only [7]. Using data from the Adult Tobacco Survey in India in 2009-2010 and 2016-2017 found among older adults (≥60 years) a prevalence of current tobacco use of 49.0% in 2009-2010 and 41.5% in 2016-2017 [8]. There is a lack of recent national data on the prevalence and health correlates on smoking tobacco and smokeless tobacco use among older adults in India.

As previously reviewed [5], factors associated with "current tobacco use among older adults include age, male sex, lower socioeconomic status, residence status, poor self-rated health, chronic diseases such as chronic obstructive pulmonary disease, mental health difficulties, insufficient fruits and vegetable consumption." In addition, various studies found an association between exposure to stressful events, such as discrimination [9], traumatic stress [10], lack of social support [11], low religiosity [12, 13], lower social engagement [4] and tobacco use. In studies among older adults in India, male sex, younger age, rural residence, lower socioeconomic status, and alcohol users were associated with current tobacco use [7, 8]. This study aimed to determine the prevalence and social and health correlates of smoking tobacco and smokeless tobacco use in a national community-dwelling sample in India in 2017-2018.

OUR STUDY

This secondary data analysis utilized data from the cross-sectional and nationally representative Longitudinal Ageing Study in India (LASI) Wave 1, 2017-2018; "the overall household response rate is 96%, and the overall individual response rate is 87%" [14]. In a household survey, "interview, physical measurement and biomarker data were collected from individuals aged 45 and above and their spouses, regardless of age" [14]. We restricted our analysis to those 50 years and older. Specific details on the sampling approach are found elsewhere [14]. The study was approved by the "Indian Council of Medical Research (ICMR) Ethics Committee and written informed consent was obtained from the participants" [14].

Measures

Current tobacco use was assessed from 1) "Do you currently smoke any tobacco products (cigarettes, bidis, cigars, hookah, cheroot, etc.)? and 2) Do you use smokeless tobacco (such as chewing tobacco, gutka, pan masala, etc.)?" (Yes, No) [14].

Sociodemographic variables consisted of age group (50-59, 60-69, 70-79, and 80 or more years), sex (male, female), residential status (urban, rural), and marital status (currently married vs. widowed/divorced/separated/deserted/live-in relationship/never married). Subjective socioeconomic status was assessed with the question, "Please imagine a ten-step ladder, where at the bottom are the people who are the worst off – who have the least money, least education, and the worst jobs or no jobs, and at the top of the ladder are the people who are the best off – those who have the most money, most education, and best jobs. Please indicate the number [1-10] on the rung on the ladder where you would place yourself." [14]. Steps 1 to 3 on the socioeconomic ladder were defined as low, 4-5 as medium, and 6-10 as high socioeconomic status.

Stressors included stressful events and discrimination experiences.

Life event stressors assessed included 1) ill-treatment ("Have you felt that you were ill-treated in the past year?" Yes/No), 2) victim of violent crime ("In the last 12 months, have you been the victim of a violent crime, such as assault/mugging/ threat to life/others?" (Yes/No), 3) disaster exposure causing health effects ("In the last five years, has your health been severely affected by disasters such as floods, landslides, extreme cold and hot weather, cyclone/typhoons, droughts, earthquakes, tsunamis, or any other natural calamities?" (Yes/No), and 4) man-made incident causing health effects ("In the last five years, has your health been severely affected by man-made incidents such as riots, terrorism, building collapses, fires, traffic accidents or any other man-made incidents?" (Yes/No) [14]. Any affirmative response was coded with 1 and none=0.

Discrimination experiences were assessed with the six-item Everyday Discrimination Scale (EDS) (Short version) [15]. Response options ranged from 1="never" to 6="almost every day," and were dichotomised to 'never'=0 and 'ever' (collapsing those reporting 'less than once a year' or greater into one category)=1). Total responses were trichotomized into 0, 1-2, and 3-6 discrimination experiences. Cronbach's alpha for the EDS in this study was 0.86.

Social support included spirituality/religiosity, non-organisational religiosity and social network.

Spirituality/religiosity was measured with four items from the Daily Spiritual Experience Scale (DSES) [16], 1) "Do you think that you have a feeling of deep inner peace?" 2) "Do you think that you are spiritually touched by the beauty of creation?" 3) "Do you think that you are thankful for whatever you received in your life?" and 4) "Do you think that you are selflessly caring for others?" Responses ranged from 1=never to 5=every day in a week, and the summed scores were trichotomized to 4-7=low, 8-11=medium, and 12-20=high. Cronbach's alpha for the DSES in this study was 0.86.

Social engagement was measured with 11 items, e.g., "Eat-out-of-house (restaurant/hotel)" [14]. Responses were coded 1= daily to at least once a month and 0=rarely/once a year or never (Cronbach's alpha 0.67). Responses were trichotomized into 0=low, 1=medium, and 2-8=high social engagement.

Health factor variables included self-rated health status, life satisfaction, body mass index, physical activity, alcohol use, hypertension, diabetes, angina, arthritis or rheumatism, any bone or joint diseases, lung disease and major depressive disorder.

Self-rated health status was sourced from the question, "In general, would you say your health is excellent, very good, good, fair, or poor?" Responses were coded as "1=poor, 2=fair, 3=good, 4=very good and 5=excellent" [14].

Life satisfaction was assessed with the item, "Please, think about your life as a whole. How satisfied are you with it? Are you completely satisfied, very satisfied, somewhat satisfied, not very satisfied, or not at all satisfied?" [14]. Responses were grouped into 1 (low)=not very satisfied or not at all satisfied, and 0=somewhat satisfied or very satisfied or completely satisfied.

Anthropometry: "Height and weight of adults were measured using the Seca 803 digital scale." [14]. "Body Mass Index=BMI was calculated according to Asian criteria: underweight (<18.5 kg/m^2), normal weight (18.5-22.9 kg/m^2), overweight (23.0-24.9 kg/m^2), class I obesity (25.0-29.9 kg/m^2), and class II obesity (≥30.0 kg/m^2)" [17].

Vigorous physical activity. " For vigorous activity, respondents were asked about their involvement in running or jogging, swimming, going to a health centre/gym, cycling, digging with a spade or shovel, heavy lifting, chopping, farm work, fast bicycling, and cycling with load." [14]. Responses were trichotomized into 1=hardly ever/never, 2=less than twice a week, and 3=more than once a week [18].

Lifetime alcohol use was assessed with the question, "Have you ever consumed any alcoholic beverages such as beer, wine, liquor, country liquor, etc?" (Yes, No) [14].

Hypertension or raised blood pressure (BP) was defined as "systolic BP ≥140 mm Hg and/or diastolic BP ≥90 mm Hg (based on the last two averaged of three readings) or where the participant is currently on antihypertensive medication" [19].

Any bone or joint diseases, diabetes, and chronic lung disease were assessed by self-reported health care provider diagnosis [14].

Angina was assessed with the "World Health Organization's Rose angina questionnaire" [20], defined based on "discomfort at walking uphill or hurrying, or at an ordinary pace on level ground. Furthermore, the pain should be located at the sternum or in the left chest and arm, causing the patient to stop or slow down, and the pain should resolve within 10 minutes when the patient stops or slows down" [21].

Major depressive disorder in the past 12 months was assessed with the Health and Retirement Study (HRS) Composite International Diagnostic Interview short form (CIDI-SF) [22], using criteria of the Diagnostic and Statistical Manual of Mental Disorders (DSM) [23]. Study respondents were required to "endorse either anhedonia or depressed mood for most of the day for most of a 2-week period or more," and those who fulfilled this criterion "completed an additional seven symptoms: lost interest, feeling tired, change in weight, trouble with sleep, trouble concentrating, feeling down, and thoughts of death" [24]. "Those with a score ≥3 were considered to meet the criteria for having MDD in the previous 12 months; MDD symptomology scores ranged from 0 to 7" [24].

Data analysis

Descriptive statistics were applied to describe health status, sociodemographic information, and tobacco use. Adjusted logistic regression was utilized to assess the predictors of current tobacco, use, current smoking tobacco, and current smokeless tobacco use. $P < 0.05$ was accepted as significant, missing values were excluded, and no multi-collinearity was found. Statistical analyses were conducted using STATA software version 15.0 (Stata Corporation, College Station, TX, USA), taking the complex study design into account.

FINDINGS

The sample included 52,393 older adults (50 years and older), with a median age of 62 years (14 years interquartile range), 53.3% were female and 46.7% male. Majority (70.1%) of participants were married, 69.0% were residing in rural areas, and 38.2% had low subjective socioeconomic status. Almost one in ten participants (9.1%) had experienced stressful life events and 17.3% had discrimination experiences. In terms of social support, 35.0% of the older adults had high spirituality or religiosity, and 29.6% had high social engagement.

Almost half (43.3%) rated their health status as fair or poor, 12.0% had low life satisfaction. 45.4% had hypertension, 8.9% angina, 13.4% had diabetes, 17.6% arthritis, 7.5% lung disease, 39.8% overweight/obesity, 14.9% had ever engaged in alcohol use, and 37.7% engaged in vigorous physical activity. The prevalence of current tobacco use was 33.0%, 13.7% current smoking tobacco, and 21.0% current smokeless tobacco use (see Table 1).

Table 1. Sample and tobacco use characteristics among older adults in India, 2017-2018

Variable	Sample	Current tobacco use	Current smoking tobacco	Current smokeless tobacco use
	N (%)	%	%	%
Sociodemographic factors				
All	52393	33.0	13.7	21.0
Age in years				
50-59	20916 (38.1)	31.8	13.5	20.3
60-69	18979 (36.2)	34.4	14.3	21.8
70-79	9108 (18.7)	33.5	13.9	21.1
≥80	3390 (7.0)	30.8	11.0	20.9
Sex				
Female	27815 (53.3)	18.0	3.0	15.2
Male	24578 (46.7)	50.2	26.0	27.7
Marital status				
Not married	15151 (29.9)	27.3	8.4	19.8
Married	37236 (70.1)	35.4	15.9	21.6
Subjective socioeconomic status				
Low	17462 (38.2)	39.6	16.2	25.8
Medium	20070 (37.4)	32.0	13.3	20.3
High	13176 (24.4)	24.8	10.5	15.3
Residence				
Rural	34099 (69.0)	38.4	16.0	24.5
Urban	18294 (31.0)	20.8	8.4	13.2
Stressors				
Stressful events	3986 (9.1)	39.3	16.5	25.4
Discrimination experiences				
Low (0)	43281 (82.7)	33.0	13.5	21.3
Medium (1-2)	4483 (10.7)	34.2	14.0	22.2
High (3-6)	3151 (6.6)	34.2	17.1	19.0
Social support				
Spirituality/Religiosity				
Low	14474 (31.7)	36.4	14.8	23.4
Moderate	16896 (33.3)	33.2	14.3	20.9
High	19520 (35.0)	30.1	12.2	19.4
Social engagement				
Low	19995 (41.3)	34.3	14.0	22.2
Moderate	15547 (29.1)	33.4	13.3	21.7
High	16100 (29.6)	31.1	13.8	18.8

Variable	Sample	Current tobacco use	Current smoking tobacco	Current smokeless tobacco use
	N (%)	%	%	%
Health factors				
Self-rated health status (low/fair)	21248 (43.3)	34.3	14.3	21.9
Life satisfaction (low)	5309 (12.0)	37.1	16.2	23.2
Body mass index				
Normal	17179 (37.2)	37.4	15.5	23.8
Underweight	9428 (23.0)	47.2	22.3	28.0
Overweight/Obesity	20039 (39.8)	22.4	7.7	15.6
Vigorous physical activity				
Never	32762 (62.3)	27.4	10.9	17.5
Once/week	4262 (8.8)	37.7	16.7	23.4
>once/week	14930 (28.9)	43.6	18.7	27.9
Ever alcohol use	9346 (14.9)	67.3	34.6	38.6
Hypertension	22826 (45.4)	29.1	11.1	19.2
Diabetes	7423 (13.4)	21.0	8.0	14.1
Angina	4510 (8.9)	33.7	13.5	22.0
Any bone or joint diseases	8329 (17.6)	29.1	11.1	19.4
Chronic lung disease	3297 (7.5)	32.0	15.2	18.4
Major depressive disorder	3263 (8.0)	34.8	13.4	23.3

Associations with tobacco use categories

In adjusted logistic regression analysis, male sex, stressful life events, underweight, vigorous physical activity, lifetime alcohol use and major depressive disorder were positively associated with current tobacco use, while older age (≥80 years), married, higher subjective socioeconomic status, urban residence, spirituality or religiosity, overweight/obesity, hypertension, diabetes, and lung disease were negatively associated with current tobacco use. While current smoking tobacco decreased with age, current smokeless tobacco use did not significantly decrease with age. Having multiple types of discrimination experiences increased odds of current smoking tobacco but decreased odds of current smokeless tobacco use. Higher social support (spirituality/religiosity and social engagement) decreased the odds of current smokeless tobacco use. Low or fair self-rated health status was positively associated with current smoking tobacco (see Table 2).

Table 2. Associations with current tobacco use categories

Variable	Current tobacco use	Current smoking tobacco	Current smokeless tobacco use
	AOR (95% CI)	AOR (95% CI)	AOR (95% CI)
Sociodemographic factors			
Age in years			
50-59	1 (Reference)	1 (Reference)	1 (Reference)
60-69	0.98 (0.90, 1.06)	0.92 (0.83, 1.02)	1.01 (0.92, 1.10)
70-79	0.90 (0.81, 1.00)	0.80 (0.70, 0.92)**	1.00 (0.89, 1.12)
≥80	0.78 (0.65, 0.93)**	0.59 (0.47, 0.75)***	1.00 (0.84, 1.20)
Sex			
Female	1 (Reference)	1 (Reference)	1 (Reference)
Male	4.43 (4.05, 4.84)***	10.59 (9.37, 11.96)***	1.89 (1.72, 2.07)***
Marital status			
Not married	1 (Reference)	1 (Reference)	1 (Reference)
Married	0.85 (0.78, 0.93)***	0.99 (0.87, 1.12)	0.83 (0.77, 0.92)***
Subjective socioeconomic status	1 (Reference)	1 (Reference)	1 (Reference)
Low	0.79 (0.73, 0.86)***	0.87 (0.78, 0.97)*	0.82 (0.75, 0.89)***
Medium	0.65 (0.59, 0.72)***	0.80 (0.70, 0.91)***	0.67 (0.60, 0.74)***
High			
Residence			
Rural	1 (Reference)	1 (Reference)	1 (Reference)
Urban	0.61 (0.56, 0.68)***	0.73 (0.64, 0.83)***	0.64 (0.57, 0.70)***
Stressors			
Stressful events	1.20 (1.06, 1.36)**	1.08 (0.93, 1.25)	1.21 (1.08, 1.37)**
Discrimination experiences	1 (Reference)	1 (Reference)	1 (Reference)
Low (0)	0.94 (0.82, 1.08)	0.95 (0.82, 1.11)	0.95 (0.84, 1.09)
Medium (1-2)	0.89 (0.78, 1.01)	1.18 (1.00, 1.39)*	0.76 (0.66, 0.87)***
High (3-6)			
Social support			
Spirituality/Religiosity			
Low	1 (Reference)	1 (Reference)	1 (Reference)
Moderate	0.90 (0.82, 0.98)*	0.98 (0.88, 1.10)	0.90 (0.82, 0.99)*
High	0.83 (0.75, 0.91)***	0.89 (0.80, 1.00)	0.88 (0.79, 0.97)**
Social engagement			
Low	1 (Reference)	1 (Reference)	1 (Reference)
Moderate	0.97 (0.89, 1.05)	0.95 (0.85, 1.06)	0.99 (0.91, 1.08)
High	0.92 (0.84, 1.02)	1.00 (0.89, 1.14)	0.90 (0.81, 1.00)*

Variable	**Current tobacco use**	**Current smoking tobacco**	**Current smokeless tobacco use**
	AOR (95% CI)	**AOR (95% CI)**	**AOR (95% CI)**
Health factors			
Self-rated health status (low/fair)	1.08 (1.00, 1.17)	1.12 (1.01, 1.23)*	1.02 (0.94, 1.11)
Life satisfaction (low)	1.01 (0.90, 1.14)	1.13 (0.98, 1.31)	0.95 (0.85, 1.07)
Body mass index			
Normal	1 (Reference)	1 (Reference)	1 (Reference)
Underweight	1.41 (1.28, 1.54)***	1.56 (1.40, 1.74)***	1.11 (1.01, 1.22)*
Overweight/Obesity	0.68 (0.63, 0.75)***	0.66 (0.59, 0.75)***	0.77 (0.71, 0.85)***
Vigorous physical activity			
Never	1 (Reference)	1 (Reference)	1 (Reference)
Once/week	1.20 (1.06, 1.36)**	1.10 (0.94, 1.28)	1.20 (1.05, 1.37)**
>once/week	1.30 (1.19, 1.42)***	1.04 (0.93, 1.15)	1.37 (1.26, 1.50)***
Ever alcohol use	2.98 (2.71, 3.29)***	2.02 (1.82, 2.23)***	2.02 (1.84, 2.22)***
Hypertension	0.92 (0.85, 0.99)*	0.88 (0.80, 0.97)*	0.97 (0.89, 1.05)
Diabetes	0.73 (0.65, 0.83)***	0.77 (0.65, 0.91)**	0.81 (0.71, 0.93)**
Angina	1.09 (0.96, 1.23)	1.08 (0.97, 1.27)	1.07 (0.94, 1.22)
Any bone or joint diseases	1.04 (0.94, 1.15)	0.97 (0.85, 1.10)	1.06 (0.95, 1.17)
Chronic lung disease	0.83 (0.72, 0.96)*	1.00 (0.84, 1.19)	0.77 (0.66, 0.89)***
Major depressive disorder	1.15 (1.02, 1.32)*	1.02 (0.86, 1.20)	1.17 (1.03, 1.34)*

AOR=Adjusted Odds Ratio; CI=Confidence Interval; ***$p<0.001$; ** $p<0.01$; *$p<0.05$.

DISCUSSION

In this national 2017-2018 India LASI survey among community-dwelling older adults (≥50 years), the prevalence of current tobacco use was 33.0%, 13.7% current smoking tobacco, and 21.0% current smokeless tobacco use, which seems higher than in the 2007 India national survey of older adults (≥50 years) (49.4% current tobacco use) [6] and in the 2011 seven states study in India among older adults (≥60 years) (27.8% current tobacco use) [7], but lower than in the Adult Tobacco Survey India 2009-2010 and 2016-2017 for older adults (≥60 years) (49.0% in 2009-2010 and 41.5% in 2016-2017 [8]. The found prevalence of current tobacco use (33.0%) among older adults in India is much lower than data from a systematic review on tobacco use among the elderly (13%) [3]. It appears that in several types of surveys in India a reduction of tobacco use has occurred, which may be attributed to tobacco control measures at national and subnational levels in India [25].

In line with other studies, especially in middle-income countries [6-8, 26-28], men were significantly more likely to engage in current tobacco use, in particular in current smoking and to a lessor extent in smokeless tobacco use than women, reflecting social and cultural norms [5]. Current smoking tobacco significantly decreased from 60-69 year-olds to 70-79 year-olds and 80 years and above, while current smokeless tobacco use did not significantly decrease with age. It is possible that those 70 years and older more frequently quit smoking than smokeless tobacco use due to increased awareness of the dangers to health of smoking [27]. More efforts should directed to quit smokeless tobacco use too in India.

Consistent with previous research [7, 8, 27, 29], this study showed an association between lower socioeconomic status and current tobacco use, smoking and smokeless tobacco use. While some previous research [6], found a higher prevalence of current tobacco use in urban than in rural areas, this study showed the reverse, which is consistent with previous research among older adults in India [7, 8] and in Ghana [27] and in Indonesia [5].

Consistent with some previous research [9, 10], this study found a positive association between exposure to stressful events and current tobacco use, and between exposure to discrimination experiences and current smoking tobacco. However, a negative association was found between discrimination experiences and current smokeless tobacco use. In this line, major depressive disorder was significantly positively associated with tobacco use in this study, which is similar to results from a study among older adults in Indonesia [5] and Ireland [30].

In agreement with some previous research findings [11-13, 26, 31], this study showed that higher social support (spirituality/religiosity and social engagement) were found protective against tobacco use. This could mean that increasing social support and social engagement in older adults may be a way of reducing tobacco use [31]. Lifetime alcohol use was in this study highly significantly associated with current tobacco use, which confirms previous research findings [7, 8, 32, 33].

Poorer self-rated health status was only associated with current tobacco smoking in this study, and no association between low life satisfaction and any of the tobacco use categories was found, unlike in a study among older adults in Ghana that found lower life satisfaction to be associated with tobacco use [27]. Overweight/Obesity was negatively associated with tobacco use among older adults in India, as previously found in Indonesia [5], China [34] and South Africa [28] and may be related to the appetite suppressing effects of nicotine [35]. On the other hand, underweight was positively associated with tobacco use, which is consistent with previous research in China [34] and may be related to increased food insecurity [36].

Like in some previous studies [5] among older adults, certain chronic conditions (hypertension, diabetes and lung disease) were in this study negatively associated with current tobacco use. It is possible that due to having been diagnosed with certain conditions tobacco users quit tobacco use [5, 29]. Tobacco use may exacerbate existing chronic conditions in the increasingly ageing older population in India, calling for a critical need for tobacco cessation programming [27].

Study limitations include the cross-sectional design, the assessment of some variables, including tobacco use, by self-report, and that certain relevant variables, such as assessing knowledge on tobacco health, were not assessed.

CONCLUSION

One in three older adults reported current tobacco use in India, and several associated factors were identified, such as younger age, male sex, not married, rural residence, low subjective socioeconomic status, stressful life events, low spirituality/religiosity, underweight, vigorous physical activity, lifetime alcohol use and major depressive disorder that could assist in programmes promoting the prevention and control of tobacco use in this population.

ACKNOWLEDGMENTS

The Longitudinal Aging Study in India Project is funded by the Ministry of Health and Family Welfare, Government of India, the National Institute on Aging (R01 AG042778, R01 AG030153), and United Nations Population Fund, India.

REFERENCES

[1] World Health Organization. Tobacco factsheet, 2020. URL: https://www.who.int/news-room/fact-sheets/detail/tobacco.

[2] Centers for Disease Control and Prevention (CDC). Smoking and tobacco use: Health effects, 2018. URL: https://www.cdc.gov/tobacco/basic_information/health_effects/index.htm.

[3] Marinho V, Laks J, Coutinho ES, Blay SL. Tobacco use among the elderly: a systematic review and meta-analysis. Cad Saude Publica 2010;26(12):2213-33.

[4] Bratzler DW, Oehlert WH, Austelle A. Smoking in the elderly: It's never too late to quit. J Okla State Med Assoc 2002;95:185-91.

[5] Pengpid S, Peltzer K. Prevalence and predictors of current and former tobacco use among older adults in Indonesia. Asian Pac J Cancer Prev 2019;20(2):395-401.

[6] He W, Muenchrath M, Kowal P. Shades of gray: A cross-country study of health and well-being of the older populations in SAGE countries, 2007-2010. Washington, DC: US Census Bureau, 2012.

[7] Mini GK, Sarma PS, Thankappan KR. Pattern of tobacco use and its correlates among older adults in India. Asian Pac J Cancer Prev 2014;15:6195-8.

[8] Mbulo L, Murty KS, Zhao L, Smith T, Palipudi K. Tobacco use and secondhand smoke exposure among older adults in India. J Aging Health 2021:8982643211000489. doi: 10.1177/08982643211000489.

[9] Vu M, Li J, Haardörfer R, Windle M, Berg CJ. Mental health and substance use among women and men at the intersections of identities and experiences of discrimination: insights from the intersectionality framework. BMC Public Health 2019;19(1):108. doi: 10.1186/s12889-019-6430-0.

[10] Pericot-Valverde I, Elliott RJ, Miller ME, Tidey JW, Gaalema DE. Posttraumatic stress disorder and tobacco use: A systematic review and meta-analysis. Addict Behav 2018;84:238-247. doi: 10.1016/j.addbeh.2018.04.024.

[11] Boateng-Poku A, Benca-Bachman CE, Najera DD, Whitfield KE, Taylor JL, Thorpe RJ Jr, et al. The role of social support on the effects of stress and depression on African

American tobacco and alcohol use. Drug Alcohol Depend 2020;209:107926. doi: 10.1016/j.drugalcdep.2020.107926.

[12] Abdel-Hady D, El-Gilany AH. Tobacco use and its associated factors among older people: a community-based study in Egypt. East Mediterr Health J 2020;26(1):68-74. doi: 10.26719/2020.26.1.68.

[13] Martinez EZ, Giglio FM, Terada NAY, da Silva AS, Zucoloto ML. Smoking prevalence among users of primary healthcare units in Brazil: The role of religiosity. J Relig Health 2017;56(6):2180-93. doi: 10.1007/s10943-017-0389-x.

[14] International Institute for Population Sciences (IIPS), NPHCE, MoHFW, Harvard TH Chan School of Public Health (HSPH) and the University of Southern California (USC). Longitudinal Ageing Study in India (LASI) Wave 1, 2017-18, India Report. Mumbai: International Institute for Population Sciences, 2020.

[15] Sternthal MJ, Slopen N, Williams DR. Racial disparities in health: How much does stress really matter? Du Bois Rev 2011;8(1):95-113. doi: 10.1017/S1742058 X11000087.

[16] Underwood LG, Teresi JA. The daily spiritual experience scale: development, theoretical description, reliability, exploratory factor analysis, and preliminary construct validity using health-related data. Ann Behav Med 2002;24(1):22-33. doi: 10.1207/S15324796ABM2401_04.

[17] Wen CP, David Cheng TY, Tsai SP, Chan HT, Hsu HL, Hsu CC, et al. Are Asians at greater mortality risks for being overweight than Caucasians? Redefining obesity for Asians. Public Health Nutr 2009;12(4):497-506. doi: 10.1017/S1368980008002802.

[18] Lübs L, Peplies J, Drell C, Bammann K. Cross-sectional and longitudinal factors influencing physical activity of 65 to 75-year-olds: a pan European cohort study based on the survey of health, ageing and retirement in Europe (SHARE). BMC Geriatr 2018;18(1):94. doi: 10.1186/s12877-018-0781-8.

[19] Chobanian AV, Bakris GL, Black HR, Cushman WC, Green LA, Izzo Jr JL, et al. The seventh report of the joint national committee on prevention, detection, evaluation, and treatment of high blood pressure: the JNC 7 report. JAMA 2003;289(19):2560–71.

[20] Rose GA. The diagnosis of ischaemic heart pain and intermittent claudication in field surveys. Bull World Health Organ 1962;27:645–58.

[21] Achterberg S, Soedamah-Muthu SS, Cramer MJ, Kappelle LJ, van der Graaf Y, Algra A, et al. Prognostic value of the Rose questionnaire: a validation with future coronary events in the SMART study. Eur J Prev Cardiol 2012;19(1):5-14. doi: 10.1177/1741826710391117.

[22] Kessler RC, Andrews A, Mroczek D, Ustun B, Wittchen HU. The World Health Organization Composite International Diagnostic Interview Short-Form (CIDI-SF). Int J Methods Psychiatr Res 1998;7:171–85.

[23] American Psychiatric Association. Diagnostic and statistical manual of mental disorders (DSM-5), 5th ed. Washington, DC: American Psychiatric Publishing, 2013.

[24] Steffick D. Documentation of affective functioning measures in the Health and Retirement Study, 2000. URL: http://hrsonline. isr.umich.edu/sitedocs/userg/dr-005.pdf.

[25] Yadav A, Singh PK, Yadav N, Kaushik R, Chandan K, Chandra A, et al. Smokeless tobacco control in India: Policy review and lessons for high-burden countries. BMJ Glob Health 2020;5(7):e002367. doi: 10.1136/bmjgh-2020-002367.

[26] Peltzer K, Pengpid S. Prevalence and correlates of past and current tobacco use among a nationally representative sample of older adults in Mexico. Int J Disabil Hum Dev 2020;19(3) 543-8.

[27] Yawson AE, Baddoo A, Hagan-Seneadza NA, Calys-Tagoe B, Hewlett S, Dako-Gyeke P, et al. Tobacco use in older adults in Ghana: sociodemographic characteristics, health risks and subjective wellbeing. BMC Public Health 2013;13:979. doi: 10.1186/1471-2458-13-979.

[28] Peltzer K, Phaswana-Mafuya N. Tobacco use and associated factors in older adults in South Africa. J Psychol Afr 2012;22:283–8.

[29] Pang S, Subramaniam M, Abdin E, Lee SP, Chua BY, Shafie SB, et al. Prevalence and predictors of tobacco use in the elderly. Int J Geriatr Psychiatry 2016;31:716-22.

[30] Burns A, Strawbridge JD, Clancy L, Doyle F. Exploring smoking, mental health and smoking-related disease in a nationally representative sample of older adults in Ireland - A retrospective secondary analysis. J Psychosom Res 2017;98:78-86.

[31] Lin EY, Witten K, Casswell S, You RQ. Neighbourhood matters: perceptions of neighbourhood cohesiveness and associations with alcohol, cannabis and tobacco use. Drug Alcohol Rev 2012;31(4):402-12. doi: 10.1111/j.1465-3362.2011.00385.x.

[32] Blazer DG, Wu LT. Patterns of tobacco use and tobacco-related psychiatric morbidity and substance use among middle-aged and older adults in the United States. Aging Ment Health 2012;16:296-304.

[33] Dani JA, Harris RA. Nicotine addiction and comorbidity with alcohol abuse and mental illness. Nat Neurosci 2005;8:1465-70.

[34] Wang Q. Smoking and body weight: evidence from China health and nutrition survey. BMC Public Health 2015;15:1238. doi: 10.1186/s12889-015-2549-9.

[35] Mineur YS, Abizaid A, Rao Y, Salas R, DiLeone RJ, Gündisch D, et al. Nicotine decreases food intake through activation of POMC neurons. Science 2011;332(6035):1330-2. doi: 10.1126/science.1201889.

[36] Pengpid S, Vonglokham M, Kounnavong S, Sychareun V, Peltzer K. The prevalence of underweight and overweight/obesity and its correlates among adults in Laos: a cross-sectional national population-based survey, 2013. Eat Weight Disord 2020;25(2):265-73. doi: 10.1007/s40519-018-0571-5.

In: Social and Health Issues … ISBN: 978-1-53619-937-6
Editors: S Pengpid, K Peltzer et al.

Chapter 19

PREVALENCE AND CORRELATES OF HEAVY EPISODIC DRINKING AMONG MIDDLE-AGED AND OLDER ADULTS IN INDIA: RESULTS OF A NATIONAL SURVEY IN 2017-2018

Karl Peltzer[1,2], MA Clin Psych, PhD, Dr Habil and Supa Pengpid[1,3,*], MPH, DrPH, MBA
[1]Department of Research Administration and Development, University of Limpopo, Turfloop, South Africa
[2]Department of Psychology, College of Medical and Health Science, Asia University, Taichung, Taiwan
[3]ASEAN Institute for Health Development, Mahidol University, Salaya, Phutthamonthon, Nakhon Pathom, Thailand

---

[*] *Correspondence*: Professor Supa Pengpid, ASEAN Institute for Health Development, Mahidol University, 25/25 Phutthamonthon Road 4, Salaya, Phutthamonton, Nakhon Pathom 73170, Thailand. Email: supaprom@yahoo.com.

ABSTRACT

In this chapter we estimate the prevalence and correlates of heavy episodic drinking (HED) among middle-aged and older adults in India. The study included 72,262 individuals (45 years and older) from the cross-sectional 2017-2018 Longitudinal Ageing Study in India (LASI) Wave 1. Results indicate a prevalence of HED of 2.9%, 6.1% among men and 0.5% among women. In adjusted logistic regression analysis, male sex (Adjusted Odds Ratio = AOR: 7.87, 95% Confidence Interval = CI: 5.97-10.36), Christian (AOR: 2.28, 95% CI: 1.76-2.96), Sikh (AOR: 3.79, 95% CI: 2.87-5.01), current tobacco use (AOR: 3.87, 95% CI: 3.23-4.63), and high discrimination experiences (AOR: 1.66, 95% CI: 1.11-2.46) were positively associated with HED. Older age (≥70 years) (AOR: 0.47, 95% CI: 0.36-0.60), higher education (≥10 years) (AOR: 0.61, 95% CI: 0.48-0.78), Muslim (AOR: 0.10, 95% CI: 0.06-0.17), daily prayer (AOR: 0.61, 95% CI: 0.51-0.73), and overweight/obesity (AOR: 0.72, 95% CI: 0.60-0.87) were negatively associated with HED. In addition, in unadjusted analyses, lower subjective socioeconomic status, married, underweight, and vigorous physical activity were positively associated with HED. A low prevalence of HED was found and several associated factors were identified.

INTRODUCTION

"Harmful alcohol use is a significant contributor to the global burden of disease" [1]. "Heavy episodic drinking (HED) is defined as drinking at least 60 grams or more of pure alcohol on at least one occasion in the past 30 days" [2]. HED is a "major indicator for the acute effects of alcohol consumption, such as injury" [2]. "Worldwide, 18.2% of persons 15 years and older were estimated to engage in HED in 2016" [3]. In India, "nationally, about 14.6% of the population (between 10 and 75 years of age) consumes alcohol and excessive alcohol consumption is around 2.7%" [4]. In a study among adults (≥15 years) in five states in India in 2014, 7.3% had HED among current drinkers, and 2.8% had HED among the total population [5]. There is a lack of recent national community-dwelling studies on HED among middle-aged and older adults in India.

In national population-based surveys in low- and middle-income countries, the prevalence of HED among the general adult population was 12.5% in Ethiopia [6], 12.8% in Kenya [7], 14.1% in South Africa [8], 24.1% in Ecuador [9] and 5.7% in Malaysia [10]. As reviewed previously [7], risk factors for HED may include “being male, middle age, specific ethnic groups, lower socioeconomic status, cardio-metabolic risk, hypertension, and comorbidities with tobacco use.” The study aimed to assess the prevalence and correlates of HED among middle-aged and older adults in a national community-dwelling survey in India in 2017-2018.

OUR STUDY

This secondary data analysis utilized nationally representative cross-sectional data of the Longitudinal Ageing Study in India (LASI) Wave 1, 2017-2018; the individual response rate was almost 90% [11]. Using a household survey, interview and physical measurement data were collected from middle-aged and older adults (≥45 years, spouses, regardless of age). More specific sampling details are shown elsewhere [11]. The Indian Council of Medical Research (ICMR) Ethics Committee approved the study and written, or oral informed consent was obtained from the participants [11].

Measures

Heavy episodic alcohol use was measured with the item, “In the last 3 months, how frequently on average, have you had at least 5 or more drinks on one occasion?” [11] and defined as “one to three days per month, one to four days per week, five or more days per week, or daily.”

Independent variables

Sociodemographic variables included sex, years of education, age, residential, and marital status [11]. Socioeconomic status was sourced from the item, "Please imagine a ten-step ladder, where at the bottom are the people who are the worst off – who have the least money, least education, and the worst jobs or no jobs, and at the top of the ladder are the people who are the best off – those who have the most money, most education, and best jobs. Please indicate the number given (1-10) on the rung on the ladder where you would place yourself" [11]. Subjective socioeconomic status was trichotomized into poor = steps 1 to 3, medium steps 4-5, and high steps 6-10.

Religious affiliation was sourced from the question, "What is your religion?" Response options were "None, Hindu, Muslim, Christian, Sikh, Buddhist/neo-Buddhist, Jain, Jewish, Parsi/Zoroastrian and Other, please specify…" [11].

Nonorganizational religiosity was assessed with the question, "In the past year, how often have you done pooja or prayer?" Response options ranged from 1 = not at all to 6 = every day [11].

Discrimination experiences were assessed with the six-item Everyday Discrimination Scale (EDS) (Short version) [12]. Response options ranged from 1 = "never" to 6 = "almost every day", and were dichotomised to 'never' = 0 and 'ever' (collapsing those reporting 'less than once a year' or greater into one category) = 1; Cronbach's alpha for the EDS in this study was 0.86.

Anthropometry: "Height and weight of adults were measured using the Seca 803 digital scale." [11]. "Body Mass Index = BMI was calculated according to Asian criteria: underweight (< 18.5 kg/m^2), normal weight (18.5-22.9 kg/m^2), overweight (23.0-24.9 kg/m^2), class I obesity (25.0-29.9 kg/m^2), and class II obesity (≥30.0 kg/m^2)" [13].

Current tobacco use was sourced from two items, 1) "Do you currently smoke any tobacco products (cigarettes, bidis, cigars, hookah, cheroot, etc.)? and 2) Do you use smokeless tobacco (such as chewing tobacco, gutka, pan masala, etc.)?" (Yes, No) [11].

Vigorous physical activity. " For vigorous activity, respondents were asked about their involvement in running or jogging, swimming, going to a health centre/gym, cycling, digging with a spade or shovel, heavy lifting, chopping, farm work, fast bicycling, and cycling with loads" [11]. Responses were trichotomized into 1 = hardly ever/never, 2 = less than twice a week, and 3 = more than once a week [14].

Data analysis

Descriptive statistics were used to describe the sample and HED prevalence. Unadjusted and adjusted logistic regression was used to estimate the prevalence of HED. Missing values are excluded from the analysis, and $p < 0.05$ was accepted as significant. Considering the complex study design, statistical analysis was conducted using STATA software version 15.0 (Stata Corporation, College Station, TX, USA).

FINDINGS

The sample comprised 72,262 middle-aged and older adults (≥45 years) from India. Table 1 shows details of the sample characteristics. Among those participants who reported having experienced discrimination, the perceived reasons were age 48.9%, financial status 41.8%, caste 12.9%, gender 9.3%, other 8.9%, other aspects of physical appearance 6.3%, religion 5.3%, physical disability 3.9%, and weight 1.6%. The prevalence of HED was 2.9%, 6.1% among men and 0.5% among women (see Table 1).

Associations with HED

In adjusted logistic regression analysis, male sex (Adjusted Odds Ratio = AOR: 7.87, 95% Confidence Interval = CI: 5.97-10.36), Christian (AOR: 2.28, 95% CI: 1.76-2.96), Sikh (AOR: 3.79, 95% CI: 2.87-5.01), current tobacco use (AOR: 3.87, 95% CI: 3.23-4.63), and high discrimination experiences (AOR: 1.66, 95% CI: 1.11-2.46) were positively associated with HED. Older age (≥70 years) (AOR: 0.47, 95% CI: 0.36-0.60), higher education (≥10 years) (AOR: 0.61, 95% CI: 0.48-0.78), Muslim (AOR: 0.10, 95% CI: 0.06-0.17), daily prayer (AOR: 0.61, 95% CI: 0.51-0.73),

Table 1. Sample characteristics of middle-aged and older adults in India, 2017-2018

Variable	**Sample**	**Heavy episodic drinking**		
		All	**Male**	**Female**
	N (%)	%	%	%
All	**72262**	**2.9**	**6.1**	**0.5**
Age in years				
45-59	40785 (54.1)	3.1	7.5	0.5
60-69	18979 (26.8)	3.1	5.8	0.7
70 or more	12499 (19.0)	1.9	3.5	0.4
Sex				
Female	41685 (58.0)			
Male	30577 (42.0)			
Education in years				
0	33213 (49.5)	2.9	8.1	0.8
1-4 years	8056 (10.8)	3.5	6.5	0.2
5-9 years	16911 (21.1)	3.2	6.0	0.1
≥10 years	14079 (18.5)	2.1	3.4	0.1
Socioeconomic status				
Low	23625 (37.2)	3.6	7.5	0.8
Medium	28380 (38.7)	2.8	6.2	0.3
High	18134 (24.1)	2.2	4.7	0.3
Marital status				
Not married	16852 (24.4)	1.8	5.5	0.8
Married	55401 (75.6)	3.2	6.2	0.4
Residence status				
Rural	46539 (68.2)	3.2	6.6	0.7
Urban	25723 (31.8)	2.1	4.9	0.2
Religious affiliation				
Hindu	52983 (81.9)	3.0	6.5	0.5
Muslim	8668 (11.7)	0.3	0.7	0.0
Christian	7216 (3.0)	5.7	12.7	1.5
Sikh	1999 (1.8)	5.2	11.8	0.0
Other or none	1392 (1.7)	5.6	10.0	2.3

Variable	Sample	Heavy episodic drinking		
		All	Male	Female
	N (%)	%	%	%
Discrimination experiences				
0	60008 (82.7)	2.7	5.8	0.5
1-2	6126 (10.7)	3.4	7.3	0.6
3-6	4247 (6.6)	6.3	12.4	1.2
Done pooja or prayer				
1-3 times/month or ≥1 times/ year or not at all	19844 (31.3)	4.9	8.6	1.1
Once/week or ≥1/week	23427 (33.8)	3.8	7.8	0.7
Every day	27089 (34.9)	1.7	4.1	0.2
Body mass index				
Normal	23447 (36.7)	3.4	6.6	0.7
Under	11644 (20.8)	4.1	8.0	0.9
Overweight/obese	29497 (42.5)	1.6	4.1	0.3
Current tobacco use	21071 (30.4)	7.0	9.3	1.9
Vigorous physical activity				
Hardly ever/never	43224 (58.9)	2.1	5.5	0.3
≤Once a week	6183 (9.1)	3.5	6.8	0.4
>Once a week	22210 (32.0)	4.2	6.8	1.0

and overweight/obesity (AOR: 0.72, 95% CI: 0.60-0.87) were negatively associated with HED. In addition, in unadjusted analyses, lower subjective socioeconomic status, married, underweight, and vigorous physical activity were positively associated with HED (see Table 2).

Table 2. Associations with heavy episodic drinking among middle-aged and older adults in India, 2017-2018

Variable	COR (95% CI)	AOR (95% CI)
Age in years)		
45-59	1 (Reference)	1 (Reference)
60-69	0.99 (0.84, 1.18)	0.81 (0.68, 0.96)*
70 or more	0.60 (0.48, 0.75)***	0.47 (0.36, 0.60)***
Sex		
Female	1 (Reference)	1 (Reference)
Male	12.90 (10.07, 16.51)***	7.87 (5.97, 10.36)***
Education in years		
0	1 (Reference)	1 (Reference)
1-4 years	1.22 (0.98, 1.50)	0.81 (0.66, 1.01)
5-9 years	1.12 (0.93, 1.35)	0.76 (0.63, 0.92)**
≥10 years	0.73 (0.58, 0.91)**	0.61 (0.48, 0.78)***

Table 2. (Continued)

Variable	COR (95% CI)	AOR (95% CI)
Socioeconomic status		
Low	1 (Reference)	1 (Reference)
Medium	0.77 (0.65, 0.92)**	0.95 (0.81, 1.13)
High	0.60 (0.49, 0.74)***	0.96 (0.78, 1.17)
Marital status		
Not married	1 (Reference)	1 (Reference)
Married	1.80 (1.47, 2.20)***	0.93 (0.74, 1.18)
Residence status		
Rural	1 (Reference)	1 (Reference)
Urban	0.64 (0.50, 0.83)***	1.11 (0.87, 1.42)
Religion		
Hindu	1 (Reference)	1 (Reference)
Muslim	0.09 (0.06, 0.15)***	0.10 (0.06, 0.17)***
Christian	1.94 (1.13, 3.33)*	2.28 (1.76, 2.96)***
Sikh	1.74 (1.37, 2.22)***	3.79 (2.87, 5.01)***
Other or none	1.90 (1.22, 2.97)**	2.30 (1.37, 3.88)**
Discrimination experiences		
0	1 (Reference)	1 (Reference)
1-2	1.28 (1.03, 1.58)*	1.27 (1.02, 1.58)*
3-5	2.43 (1.48, 4.01)***	1.66 (1.11, 2.46)*
Done pooja or prayer		
1-3 times/month/≥1 times/ year/not at all	1 (Reference)	1 (Reference)
Once/week or ≥1/week	0.76 (0.62, 0.95)*	1.00 (0.82, 1.22)
Every day	0.33 (0.28, 0.39)***	0.61 (0.51, 0.73)***
Body mass index		
Normal	1 (Reference)	1 (Reference)
Under	1.21 (1.02, 1.44)*	1.07 (0.90, 1.28)
Overweight/obese	0.46 (0.39, 0.55)***	0.72 (0.60, 0.87)***
Current tobacco use	6.71 (5.44, 8.30)***	3.87 (3.23, 4.63)***
Vigorous physical activity		
Hardly ever/never	1 (Reference)	1 (Reference)
≤Once a week	1.68 (1.32, 2.14)***	1.10 (0.86, 1.40)
>Once a week	2.01 (1.69, 2.39)***	1.10 (0.92, 1.31)

UOR = Unadjusted Odds Ratio; AOR = Adjusted Odds Ratio; CI = Confidence Interval;
***$p < 0.001$, **$p < 0.01$, *$p < 0.05$.

Discussion

In a large national middle-aged and older adult (≥45 years) sample in India in 2017-2018, the prevalence of HED (2.9%) is similar to a previous study in five states among the general adult population in India (2.8%) [5], but lower than in other low- and middle-income countries, such as in Ethiopia (12.5%) [6], in Kenya (12.8%) [7], in South Africa (14.1%) [8], in Ecuador (24.1%) [9] and in Malaysia (5.7%) [10]. Religion contributed to significant differences in the prevalence of HED. Compared to Hindus, Muslims had significantly lower, and Christians and Sikhs had significantly higher rates of HED. Consistent with research in Southeast Asia [15], non-organised religious activity (prayer) was protective against HED in this study. Experiencing different types of discrimination was in this study significantly associated with higher rates of HED. Similar results were found among African American youth [16], and in national study among adults in China [17].

In agreement with previous studies [18-20], this study found that men and middle-aged persons (45-59 years) were more likely to engage in HED. These sex differences may be related to specific norms that for example associate alcohol use with masculinity [6, 21]. Older age was negatively associated with HED in this study, which may be expected as the tolerance towards alcohol decreases with older age [22]. Consistent with previous research [19, 23, 24], this survey showed an association between lower education and, in unadjusted analysis lower subjective socioeconomic status and HED.

In line with previous research findings [7, 19, 24], this investigation showed stark associations between current tobacco use and HED. An explanation for the strong link between HED and tobacco use may be related to the risk of HED and nicotine co-dependence [25]. As a result, smoking cessation programmes should be offered to persons with HED. In a study among the general adult population in a high-income country, South Korea [26], underweight was negatively and overweight/obesity was positively associated with problem drinking, while in this study overweight/obesity was negatively and underweight in unadjusted analysis positively associated with HED.

Regarding alcohol policy in India, "although the prohibition of alcohol use is encouraged in the Constitution of India, alcohol policy is a state subject. States are having full control of alcohol-related legislation, excise rates, and the production, distribution, and sale of alcohol." [27]. Some states have a complete ban on alcohol use, in other states the minimum legal drinking age differs from 18 to 25 years; "other laws related to the regulation of alcohol use like hours of sales, drunken driving and sale to minors are regularly breached" [27]. In the middle-income country, India, the primary health care system is the first contact of patients, where low-cost evidence-based brief intervention should be provided for HED [27].

Study limitations include that most data were collected by self-report, including alcohol use. It is possible that in India the socially undesirable behaviour of alcohol use was underreported. In addition, the cross-sectional study design hinders us to draw causative conclusions.

Conclusion

In this national survey among middle-aged and older adults in India in 2017-2018, a low prevalence of HED (2.9%) was found. Results suggest that social and demographic factors (male sex, middle-aged, lower education, Christian, Sikh, and discrimination experiences) and health factors (current tobacco use) identified should be taken into account in public health interventions on HED.

Acknowledgments

The Longitudinal Aging Study in India Project is funded by the Ministry of Health and Family Welfare, Government of India, the National Institute on

Aging (R01 AG042778, R01 AG030153), and United Nations Population Fund, India.

REFERENCES

[1] NCD Risk Factor Collaboration (NCD-RisC). Worldwide trends in diabetes since 1980: A pooled analysis of 751 population-based studies with 4.4 million participants. Lancet 2016;387(10027):1513-30. doi: 10.1016/S0140-6736(16)00618-8.

[2] World Health Organization. Heavy episodic drinking among drinkers. Situation and trends, 2020. URL: https://www.who.int/gho/alcohol/consumption_patterns/heavy_episodic_drinkers_text/en/#:~:text=Heavy%20episodic%20drinking%2C%20or%20HED,in%20the%20past%2030%20days.&text=Worldwide%2C%20about%207.5%25%20of%20drinkers,monthly%20heavy%20episodic%20drinking%20occasions.

[3] World Health Organization. Global status report on alcohol and health 2018. Geneva: World Health Organization, 2018. URL: https://apps.who.int/iris/bitstream/handle/10665/274603/9789241565639-eng.pdf?ua = 1.

[4] Ministry of Social Justice and Empowerment (MoSJE). Magnitude of substance use in India. National Drug Dependence Treatment Centre (NDDTC) and All India Institute of Medical Sciences (AIIMS). New Delhi: Government of India, 2019.

[5] Kumar K, Kumar S, Singh AK. Prevalence and socio-demographic correlates of alcohol consumption: Survey findings from five states in India. Drug Alcohol Depend 2018;185:381-90. doi: 10.1016/j.drugalcdep.2017.12.024.

[6] Getachew T, Defar A, Teklie H, Gonfa G, Bekele A, Bekele A, et al. Magnitude and predictors of excessive alcohol use in Ethiopia: Findings from the 2015 national non-communicable diseases STEPS survey. Ethiop J Health Dev 2017;31(Spec Issue):312-9.

[7] Pengpid S, Peltzer K. Alcohol use among adults in Kenya: results from the national non-communicable diseases risk factor survey, 2015. J Psychol Afr 2019;29(1):49-53. doi: 10.1080/14330237.2019.1568728.

[8] Vellios NG, Van Walbeek CP. Self-reported alcohol use and binge drinking in South Africa: Evidence from the National Income Dynamics Study, 2014 - 2015. S Afr Med J 2017;108(1):33-9. doi: 10.7196/SAMJ.2017.v108i1.12615.

[9] Pengpid S, Peltzer K. Prevalence and correlates of heavy episodic alcohol consumption among adults in Ecuador: Results of the first national STEPS survey in 2018. Int J Environ Res Public Health 2020;17(23):9017. doi: 10.3390/ijerph17239017.

[10] Hatta M, Balkish MN, Rozanim K, Hamizatul AH, Ali BA, Ahmad NBA et al. How severe is binge drinking in Malaysia and who are at risk? J Alcohol Drug Depend 2013;1:131. doi:10.4172/2329-6488.1000131.

[11] International Institute for Population Sciences (IIPS), NPHCE, MoHFW, Harvard TH Chan School of Public Health (HSPH) and the University of Southern California (USC). Longitudinal Ageing Study in India (LASI) Wave 1, 2017-18, India Report. Mumbai: International Institute for Population Sciences, 2020.

[12] Sternthal MJ, Slopen N, Williams DR. Racial disparities in health: How much does stress really matter? Du Bois Rev 2011;8(1):95-113. doi: 10.1017/S1742058X1 1000087.

[13] Wen CP, David Cheng TY, Tsai SP, Chan HT, Hsu HL, Hsu CC, et al. Are Asians at greater mortality risks for being overweight than Caucasians? Redefining obesity for Asians. Public Health Nutr 2009;12(4):497-506. doi: 10.1017/S1368980008002802.

[14] Lübs L, Peplies J, Drell C, Bammann K. Cross-sectional and longitudinal factors influencing physical activity of 65 to 75-year-olds: A pan European cohort study based on the survey of health, ageing and retirement in Europe (SHARE). BMC Geriatr 2018;18(1):94. doi: 10.1186/s12877-018-0781-8.

[15] Yi S, Ngin C, Peltzer K, Pengpid S. Health and behavioral factors associated with binge drinking among university students in nine ASEAN countries. Subst Abuse Treat Prev Policy 2017;12(1):32. doi: 10.1186/s13011-017-0117-2.

[16] Madkour AS, Jackson K, Wang H, Miles TT, Mather F, Shankar A. Perceived discrimination and heavy episodic drinking among African-American youth: Differences by age and reason for discrimination. J Adolesc Health 2015;57(5):530-6. doi: 10.1016/j.jadohealth.2015.07.016.

[17] Gu J, Ming X. Perceived social discrimination, socioeconomic status, and alcohol consumption among Chinese adults: A nationally representative study. Int J Environ Res Public Health 2020;17(17):6043. doi: 10.3390/ijerph17176043.

[18] Helzer JE, Burnamm A, McEvoy LT. Alcohol abuse and dependence. In: Robins LN, Regier DA, eds. Psychiatric disorders in America: The epidemiologic catchment area study. New York: Free Press/MacMillan, 1991:81-115.

[19] Peltzer K, Davids A, Njuho P. Alcohol use and problem drinking in South Africa: findings from a national population-based survey. Afr J Psychiatry 2011;14(1):30-7. doi: 10.4314/ajpsy.v14i1.65466.

[20] Pires J, Padrão P, Damasceno A, Silva-Matos C, Lunet N. Impact of different reference period definitions in the quantification of alcohol consumption: results from a nationwide STEPS survey in Mozambique. Alcohol Alcohol 2012;47(3):328-33. doi: 10.1093/alcalc/ags003.

[21] Kabwama SN, Ndyanabangi S, Mutungi G, Wesonga R, Bahendeka SK, Guwatudde D. Alcohol use among adults in Uganda: Findings from the countrywide non-communicable diseases risk factor cross-sectional survey. Glob Health Action 2016;9:31302. doi: 10.3402/gha.v9.31302.

[22] Institute of Alcohol Studies. Older people's drinking habits, 2017. URL: http://www.ias.org.uk/Alcohol-knowledge-centre/Alcohol-and-older-people/Factsheets/Older-peoples-drinking-habits-Very-little-very-often.aspx.

[23] Pillai A, Nayak MB, Greenfield TK, Bond JC, Nadkarni A, Patel V. Patterns of alcohol use, their correlates, and impact in male drinkers: a population-based survey from Goa, India. Soc Psychiatry Psychiatr Epidemiol 2013;48(2):275-82. doi: 10.1007/s00127-012-0538-1.

[24] Katulanda P, Ranasinghe C, Rathnapala A, Karunaratne N, Sheriff R, Matthews D. Prevalence, patterns and correlates of alcohol consumption and its' association with tobacco smoking among Sri Lankan adults: A cross-sectional study. BMC Public Health 2014;14:612. doi: 10.1186/1471-2458-14-612.

[25] Diehl A, Scherbaum N. Nikotinabhängigkeit als komorbide Störung bei Alkoholabhängigkeit--Epidemiologie, Atiologie und Therapie. Fortschr Neurol Psychiatr 2008;76(1):14-20. [German] doi: 10.1055/s-2007-980076.

[26] Chang AK, Choi JY. Factors influencing BMI classifications of Korean adults. J Phys Ther Sci 2015;27(5):1565-70. doi: 10.1589/jpts.27.1565.

[27] Eashwar VMA, Umadevi R, Gopalakrishnan S. Alcohol consumption in India- An epidemiological review. J Family Med Prim Care 2020;9(1):49-55. doi:10.4103/jfmpc.jfmpc_873_19.

In: Social and Health Issues … ISBN: 978-1-53619-937-6
Editors: S Pengpid, K Peltzer et al.

Chapter 20

Prevalence and Correlates of Loneliness among a Nationally Representative Population-Based Sample of Middle-Aged and Older Adults in India

Supa Pengpid[1,2], MPH, DrPH, MBA
and Karl Peltzer[2,3,*], MA Clin Psych, PhD, Dr Habil
[1]ASEAN Institute for Health Development, Mahidol University, Salaya, Phutthamonthon, Nakhon Pathom, Thailand
[2]Department of Research Administration and Development, University of Limpopo, Turfloop, South Africa
[3]Department of Psychology, College of Medical and Health Science, Asia University, Taichung, Taiwan

* *Correspondence*: Professor Karl Peltzer, Department of Research Administration and Development, University of Limpopo, Turfloop Campus, Private Bag X1106, Sovenga 0727, South Africa. Email: kfpeltzer@gmail.com.

Abstract

In this chapter we wanted to determine the prevalence and correlates of loneliness in middle-aged and older adults in India. The sample included 72,262 middle-aged and older adults from the cross-sectional 2017-2018 Longitudinal Ageing Study in India (LASI) Wave 1. Loneliness was assessed with a single item. Results indicate that the prevalence of moderate loneliness was 20.5%, and severe loneliness was 13.3%. In adjusted multinominal logistic regression analysis, food insecurity, discrimination experiences, exposure to life event stressors, unsafe home, low life satisfaction, multimorbidity, functional disability and poor distant vision were positively and being married, high spirituality/religiosity, and medium attendance of religious services, were negatively associated with severe loneliness. In addition, no schooling and poor childhood health were positively associated with moderate loneliness. More than one in ten middle-aged and older adults in India reported severe loneliness. Several risk and protective factors were identified, which can be targeted in public health interventions.

Introduction

Loneliness is a "distressing feeling that accompanies the perception that one's social needs are not being met by the quantity or especially the quality of one's social relationships" [1] and may be a "common phenomenon in old age due to changes in the quality and quantity of social relationships" [2, 3]. "Loneliness and isolation have a detrimental effect on health in old age." [4] The prevalence of loneliness among older adults in 11 European countries has been found to be common, ranging from 10% in France and Norway to more than 30% in Bulgaria [5]. In a middle-income country, South Africa, the prevalence of self-reported loneliness was among older adults 9.9% [6], almost 10% of 70 to 74 year-olds in Indonesia reported occasionally or all of the time to be lonely [7], in Malaysia 32.5% of older adults (≥60 years) reported sometimes feeling lonely, and 20.9% always feeling lonely [8], and in a study among older adults (≥50 years) in Mexico, 12.3% reported loneliness [9]. In a study among rural older adults (N=897) in India, the prevalence of loneliness was 48% (measured with a 3-item scale) [10] and in a national community-dwelling survey among older adults (≥50 years) in India in 2007, 18% reported loneliness [11]. There is scarce information on more recent national estimates of loneliness and its correlates among older adults in India.

Several risk factors associated with loneliness have been identified [7, 12], including sex, age, lower socioeconomic status, functional disability, negative life events, adverse childhood experiences and multimorbidity and several protective factors include social support, being married, social support and social engagement. This study aimed to determine the prevalence and correlates of loneliness among middle-aged and older adults in a national population survey in India in 2017-2018.

OUR STUDY

This secondary data analysis utilized data from the cross-sectional and nationally representative Longitudinal Ageing Study in India (LASI) Wave 1, 2017-2018; "the overall household response rate is 96%, and the overall individual response rate is 87%." [13]. In a household survey, "interview, physical measurement and biomarker data were collected from individuals aged 45 and above and their spouses, regardless of age." [13]. Specific details on the sampling approach are found elsewhere elsewhere [13]. The study was approved by the "Indian Council of Medical Research (ICMR) Ethics Committee and written informed consent was obtained from the participants" [13].

Measures

The loneliness item asked for "How often did you feel lonely in the past week?" Response options were coded into no loneliness: "1=rarely or none of the time (<1 day), moderate loneliness: 2=sometimes or 1–2 days/week, and severe loneliness: 3=occasionally or all the time or 3–7 days/week)."[14].

Sociodemographic variables consisted of education (none and ≥1 years), age, sex (male, female), marital status (currently married vs. widowed/divorced/separated/deserted/live-in relationship/never married), and residence (rural, urban) [13].

Stressors

Food insecurity was assessed with four questions, 1) "In the last 12 months, did you ever reduce the size of your meals or skip meals because there was not enough food at your household? (Yes/No) 2) In the last 12 months, were you hungry but didn't eat because there was not enough food at your household? (Yes/No) 3) In the past 12 months, did you ever not eat for a whole day because there was not enough food in your household? and 4) Do you think that you have lost weight in the last 12 months because there was not enough food in your household?" [13]. Any positive response to the four questions was scored as one.

Discrimination experiences were assessed with the six-item Everyday Discrimination Scale (EDS) (Short version) [15]. Response options ranged from 1="never" to 6="almost every day," and were dichotomised to 'never'=0 and 'ever' (collapsing those reporting 'less than once a year' or greater into one category)=1; Cronbach's alpha for the EDS in this study was 0.86.

Life event stressors were assessed with four items: 1) ill-treatment ("Have you felt that you were ill-treated in the past year?" Yes/No), 2) victim of violent crime ("In the last 12 months, have you been the victim of a violent crime, such as assault/mugging/threat to life/others?" (Yes/No), 3) disaster exposure causing health effects ("In the last five years, has your health been severely affected by disasters such as floods, landslides, extreme cold and hot weather, cyclone/typhoons, droughts, earthquakes, tsunamis, or any other natural calamities?" (Yes/No), and 4) man-made incident causing health effects ("In the last five years, has your health been severely affected by man-made incidents such as riots, terrorism, building collapses, fires, traffic accidents or any other man-made incidents?" (Yes/No) [13]. Any affirmative response was coded with one.

Poor childhood health was assessed with the question, "Would you say your childhood health was very good, good, fair, poor or very poor on the basis of what you remember, or what you heard or perceived from your parents?") (coded poor or very poor=1) [13].

Unsafe home was measured with the item, "In general, how safe from crime and violence do you feel when you are alone at home?" (coded complete safe or safe=0, and not very safe or not safe at all=1) [13].

Social support

Intrinsic religiosity was measured with four items from the Daily Spiritual Experience Scale (DSES) [16], 1) "Do you think that you have a feeling of deep inner peace?" 2) "Do you think that you are spiritually touched by the beauty of creation?" 3) "Do you think that you are thankful for whatever you received in your life?" and 4) "Do you think that you are selflessly caring for others?" Responses ranged from 1=never to 5=every day in a week, and the summed scores were trichotomized to 4-7=low, 8-11=medium, and 12-20=high. Cronbach's alpha for the DSES in this study was 0.86.

Organizational religiosity was assessed with the question, "In the past year, how often have you attended religious services (at a temple/mosque/church, etc.)?" Response options were grouped into 1 (low)=not at all, 2 (medium)=1-3 times a month or 1 or more times a year, and 3(high)=once a week or more than once a week or every day [13].

Life satisfaction was assessed with the item, "Please, think about your life as a whole. How satisfied are you with it? Are you completely satisfied, very satisfied, somewhat satisfied, not very satisfied, or not at all satisfied?" [13]. Responses were grouped into 1 (low)=not very satisfied or not at all satisfied, 2 (medium)=somewhat satisfied, and 3 (high)=very satisfied or completely satisfied.

Chronic conditions were sourced from the item, "Has any health professional ever told you that you have…?": 1) "Hypertension or high blood pressure (Yes/No); 2) Diabetes or high blood sugar; 3) Cancer or malignant tumor; 4) Chronic lung disease such as asthma, chronic obstructive pulmonary disease/Chronic bronchitis or other chronic lung problems; 5) Chronic heart diseases such as Coronary heart disease (heart attack or Myocardial Infarction), congestive heart failure, or other chronic heart problems; 6) Stroke; 7) Arthritis or rheumatism, Osteoporosis or other bone/joint diseases, and 8) High cholesterol." (Yes/No). [13]. Responses were summed and trichotomized into 0, 1, 2 or more chronic conditions.

Functional disability was assessed with six items of Activities of Daily Living (ADL) and seven items of Instrumental Activities of Daily Living (IADL) [17, 18]; (Cronbach alpha 0.89). Responses were "Yes/No" and were trichotomized into 0,1, or ≥2 ADL/IADL items.

Vision was assessed with two questions, 1) "How good is your eyesight for seeing things at a distance, like recognizing a person across the street (or 20 meters away), whether or not you wear glasses, contacts, or corrective lenses?" And 2) "How good is your eyesight for seeing things up close, like reading an ordinary newspaper print whether or not you wear glasses, contacts, or corrective lenses?" [13]. Responses ranged from 1=very good to 5=very poor, and poor near or far vision was classified as "poor or very poor."

Hearing loss was sourced from the item. "Have you ever been diagnosed with any hearing or ear-related problem or condition?" (Yes, No) [13].

Data analysis

Considering the clustered study design, data analyses were conducted with "STATA software version 15.0 (Stata Corporation, College Station, TX, USA)." Adjusted multinominal logistic regression was used to calculate predictors of moderate and severe loneliness, with no loneliness as the reference category. P values of below 0.05 were accepted as significant and missing values were excluded from the analysis.

Findings

The sample included 72,262 middle-aged and older adults (45 years and older), 58.0% were female and 42.0% male. Almost half of the participants (49.5%) had no formal education, 75.6% were married, and 68.2% were residing in rural areas. One in ten participants (9.7%) had food insecurity, 14.1% had discrimination experiences, 9.0% had experienced life event stressors, 1.6% had poor childhood health, and 13.9% felt unsafe at home. Further, the sample characteristics are shown in Table 1. The prevalence of moderate loneliness was 20.5%, and severe loneliness 13.3% (see Table 1).

Table 1. Sample and loneliness characteristics of middle-aged and older adults in India, 2017-2018

Variable	Sample	Loneliness in the past week		
		<1 day	1–2 days	3–7 days
	N (%)	%	%	%
Sociodemographic factors				
All	72262	66.1	20.5	13.3
Age in years				
45-59	40785 (54.1)	68.9	19.1	12.0
60-69	18979 (26.8)	64.2	21.3	14.4
70 or more	12498 (19.0)	60.5	23.8	15.7
Sex				
Female	41685 (58.0)	64.1	21.1	14.8
Male	30577 (42.0)	69.0	19.7	11.3
Education				
Some	39046 (50.5)	69.9	18.3	11.8
No schooling	33213 (49.5)	62.3	22.9	14.9
Marital status				
Not married	16852 (24.4)	52.2	25.7	22.1
Married	55401 (75.6)	70.6	18.9	10.5
Residential status				
Rural	46539 (68.2)	65.4	21.5	13.2
Urban	25723 (31.8)	67.8	18.5	13.7

Table 1. (Continued)

Variable	Sample	Loneliness in the past week		
		<1 day	1–2 days	3–7 days
	N (%)	%	%	%
Stressors				
Food insecurity	5806 (9.7)	47.6	27.7	24.6
Discrimination experiences				
0	60008 (82.7)	69.4	19.3	11.3
1-2	6126 (10.7)	53.6	26.0	20.4
3-6	4247 (6.6)	32.4	33.6	33.9
Life event stressors	5345 (9.0)	52.4	26.6	21.0
Poor childhood health	1068 (1.6)	53.5	30.8	15.7
Unsafe home	8860 (13.9)	46.1	25.9	28.0
Social support				
Spirituality/religiosity				
Low	19844 (31.3)	64.6	20.2	15.2
Medium	23427 (33.8)	65.5	21.0	13.6
High	27089 (34.9)	68.1	20.5	11.4
Religious service				
Low	36760 (53.8)	62.1	21.4	16.5
Medium	25196 (32.2)	68.0	20.0	12.0
High	10169 (14.0)	66.6	20.7	12.6
Life satisfaction				
Low	6793 (11.1)	44.9	29.5	25.6
Medium	28591 (40.9)	63.9	22.1	14.0
High	36165 (48.1)	72.9	17.2	9.9
Health status				
Chronic conditions				
0	39715 (55.0)	68.4	19.7	11.9
1	19336 (26.9)	65.3	21.1	13.6
2 or more	12991 (18.1)	60.3	22.5	17.2
Functional disability				
ADL & IADL=0	46762 (60.7)	70.5	18.0	11.4
ADL & IADL=1	7425 (10.5)	66.0	21.8	12.2
ADL & IADL=2 or more	17700 (28.8)	56.6	25.5	17.9
Poor distant vision	9756 (14.2)	56.1	26.0	17.9
Poor near vision	11866 (16.8)	60.2	23.8	16.0
Hearing loss	4874 (6.6)	60.5	21.1	18.4

Associations with moderate and severe loneliness

In adjusted multinominal logistic regression analysis, food insecurity, discrimination experiences, exposure to life event stressors, unsafe home, low life satisfaction, multimorbidity, functional disability and poor distant vision were positively and being married, high spirituality/religiosity, and medium attendance of religious services, were negatively associated with severe loneliness. In addition, no schooling and poor childhood health were positively associated with moderate loneliness (see Table 2).

Table 2. Associations with moderate and severe loneliness

Variable	Moderate loneliness ARRR (95% CI)	Severe loneliness ARRR (95% CI)
Sociodemographic factors		
Age in years		
45-59	1 (Reference)	1 (Reference)
60-69	0.98 (0.90, 1.07)	0.97 (0.84, 1.10)
70 or more	0.93 (0.83, 1.05)	0.90 (0.78, 1.03)
Sex		
Female	1 (Reference)	1 (Reference)
Male	1.02 (0.93, 1.12)	0.91 (0.80, 1.05)
Education		
Some	1 (Reference)	1 (Reference)
No schooling	1.12 (1.02, 1.23)*	1.00 (0.86, 1.16)
Marital status		
Not married	1 (Reference)	1 (Reference)
Married	0.60 (0.55, 0.66)***	0.40 (0.35, 0.46)***
Residential status		
Rural	1 (Reference)	1 (Reference)
Urban	0.93 (0.84, 1.03)	1.07 (0.91, 1.26)
Stressors		
Food insecurity	1.42 (1.25, 1.62)***	1.80 (1.56, 2.08)***
Discrimination experiences		
0	1 (Reference)	1 (Reference)
1-2	1.42 (1.19, 1.70)***	1.79 (1.52, 2.10)***
3-5	3.15 (2.72, 3.65)***	5.20 (4.42, 6.13)***
Life event stressors	1.27 (1.11, 1.44)***	1.34 (1.16, 1.55)***
Poor childhood health	1.52 (1.09, 2.11)*	1.06 (0.78, 1.44)
Unsafe home	1.31 (1.03, 1.66)*	1.78 (1.25, 2.53)***

Table 2. (Continued)

Variable	Moderate loneliness ARRR (95% CI)	Severe loneliness ARRR (95% CI)
Social support		
Spirituality/religiosity		
Low	1 (Reference)	1 (Reference)
Medium	1.08 (0.98, 1.19)	0.95 (0.80, 1.13)
High	1.04 (0.96, 1.13)	0.80 (0.70, 0.91)***
Attendance of religious service		
Low	1 (Reference)	1 (Reference)
Medium	0.93 (0.85, 1.01)	0.77 (0.64, 0.94)*
High	1.04 (0.93, 1.15)	0.88 (0.71, 1.10)
Life satisfaction (low)	1.75 (1.52, 2.02)***	2.16 (1.91, 2.45)***
Health status		
Chronic conditions		
0	1 (Reference)	1 (Reference)
1	1.04 (0.96, 1.12)	1.07 (0.94, 1.21)
2 or more	1.14 (1.00, 1.29)*	1.30 (1.08, 1.56)**
Functional disability		
0	1 (Reference)	1 (Reference)
1	1.17 (1.06, 1.29)***	0.99 (0.86, 1.13)
2 or more	1.38 (1.25, 1.53)***	1.26 (1.11, 1.43)***
Poor distant vision	1.24 (1.11, 1.37)***	1.25 (1.09, 1.43)***
Poor near vision	1.01 (0.92, 1.11)	1.01 (0.89, 1.14)
Hearing loss	0.89 (0.75, 1.05)	1.15 (0.90, 1.48)

ARRR=Adjusted Relative Risk Ratio; CI=Confidence Interval; ***$p<0.001$, **$p<0.01$, *$p<0.05$.

Discussion

In this nationally representative sample of middle-aged and older adults in India in 2017-2018, the prevalence of loneliness (20.5% moderate and 13.3% severe), seems higher than in several previous studies, including in 2007 in India (18%, ≥50 years) [11], in Mexico (12.3%, ≥50 years) [9], South Africa (9.9%, ≥50 years) [6], and lower than in Malaysia (53.4%) [8], and lower than in a local study in India (48%) [10]. Differences in the prevalence of loneliness may be attributed to different measures of loneliness. "Promising interventions targeting loneliness and social isolation among older adults may include new technologies and community engaged arts" [19].

This study found that various stressors, including food insecurity, having no education, discrimination experiences, experiences of stressful life events, unsafe home, and poor childhood health were associated with moderate and/or severe loneliness. These results are consistent with previous research findings [6, 7, 12]. Based on the Health and Retirement Study (HRS) in the USA, "discrimination based on race, ancestry, sex, and sexual orientation was associated with greater loneliness" [20]. It is possible that older adults with food insecurity "have less resources and opportunities that could prevent them becoming lonely" [12]. Unlike some previous studies [21], this study did not find an association between rural residence and loneliness as well as sex and loneliness [12].

In line with previous results [6, 7, 11, 12], being separated, divorced, widowed, or never married increased the odds of loneliness significantly in this study. Consistent with previous research [7, 22, 23], this study showed that measures of social support (spirituality/religiosity, attendance of religious services and life satisfaction) were protective against loneliness. Having multiple chronic conditions, functional disability and poor distant vision increased the odds of loneliness in this study. These results were found previously [6, 7, 12] and "may be explained by the limiting effect of having chronic conditions and/or having functional disability on the participation and performance of specific activities" [6, 7, 24].

Study limitations include the cross-sectional design, the assessment of some variables by self-report, and loneliness was only assessed with one item. However, some research seems to indicate "a high correlation between single-item and multi-item loneliness indices." [25] Some questions, e.g., on living status (living alone, etc.), were not included in this study and should be incorporated in further investigations.

Conclusion

More than one in ten middle-aged and older adults in India reported severe loneliness. Several risk factors, such as food insecurity, discrimination experiences, exposure to life event stressors, unsafe home, low life satisfaction, multimorbidity, functional disability, poor distant vision, not married, low spirituality/religiosity, and no attendance of religious services, were identified, which can be targeted in public health interventions.

Acknowledgments

The Longitudinal Aging Study in India Project is funded by the Ministry of Health and Family Welfare, Government of India, the National Institute on Aging (R01 AG042778, R01 AG030153), and United Nations Population Fund, India.

References

[1] Hawkley LC, Cacioppo JT. Loneliness matters: a theoretical and empirical review of consequences and mechanisms. Ann Behav Med 2010;40:218–27. https://doi.org/10.1007/s12160-010-9210-8.

[2] Qualter P, Vanhalst J, Harris R, Van Roekel E, Lodder G, Bangee M, et al. Loneliness across the life span. Perspect Psychol Sci 2015;10:250-64.

[3] Luanaigh CO, Lawlor BA. Loneliness and the health of older people. Int J Geriatric Psychiatry 2008:23(12):1213-21. doi: 10.1002/gps.2054.

[4] Courtin E, Knapp M. Social isolation, loneliness and health in old age: a scoping review. Health Soc Care Community 2017;25(3):799-812. doi: 10.1111/hsc.12311.

[5] Hansen T, Slagsvold B. Late-life loneliness in 11 European countries: Results from the generations and gender survey. Soc Indic Res 2016;129:445-64. doi:10.1007/s11205-015-1111-6.

[6] Phaswana-Mafuya N, Peltzer K. Loneliness and health among older adults in South Africa. Glob J Health Sci 2017;9(12):doi:10.5539/gjhs.v9n12p1.

[7] Peltzer K, Pengpid S. Loneliness correlates and associations with health variables in the general population in Indonesia. Int J Ment Health Syst 2019;13:24. https://doi.org/10.1186/s13033-019-0281-z.

[8] Teh JK, Tey NP, Ng ST. Family support and loneliness among older persons in multiethnic Malaysia. ScientificWorldJournal 2014;2014:654382. doi: 10.1155/2014/654382.

[9] Peltzer K, Pengpid S. Prevalence and correlates of loneliness among a nationally representative population-based sample of older adults in Mexico. Int J Disabil Hum Dev 2020;19(3):581-8.

[10] Chokkanathan S. Prevalence of and risk factors for loneliness in rural older adults. Australas J Ageing 2020;39(4):e545-51. doi: 10.1111/ajag.12835.

[11] Srivastava S, Ramanathan M, Dhillon P, Maurya C, Singh SK. Gender differentials in prevalence of loneliness among older adults in India: An Analysis from WHO Study on Global AGEing and Adult Health. Ageing Int 2020. https://doi.org/10.1007/s12126-020-09394-7.

[12] Cohen-Mansfield J, Hazan H, Lerman Y, Shalom V. Correlates and predictors of loneliness in older-adults: a review of quantitative results informed by qualitative insights. Int Psychogeriatr 2016;28(4):557-76. doi: 10.1017/S1041610215001532.

[13] International Institute for Population Sciences (IIPS), NPHCE, MoHFW, Harvard TH Chan School of Public Health (HSPH) and the University of Southern California (USC). Longitudinal Ageing Study in India (LASI) Wave 1, 2017-18, India Report. Mumbai: International Institute for Population Sciences, 2020.

[14] Andresen EM, Malmgren JA, Carter WB, Patrick DL. Screening for depression in well older adults: evaluation of a short form of the CES-D (Center for Epidemiologic Studies Depression Scale). Am J Prev Med 1994;10(2):77-84.

[15] Sternthal MJ, Slopen N, Williams DR. Racial disparities in health: How much does stress really matter? Du Bois Rev 2011;8(1):95-113. doi: 10 1017/ S1742058X11000087.

[16] Underwood LG, Teresi JA. The daily spiritual experience scale: development, theoretical description, reliability, exploratory factor analysis, and preliminary construct validity using health-related data. Ann Behav Med 2002;24(1):22-33. doi: 10.1207/S15324796ABM2401_04.

[17] Katz S, Ford AB, Moskowitz RW, Jackson BA, Jaffe MW. Studies of illness in the aged. the index of adl: a standardized measure of biological and psychosocial function. JAMA. 1963;185:914-9. doi: 10.1001/jama.1963.03060120024016.

[18] Lawton MP, Brody EM. Assessment of older people: self-maintaining and instrumental activities of daily living. Gerontologist. 1969;9(3):179-86.

[19] Poscia A, Stojanovic J, La Milia DI, Duplaga M, Grysztar M, Moscato U, et al. Interventions targeting loneliness and social isolation among the older people: An update systematic review. Exp Gerontol 2018;102:133-44. doi: 10.1016/j.exger.2017.11.017.

[20] Sutin AR, Stephan Y, Carretta H, Terracciano A. Perceived discrimination and physical, cognitive, and emotional health in older adulthood. Am J Geriatr Psychiatry 2015;23(2):171-9. doi:10.1016/j.jagp.2014.03.007.

[21] Kamiya Y, Doyle M, Henretta JC, Timonen V. Early-life circumstances and later-life loneliness in Ireland. Gerontologist 2014;54(5):773–83. https:// doi.org/10.1093/geront/gnt097.

[22] Nyqvist F, Victor CR, Forsman AK, Cattan M. The association between social capital and loneliness in diferent age groups: a populationbased study in Western Finland. BMC Public Health 2016;16:542. https ://doi.org/10.1186/s12889-016-3248-x.

[23] Victor CR, Yang K. The prevalence of loneliness among adults: a case study of the United Kingdom. J Psychol 2012;146(1–2):85–104. https:// doi.org/10.1080/ 00223980.2011.613875.

[24] Jessen MAB, Pallesen AVJ, Kriegbaum M, Kristiansen M. The association between loneliness and health—a survey-basedstudy among middleaged and older adults in Denmark. Aging Ment Health 2018;22(10):1338-43. https://doi. org/10.1080/13607863.2017.1348480.

[25] Stickley A, Koyanagi A, Leinsalu M, Ferlander S, Sabawoon W, McKee M. Loneliness and health in Eastern Europe: fndings from Moscow, Russia. Public Health 2015;129(4):403–10. https://doi.org/10.1016/j. puhe.2014.12.021.

In: Social and Health Issues ... ISBN: 978-1-53619-937-6
Editors: S Pengpid, K Peltzer et al.

Chapter 21

PERCEIVED HEALTH CARE DISCRIMINATION AMONG MIDDLE-AGED AND OLDER ADULTS IN INDIA: RESULTS OF A NATIONAL SURVEY IN 2017-2018

Karl Peltzer[1,2], MA Clin Psych, PhD, Dr Habil and Supa Pengpid[1,3,*], MPH, DrPH, MBA

[1]Department of Research Administration and Development, University of Limpopo, Turfloop, South Africa
[2]Department of Psychology, College of Medical and Health Science, Asia University, Taichung, Taiwan
[3]ASEAN Institute for Health Development, Mahidol University, Salaya, Phutthamonthon, Nakhon Pathom, Thailand

[*] *Correspondence*: Professor Supa Pengpid, ASEAN Institute for Health Development, Mahidol University, 25/25 Phutthamonthon Road 4, Salaya, Phutthamonton, Nakhon Pathom 73170, Thailand. Email: supaprom@yahoo.com.

ABSTRACT

We aimed to estimate the prevalence and correlates of perceived health care discrimination in middle-aged and older adults in a national population survey in India. The sample included 72,262 middle-aged and older adults from a cross-sectional national community-dwelling survey in India in 2017-2018. Results indicate that the prevalence of perceived health care discrimination was 5.9%. Among participants with health care discrimination, the major perceived reasons of health care discrimination included age (51.4%), followed by financial status (48.2%), caste (16.0%), and gender (10.7%). In the adjusted logistic regression analysis, male sex, food insecurity and utilization of traditional or complementary medicine practitioner were positively associated with health care discrimination, while higher education, higher subjective socioeconomic status, receipt of health insurance, Christian, Sikh and other religion were negatively associated with health care discrimination. In addition, in unadjusted analysis, scheduled tribes, other backward classes and rural residence were associated with health care discrimination. A significant proportion (5.9%) of middle-aged and older adults in India experienced health care discrimination, and several associated factors were identified that may be targeted to reduce health care discrimination.

INTRODUCTION

Perceived discrimination can be defined as "a behavioural manifestation of a negative attitude, judgment, or unfair treatment toward members of a group", such as age, gender, religion, caste, weight, physical disability, physical appearance, and financial status, and can be characterised as a form of stress [1]. Following the "Rejection-Identification Model" [2], "members of disadvantaged groups cope with the pain of attributions to prejudice by increasing identification with their disadvantaged group" [3]. There are two different types of perceived discrimination, one is referring to major lifetime experiences including singular incidents in society such as the housing or labour market, and the second type is everyday perceived discrimination including daily interpersonal hassles and insults encompassing chronic psychosocial stressors [4].

Perceived discrimination has been associated with negative mental and physical health outcomes [1]. One type of discrimination includes health care discrimination, which has also been detrimental to patient's health [5]. However, health care discrimination seems to be understudied in low- and middle-income countries, such as in India [6]. Health care discrimination seems to have been commonly experienced in several studies. For example, in a study among middle- and older age US Americans with chronic conditions the prevalence of health care discrimination was 20% among Blacks and 19% among Whites in 2014 [5], in a study among adults in the US perceived racial discrimination in health care was 10.9% among African Americans, 5.2% among Hispanics and 2% among Whites [7], and in a more recent national online survey in 2019 among adults in the US, 21.4% reported health care discrimination [6].

Major perceived reasons for health care discrimination included for "US Whites age (29%), weight or physical appearance (16%), gender (10%) and financial status (10%), and for US Hispanics age (27%), race or ancestry (23%), weight or physical appearance (14%) and financial status (14%)" [5] and in a national US online survey of those reporting experiences of discrimination, "racial/ethnic discrimination was the most common type (17.3%), followed by discrimination based on educational or income level (12.9%), weight (11.6%), sex (11.4%), and age (9.6%)" [6].

Factors associated with health care discrimination may include Blacks versus Whites [5, 7], men [5, 7], middle-aged [7], lower socioeconomic status [5], female sex, younger age, lower income [6, 7], and greater use of complementary and alternative medicine [8]. "To better understand and respond to interpersonal discrimination in the health care system, it is necessary to identify these experiences at the national level" [6]. Therefore, this study aimed to estimate the prevalence and correlates of perceived health care discrimination in middle-aged and older adults in a national population survey in India.

Our Study

National cross-sectional data from the Longitudinal Aging Study in India (LASI) Wave 1, 2017-2018 were analyzed (individual response rate 87%) [9]. "Face-to-face interviews, physical measurement and biomarker data were collected by male and female trained research teams from individuals aged 45 and above and their female spouses, regardless of age, in a household survey from 35 states and union territories of India (excluding Sikkim)" [9]. Field teams input responses directly into a laptop computer. Details of the sampling strategy have been described elsewhere [9]. The study was approved by the Indian Council of Medical Research (ICMR) Ethics Committee and written, or oral informed consent was attained from participants [9].

Measures

Health care discrimination was assessed with the Everyday Discrimination Scale (short version) [10]. In particular, respondents were asked how frequently they "received poorer services or treatment than other people from doctors or hospitals." Responses were coded as never = 0 and "less than once a year/a few times a year/a few times a month/at least once a week/almost every day" = 1). In a follow-up question, participants were asked about the potential reasons for the discrimination. Response options were "age, gender, religion, caste, weight, physical disability, other aspects of physical appearance, financial status, and other." [10].

Covariates consisted of education, age, sex, caste/tribe, religious affiliation, receipt of health insurance, urban and rural residence [9]. Subjective socioeconomic status was assessed with the question, "Please imagine a ten-step ladder, where at the bottom are the people who are the worst off – who have the least money, least education, and the worst jobs or no jobs, and at the top of the ladder are the people who are the best off – those who have the most money, most education, and best jobs. Please indicate the number (1-10) on the rung on the ladder where you would place yourself" [9]. Steps 1 to 3 on the socioeconomic ladder were defined as low, 4-5 as medium, and 6-10 as high.

Food insecurity was assessed with four questions, 1) "In the last 12 months, did you ever reduce the size of your meals or skip meals because there was not enough food at your household? (Yes, No) 2) In the last 12 months, were you hungry but didn't eat because there was not enough food at your household? 3) In the past 12 months, did you ever not eat for a whole day because there was not enough food in your household? and 4) Do you think that you have lost weight in the last 12 months because there was not enough food in your household?" (Yes, No) [9]. Any positive response to the four questions was scored as one.

Utilization of traditional and complementary medicine practitioners was assessed with two questions, 1) "In the past 12 months, have you consulted any AYUSH practitioner (Ayurveda /Yoga/Naturopathy/Unani/ Siddha /Homeopathy)? (Yes, No)" and 2) "In the past 12 months, have you consulted any Traditional /Folk healers (tribal medicine/bhopa/jhaad-fook/black magic)? (Yes, No)." [9].

Data analysis

Considering the clustered study design, data analyses were conducted with "STATA software version 15.0 (Stata Corporation, College Station, TX, USA)." Unadjusted and adjusted logistic regression analyses were used to calculate associations between independent variables and health care discrimination. Covariates were selected based on previous literature review [5-8]. *P*-values of below 0.05 were accepted as significant and missing values were excluded from the analysis.

FINDINGS

The sample included 72,262 middle-aged and older adults (45 years and older), 58.0% were female and 42.0% male. Almost half of the participants

(49.5%) had no formal education, and 68.2% were residing in rural areas.

Table 1. Sample characteristics among middle-aged and older adults in India, 2017-2018 (N = 72,262)

Variable	Variable specification	Sample	Health care discrimination
		%	
All			**5.9**
Age in years	45-59	54.1	5.7
	60-69	26.8	6.3
	70 or more	19.0	6.0
Sex	Female	58.0	5.7
	Male	42.0	6.3
Education in years	0	49.5	7.3
	1-4	10.8	6.0
	5-9	21.1	5.2
	≥10	18.5	3.4
Subjective socioeconomic status	Low	37.2	7.3
	Medium	38.7	5.5
	High	24.1	4.5
Has health insurance	No	80.3	6.3
	Yes	20.7	4.4
Caste/tribe	None of the below	18.5	5.1
	Scheduled tribe	49.5	7.3
	Scheduled caste	10.8	5.4
	Other backward class	21.1	6.1
Religious affiliation	Hindu	81.9	6.2
	Muslim	11.7	5.9
	Christian	3.0	3.6
	Sikh	1.8	1.7
	Other or none	1.7	3.8
Residence	Rural	68.2	6.4
	Urban	31.8	5.0
Food insecurity	No	90.3	5.0
	Yes	9.7	14.3
Utilization of traditional or complementary medicine	No	87.0	5.5
	Yes	13.0	8.7

One in ten participants (9.7%) had food insecurity, 37.2% had low subjective socioeconomic status, and 20.7% had health insurance. The utilization of a traditional or complementary practitioner in the past 12 months was 13.0%, and the prevalence of perceived health care discrimination was 5.9% (see Table 1).

Perceived reasons of health care discrimination

Overall, among participants with health care discrimination, the major perceived reasons of health care discrimination included age (51.4%), followed by financial status (48.2%), Caste (16.0%), and gender (10.7%). Women had a higher rate of gender as a reason for health care discrimination than men, and men reported more frequently physical disability and other aspects of physical appearance than women did (see Table 2).

Table 2. Perceived reasons of health care discrimination (multiple responses possible) (N = 3,845)

Variable	All	Male	Female
	%	%	%
Age	51.4	50.2	52.3
Gender	10.7	5.5	14.9*
Religion	5.8	6.4	5.3
Caste	16.0	16.8	15.4
Weight	2.5	2.4	2.6
Physical disability	3.9	6.1	2.1*
Other aspect of physical appearance	7.5	9.0	6.4*
Financial status	48.2	47.2	49.0
Other	4.2	4.3	4.0

$^{*}p < 0.001$

Associations with perceived health care discrimination

In the adjusted logistic regression analysis, male sex, food insecurity, and utilization of traditional or complementary medicine practitioners were positively associated with health care discrimination, while higher education, higher subjective socioeconomic status, receipt of health insurance, Christian, Sikh and other religion were negatively associated with health care discrimination. In addition, in unadjusted analysis, scheduled tribes, other backward classes and rural residence were associated with health care discrimination (see Table 3).

Table 3. Associations with health care discrimination (N = 72,262)

Variable	Variable specification	COR (95% CI)	AOR (95% CI)
Age in years	45-59	1 (Reference)	---
	60-69	1.09 (0.97, 1.23)	
	70 or more	1.06 (0.91, 1.23)	
Sex	Female	1 (Reference)	1 (Reference)
	Male	1.12 (1.00, 1.25)*	1.30 (1.15, 1.46)***
Education	0	1 (Reference)	1 (Reference)
	1-4	0.82 (0.70, 0.97)*	0.83 (0.70, 0.98)*
	5-9	0.70 (0.60, 0.81)***	0.74 (0.64, 0.87)***
	≥10	0.45 (0.39, 0.63)***	0.51 (0.42, 0.62)***
Subjective socioeconomic status	Low	1 (Reference)	1 (Reference)
	Medium	0.74 (0.66, 0.82)***	0.89 (0.79, 0.99)*
	High	0.59 (0.51, 0.70)***	0.82 (0.70, 0.96)*
Has health insurance	No	1 (Reference)	1 (Reference)
	Yes	0.67 (0.60, 0.77)***	0.72 (0.64, 0.82)***
Caste/tribe	None of the below	1 (Reference)	1 (Reference)
	Scheduled tribe	1.49 (1.29, 1.71)***	1.13 (0.97, 1.32)
	Scheduled caste	1.07 (0.89, 1.29)	0.89 (0.73, 1.09)
	Other backward classes	1.21 (1.06, 1.38)**	1.07 (0.94, 1.23)
Religious affiliation	Hindu	1 (Reference)	1 (Reference)
	Muslim	0.96 (0.82, 1.12)	0.89 (0.75, 1.05)
	Christian	0.56 (0.41, 0.78)***	0.66 (0.47, 0.93)*
	Sikh	0.26 (0.18, 0.38)***	0.26 (0.18, 0.39)***
	Other or none	0.60 (0.39, 0.93)*	0.60 (0.38, 0.95)*
Residence	Rural	1 (Reference)	1 (Reference)
	Urban	0.77 (0.67, 0.88)***	1.05 (0.89, 1.23)
Food insecurity	No	1 (Reference)	1 (Reference)
	Yes	3.19 (2.76, 3.71)***	2.84 (2.46, 3.28)***
Utilization of traditional or complementary medicine practitioners	No	1 (Reference)	1 (Reference)
	Yes	1.62 (1.42, 1.85)***	1.33 (1.17, 1.53)***

COR = Crude Odds Ratio, AOR = Adjusted Odds ratio; CI = Confidence Interval; *$p < 0.05$; **$p < 0.01$; ***$p < 0.001$

Discussion

The study aimed to estimate the prevalence and correlates of perceived health care discrimination in middle-aged and older adults in a national population survey in India in 2017-2018. Results show for the first time that the prevalence of perceived health care discrimination was 5.9% in India, which is lower than in previous studies in USA (20% among Blacks and

19% among Whites in 2014 [5], 10.9% among African Americans, 5.2% among Hispanics and 2% among Whites [7], and 21.4% in 2019) [6].

The study found, among participants with health care discrimination, the major perceived reasons of health care discrimination included age (51.4%), financial status (48.2%), caste (16.0%), and gender (10.7%). In comparison, in US surveys, similarly most common reasons for health care discrimination included age, race or ancestry, gender, and financial status. However, in US surveys a higher prevalence of discrimination against weight or physical appearance (16%) among Whites and 14% among US Hispanics was found than in this survey (9.8%). Nevertheless, the prevalence of health care discrimination identified in this investigation in India emphasises the need for further studies on the potential negative impacts of health care discrimination [6], considering the major types of perceived reasons of discrimination, as identified in this study, including, age, financial status, caste, and gender.

Consistent with previous studies [5-8], this study found an association between male sex, lower socioeconomic status (lower education, lower subjective socioeconomic status, and food insecurity), not having health insurance, use of traditional and complementary medicine and perceived health care discrimination. It is possible that discrimination is more prevalent in persons with lower socioeconomic status and not having health insurance because it is too costly to obtain medical care [7], which is also confirmed by the high prevalence of experiencing discrimination because of financial status (48.2%). Ageism in health care was the most important perceived reason of discrimination (51.4%) in this study, calling for specific strategies to address the discrimination experienced by older persons in India [11]. Persons with lower socioeconomic status are more likely to use traditional and complementary medicine than those with higher socioeconomic status in this study (analysis not shown), which may partially explain the association between traditional and complementary medicine use and perceived health care discrimination [8].

Compared to Hindus, Christians and Sikhs had lower odds of health care discrimination, and compared to none of the lower castes, scheduled tribes and other backward classes had in univariate analysis higher odds for health care discrimination. Previous studies in the US population [5, 7], also found significant differences between different racial or ancestry groups in the prevalence of health care discrimination. In an additional analysis of states in India, we found the prevalence of perceived health care discrimination was the highest in Dehli (15.3%) and Jammu and Kashmir (14.7%), highlighting the need to address health care discrimination in these identified states using localized approaches. Health care providers should be aware that a significant proportion of their patients have experienced health care discrimination, which negatively impacts on patient satisfaction, patient-care provider relationship and utilization of health care [5].

Strength and limitations of the study

Study strengths included the use of standardized measures adapted from the Health and Retirement Study and a large, nationally representative sample of middle-aged and older adults in India. The self-report of most data may have their limitations. It is possible that participants underreported health care discrimination. Health care discrimination was only assessed with one item, and future studies should include several items. Due to the cross-sectional design of the study, we were unable to determine the direction of the assessed associations.

CONCLUSION

A significant proportion (5.9%) of middle-aged and older adults in India experienced perceived health care discrimination. Factors associated with perceived health care discrimination included male sex, food insecurity, utilization of traditional or complementary medicine practitioner, lower education, lower subjective socioeconomic status, not having health insurance, and Hindus. These associated factors, together with major perceived reasons of health care discrimination (age, financial status, caste, and gender) may be targeted in an effort to reduce health care discrimination.

ACKNOWLEDGMENTS

The Longitudinal Aging Study in India Project is funded by the Ministry of Health and Family Welfare, Government of India, the National Institute on Aging (R01 AG042778, R01 AG030153), and United Nations Population Fund, India.

REFERENCES

[1] Pascoe EA, Smart Richman L. Perceived discrimination and health: a meta-analytic review. Psychol Bull 2009;135(4):531-54. doi: 10.1037/a0016059.

[2] Branscombe NR, Schmitt MT, Harvey RD. Perceiving pervasive discrimination among African-Americans: Implications for group identification and well-being. J Pers Soc Psychol 1999;77:135–49.

[3] Schmitt MT, Branscombe NR. The meaning and consequences of perceived discrimination in disadvantaged and privileged social groups. Eur Rev Soc Psychol 2002;12:167-99. doi: 10.1080/14792772143000058.

[4] Mouzon DM, Taylor RJ, Woodward A, Chatters LM. Everyday Racial Discrimination, Everyday Non-racial Discrimination, and Physical Health Among African Americans. J Ethn Cult Divers Soc Work 2017;26(1-2):68-80. doi: 10.1080/15313204.2016.1187103.

[5] Nguyen TT, Vable AM, Glymour MM, Nuru-Jeter A. Trends for reported discrimination in health care in a national sample of older adults with chronic conditions. J Gen Intern Med 2018;33(3):291-7. doi: 10.1007/s11606-017-4209-5.

[6] Nong P, Raj M, Creary M, Kardia SLR, Platt JE. Patient-reported experiences of discrimination in the US health care system. JAMA Netw Open 20201; 3(12): e2029650. doi: 10.1001/jamanetworkopen.2020.29650.

[7] Hausmann LR, Jeong K, Bost JE, Ibrahim SA. Perceived discrimination in health care and health status in a racially diverse sample. Med Care 2008;46(9):905-14. doi: 10.1097/MLR.0b013e3181792562.

[8] Shippee TP, Schafer MH, Ferraro KF. Beyond the barriers: racial discrimination and use of complementary and alternative medicine among Black Americans. Soc Sci Med 2012;74(8):1155-62. doi: 10.1016/j.socscimed.2012.01.003.

[9] International Institute for Population Sciences (IIPS), NPHCE, MoHFW, Harvard TH Chan School of Public Health (HSPH) and the University of Southern California (USC). Longitudinal Ageing Study in India (LASI) Wave 1, 2017-18, India Report. Mumbai: International Institute for Population Sciences, 2020.

[10] Sternthal MJ, Slopen N, Williams DR. Racial disparities in health: How much does stress really matter? Du Bois Rev 2011;8(1):95-113. doi: 10.1017/S1742058X11000087.

[11] Saif-Ur-Rahman KM, Mamun R, Eriksson E, He Y, Hirakawa Y. Discrimination against the elderly in health-care services: A systematic review. Psychogeriatrics 2021;21(3):418-29. doi: 10.1111/psyg.12670.

In: Social and Health Issues … ISBN: 978-1-53619-937-6
Editors: S Pengpid, K Peltzer et al.

Chapter 22

PERCEIVED WEIGHT DISCRIMINATION AMONG MIDDLE-AGED AND OLDER ADULTS IN INDIA: RESULTS OF A NATIONAL SURVEY IN 2017-2018

Supa Pengpid[1,2], MPH, DrPH, MBA
and Karl Peltzer[2,3,*], MA Clin Psych, PhD, Dr Habil
[1]ASEAN Institute for Health Development,
Mahidol University, Salaya, Phutthamonthon,
Nakhon Pathom, Thailand
[2]Department of Research Administration and Development,
University of Limpopo, Turfloop, South Africa
[3]Department of Psychology, College of Medical and Health Science,
Asia University, Taichung, Taiwan

* *Correspondence*: Professor Karl Peltzer, Department of Research Administration and Development, University of Limpopo, Turfloop Campus, Private Bag X1106, Sovenga 0727, South Africa. Email: kfpeltzer@gmail.com.

ABSTRACT

This chapter aimed to estimate the prevalence and correlates of perceived weight discrimination in middle-aged and older adults in a national population survey in India. The sample included 72,262 middle-aged and older adults from a cross-sectional national community dwelling survey in India in 2017-2018. Results indicate that the prevalence of perceived weight discrimination was 0.3%, 0.3% among women, and 0.2% among men. Among participants with weight discrimination, the major discriminatory situations were less courtesy (82.2%), followed by service setting (65.3%), and less clever (64.4%). In the adjusted logistic regression analysis, no education and food insecurity were positively associated with perceived weight discrimination, while urban residence, Muslim and Christians were negatively associated with perceived weight discrimination. In addition, in unadjusted analysis, underweight was marginally significantly associated with perceived weight discrimination, while obesity was not significantly associated with perceived weight discrimination. A low proportion (0.3%) of middle-aged and older adults in India experienced weight discrimination, and several associated factors were identified that may be targeted to reduce weight discrimination.

INTRODUCTION

Perceived discrimination can be defined as "a behavioural manifestation of a negative attitude, judgment, or unfair treatment toward members of a group", such as age, gender, religion, caste, weight, physical disability, physical appearance, and financial status, and can be characterised as a form of stress [1]. In India, among women, 20.1% are underweight (body mass index (BMI) <18.5 kg/m^2) and 36.3% are overweight or have obesity (BMI ≥ 23.0 kg/m^2) [2]. Among American College women with "under- or overweight BMIs experienced greater stigmatization for their body weight than women with average BMIs, underscoring the need for research to investigate weight discrimination across the weight spectrum" [3]. Little is known about perceived weight discrimination in a middle-income country, such as India.

In a study among adults (≥50 years) in England, 4.6% reported weight discrimination, ranging from 0.8% in persons with normal or underweight, 0.9% overweight, 6.7% class I obesity, 24.2% class II obesity and 35.1% class III obesity [4], and in USA among 25–74-year-olds the prevalence of weight/height discrimination was 5% among men and 10% among women [5]. In USA, the prevalence of perceived "weight/height discrimination increased from 7% in 1995-1996 to 12% in 2004-2006" [6], and in Germany, the overall prevalence of weight discrimination was 7.3%, 19.7% among underweight and 18.7% in obesity class II participants [7].

The proportion of participants with weight discrimination reported different discriminatory situations in England, with the highest less courtesy, followed by less clever, service setting, harassed and medical setting [4]. Factors associated with weight discrimination are younger age [5, 7], women [5, 7, 8], lower socioeconomic status [4, 5], overweight, obesity [4, 5, 7], higher BMI [5, 9], underweight [7]. To better understand and respond to weight discrimination in India, it is necessary to identify these experiences at the national level. The objective of our study was to characterize weight discrimination in a nationally representative sample of the Indian middle-aged and older adult population in terms of prevalence, primary types of discrimination, and correlates of perceived weight discrimination.

OUR STUDY

National cross-sectional data from the Longitudinal Aging Study in India (LASI) Wave 1, 2017-2018 were analyzed (individual response rate 87%) [15]. Face-to-face interviews were conducted by male and female trained research teams with individuals aged 45 and above and their female spouses, regardless of age, in a household survey from 35 states and union territories of India (excluding Sikkim). Field teams input responses directly into a laptop computer. Details of the sampling strategy have been described elsewhere [15]. The Indian Council of Medical Research (ICMR) Ethics Committee approved the study and written informed consent was attained from participants [15].

Measures

Perceived weight discrimination was assessed with the six-item Everyday Discrimination Scale (short version) [11]. Response options ranged from 1 = "never" to 6 = "almost every day", and were dichotomised to 'never' = 0 and 'ever' (collapsing those reporting 'less than once a year' or greater into one category) = 1. In a follow-up question to any of the six discrimination experiences, potential reasons were asked, including "age, gender, religion, caste, weight, physical disability, other aspects of physical appearance, financial status and other." [11]. Those who responded that any discrimination experience was due to their weight were defined as cases of perceived weight discrimination [4].

Covariates consisted of education, age, sex, caste/tribe, religious affiliation, urban and rural residence [10]. Subjective socioeconomic status was assessed with the question, "Please imagine a ten-step ladder, where at the bottom are the people who are the worst off – who have the least money, least education, and the worst jobs or no jobs, and at the top of the ladder are the people who are the best off – those who have the most money, most education, and best jobs. Please indicate the number (1-10) on the rung on the ladder where you would place yourself." [10]. Steps 1 to 3 on the socioeconomic ladder were defined as low, 4-5 as medium, and 6-10 as high.

Food insecurity was assessed with four questions, 1) "In the last 12 months, did you ever reduce the size of your meals or skip meals because there was not enough food at your household? (Yes/No) 2) In the last 12 months, were you hungry but didn't eat because there was not enough food at your household? (Yes/No) 3) In the past 12 months, did you ever not eat for a whole day because there was not enough food at your household? 4) Do you think that you have lost weight in the last 12 months because there was not enough food in your household?" [10]. Any positive response to the four questions was scored as one.

Anthropometry: "Height and weight of adults were measured using the Seca 803 digital scale." [10]. "Body Mass Index = BMI was calculated according to Asian criteria: underweight (<18.5 kg/m^2), normal weight (18.5-22.9 kg/m^2), overweight (23.0-24.9 kg/m^2), class I obesity (25.0-29.9 kg/m^2), and class II obesity (≥30.0 kg/m^2)" [12].

Data analysis

Considering the clustered study design, data analyses were conducted with "STATA software version 15.0 (Stata Corporation, College Station, TX, USA)." Unadjusted and adjusted logistic regression analyses were used to calculate associations between independent variables and perceived weight discrimination. Variables with a significance level of 0.05 in univariate analyses were subsequently included in the multivariable model. Covariates were selected based on previous literature review [4-7]. *P*-values of below 0.05 were accepted as significant and missing values were excluded from the analysis.

FINDINGS

The sample included 72,262 middle-aged and older adults (45 years and older), 58.0% were female and 42.0% male. Almost half of the participants (49.5%) had no formal education, and 68.2% were residing in rural areas. One in ten participants (9.7%) had food insecurity, and 37.2% had low subjective socioeconomic status. Regarding body weight status, 37.2% had normal weight, 23.0% underweight, 13.7% overweight, 19.7% class I obesity, and 6.4% class II obesity. The prevalence of perceived weight discrimination was 0.3%, 0.3% among women, and 0.2% among men (see Table 1).

Table 1. Sample characteristics of middle-age and older adults in India, 2017-2018 (N = 72,262)

Variable	Variable specification	Sample	Perceived weight discrimination
		%	%
All			**0.3**
Weight status	Normal	37.2	0.2
	Underweight	23.0	0.4
	Overweight	13.7	0.2
	Class I obesity	19.7	0.3
	Class II obesity	6.4	0.3
Age in years	45-59	54.1	0.3
	60-69	26.8	0.3
	70 or more	19.0	0.2
Sex	Female	58.0	0.3
	Male	42.0	0.2
Education	≥1 year	50.5	0.2
	No schooling	49.5	0.3
Subjective socioeconomic status	Low	37.2	0.3
	Medium	38.7	0.2
	High	24.1	0.3
Food insecurity	No	90.3	0.2
	Yes	9.7	0.8
Caste/tribe	None of the below	18.5	0.3
	Scheduled tribe	49.5	0.2
	Scheduled caste	10.8	0.3
	Other backward class	21.1	0.3
Religious affiliation	Hindu	81.9	0.3
	Muslim	11.7	0.1
	Christian	3.0	0.0
	Sikh	1.8	0.5
	Other or none	1.7	0.6
Residence	Rural	68.2	0.3
	Urban	31.8	0.2

Perceived weight discrimination in different discriminatory situations

Major discriminatory situations in people with weight discrimination were less courtesy (82.2%), followed by service setting (65.3%), and less clever (64.4%). Women had a higher rate of courtesy discrimination than men and men had a higher rate of harassed and medical setting discrimination (see Table 2).

Table 2. Proportion of participants reporting perceived weight discrimination in different discriminatory situations (N = 163)

Variable	All	Male	Female
	%	%	%
Less courtesy	82.2	78.2	84.4*
Service setting	65.3	64.8	65.6
Less clever	64.4	66.5	63.2
Harassed	57.5	63.4	54.2*
Medical setting	54.7	65.8	48.5*

*$p < 0.001$

Table 3. Associations with perceived weight discrimination (N = 72,262)

Variable	Variable specification	COR (95% CI)	AOR (95% CI)
Weight status (BMI)	Normal	1 (Reference)	1 (Reference)
	Underweight	1.73 (0.98, 3.07)	1.46 (0.82, 2.59)
	Overweight	0.63 (0.31, 1.30)	0.73 (0.36, 1.50)
	Class I obesity	1.04 (0.59, 1.84)	1.35 (0.79, 2.33)
	Class II obesity	1.24 (0.63, 2.41)	1.72 (0.87, 3.39)
Age in years	45-59	1 (Reference)	---
	60-69	1.00 (0.63, 1.58)	
	70 or more	0.76 (0.43, 1.35)	
Sex	Female	1 (Reference)	---
	Male	0.77 (0.52, 1.15)	
Education	≥1 year	1 (Reference)	1 (Reference)
	No schooling	1.78 (1.20, 2.65)**	1.60 (1.08, 2.38)*
Subjective socioeconomic status	Low	1 (Reference)	---
	Medium	0.85 (0.51, 1.42)	
	High	1.23 (0.79, 1.90)	
Caste/tribe	None of the below	1 (Reference)	---
	Scheduled tribe	0.68 (0.37, 1.23)	
	Scheduled caste	0.74 (0.26, 2.09)	
	Other backward classes	0.80 (0.49, 1.30)	
Religious affiliation	Hindu	1 (Reference)	1 (Reference)
	Muslim	0.43 (0.21, 0.86)*	0.40 (0.19, 0.84)*
	Christian	0.15 (0.03, 0.74)*	0.04 (0.01, 0.10)***
	Sikh	1.81 (0.87, 3.77)	1.64 (0.74, 3.63)
	Other or none	2.24 (0.40, 12.48)	2.69 (0.47, 15.49)
Residence	Rural	1 (Reference)	1 (Reference)
	Urban	0.51 (0.32, 0.79)**	0.56 (0.34, 0.91)*
Food insecurity	No	1 (Reference)	1 (Reference)
	Yes	3.54 (2.29, 5.49)***	3.02 (1.88, 4.85)***

COR = Crude Odds Ratio, AOR = Adjusted Odds ratio; CI = Confidence Interval; *$p < 0.05$; **$p < 0.01$; ***$p < 0.001$

Associations with perceived weight discrimination

In the adjusted logistic regression analysis, no education and food insecurity were positively associated with perceived weight discrimination, while urban residence, Muslim, and Christians were negatively associated with perceived weight discrimination. In addition, in unadjusted analysis, underweight was marginally significantly associated with perceived weight discrimination, while obesity was not significantly associated with perceived weight discrimination (see Table 3).

DISCUSSION

The study aimed to estimate the prevalence and correlates of perceived weight discrimination in middle-aged and older adults in a national population survey in India in 2017-2018. Results show for the first time that the prevalence of perceived weight discrimination was 0.3% in India, which is lower than in previous studies in England (4.6%, ≥50 years) [4], and in Germany (7.3%, adults) [7]. The overall prevalence of perceived weight discrimination (0.3%) only marginally increased in the underweight population (0.4%) and was the same in the obesity population (0.3%), while previous studies [4, 7] found very significant increases of perceived weight discrimination in those who were underweight (e.g., 19.7% in Germany [7] and who were obese (e.g., 18.7% in obesity class II in Germany) [7] and 24.2% class II obesity in England [4]. Results in India show that the public's stigma towards people with weight deviance was only marginally true for underweight but not for obesity, unlike in studies in high-income countries [4, 7]. This finding may indicate that in India obesity is not seen as a major problem, as a community survey in Kerala, India, showed that "50.2% of the participants did not know the seriousness of obesity as a problem of an individual's health and 31.4% that obesity is not a so serious problem to health." [13]. Some of these weight deviance differences in terms of obesity may be related to the low prevalence of class II obesity (6.4%, using Asian criteria ≥30.0 kg/m^2) in India compared to the obesity prevalence rate in some of the studied high-income countries (e.g., 31.1% ≥30.0 kg/m^2 in England) [4]. In most studies higher prevalence levels of obesity seem to be associated with higher prevalence of weight discrimination [7].

Like a study in England [4], the proportion of participants with weight discrimination reported the highest discrimination in terms of less courtesy, less clever, and service setting. Some previous studies found that weight discrimination is more prevalent at younger age [5, 7], and among women [5, 7, 8], this study did not find significant age and sex differences. Consistent with previous research [4, 5], this study showed that lower socioeconomic status (no education, food insecurity, and rural residence) increased the odds of perceived weight discrimination. Compared to Hindus, Muslims and Christians had lower odds of perceived weight discrimination, while there were no significant differences in terms of castes or tribes. Compared to people with lower socioeconomic status, people with higher socioeconomic status (having some education, not having food insecurity, and residing in urban areas) may be "less likely to experience weight discrimination due to lessor exposure to discriminatory situations or a greater sense of control" [4, 14]. Bias or stigma towards weight deviance, such as obesity and underweight, may be an important barrier to successful weight management [7], and should be addressed in public health interventions.

Strength and limitations of the study

Study strengths included the use of standardized measures adapted from the Health and Retirement Study and a large, nationally representative sample of middle-aged and older adults in India. The self-report of most data may have their limitations. It is possible that participants underreported weight discrimination. Perceived weight discrimination was only assessed with one item, and future studies should include several items. Due to the cross-sectional design of the study, we were unable to determine the direction of the assessed associations.

Conclusion

A low proportion (0.3%) of middle-aged and older adults in India experienced weight discrimination. Factors associated with perceived weight discrimination included no education, food insecurity, rural residence, Hindus, and marginally underweight. These associated factors may be targeted to reduce perceived weight discrimination.

Acknowledgments

The Longitudinal Aging Study in India Project is funded by the Ministry of Health and Family Welfare, Government of India, the National Institute on Aging (R01 AG042778, R01 AG030153), and United Nations Population Fund, India.

References

[1] Pascoe EA, Smart Richman L. Perceived discrimination and health: a meta-analytic review. Psychol Bull 2009;135(4):531-54. doi: 10.1037/a0016059.

[2] Pengpid S, Peltzer K. Prevalence and correlates of underweight and overweight/ obesity among women in India: results from the National Family Health Survey 2015-2016. Diabetes Metab Syndr Obes 2019;12:647-53. doi: 10.2147/DMSO. S206855.

[3] Davies A, Burnette CB, Mazzeo SE. Real women have (just the right) curves: investigating anti-thin bias in college women. Eat Weight Disord 2020;25(6):1711-8. doi: 10.1007/s40519-019-00812-7.

[4] Jackson SE, Steptoe A, Beeken RJ, Croker H, Wardle J. Perceived weight discrimination in England: A population-based study of adults aged ⩾50 years. Int J Obes 2015;39(5):858-64. doi: 10.1038/ijo.2014.186.

[5] Puhl RM, Andreyeva T, Brownell KD. Perceptions of weight discrimination: prevalence and comparison to race and gender discrimination in America. Int J Obes 2008;32(6):992-1000. doi: 10.1038/ijo.2008.22.

[6] Andreyeva T, Puhl RM, Brownell KD. Changes in perceived weight discrimination among Americans, 1995-1996 through 2004-2006. Obesity 2008;16(5):1129-34. doi: 10.1038/oby.2008.35.

[7] Sikorski C, Spahlholz J, Hartlev M, Riedel-Heller SG. Weight-based discrimination: an ubiquitary phenomenon? Int J Obes 2016;40(2):333-7. doi: 10.1038/ijo.2015.165.

[8] Dutton GR, Lewis TT, Durant N, Halanych J, Kiefe CI, Sidney S, et al. Perceived weight discrimination in the CARDIA study: Differences by race, sex, and weight status. Obesity 2014;22(2):530-6. doi: 10.1002/oby.20438.

[9] Stepanikova I, Baker EH, Simoni ZR, Zhu A, Rutland SB, Sims M, et al. The role of perceived discrimination in obesity among African Americans. Am J Prev Med 2017;52(1S1):S77-85. doi: 10.1016/j.amepre.2016.07.034.

[10] International Institute for Population Sciences (IIPS), NPHCE, MoHFW, Harvard TH Chan School of Public Health (HSPH) and the University of Southern California (USC). Longitudinal Ageing Study in India (LASI) Wave 1, 2017-18, India Report. Mumbai: International Institute for Population Sciences, 2020.

[11] Sternthal MJ, Slopen N, Williams DR. Racial disparities in health: How much does stress really matter? Du Bois Rev 2011;8(1):95-113. doi: 10.1017/S1742058X11000087.

[12] Wen CP, David Cheng TY, Tsai SP, Chan HT, Hsu HL, Hsu CC, et al. Are Asians at greater mortality risks for being overweight than Caucasians? Redefining obesity for Asians. Public Health Nutr 2009;12(4):497-506. doi: 10.1017/S1368980008002802.

[13] Anandhasayanam A, Kannan S, Md. Dinsar and Saranya P: Prevalence of obesity and its link between various disorders in a semi urban district in Kerala. Int J Pharm Sci Res 2016;7(9):3826-34. doi: 10.13040/IJPSR.0975-8232.7(9).3826-34.

[14] Rippon I, Kneale D, de Oliveira C, Demakakos P, Steptoe A. Perceived age discrimination in older adults. Age Ageing 2014;43(3):379-86. doi: 10.1093/ageing/aft146.

In: Social and Health Issues … ISBN: 978-1-53619-937-6
Editors: S Pengpid, K Peltzer et al.

Chapter 23

RELIGIOSITY AND WELL-BEING (SELF-REPORTED HEALTH, HAPPINESS, AND LIFE SATISFACTION) AMONG MIDDLE-AGED AND OLDER ADULTS IN INDIA: RESULTS OF A NATIONAL SURVEY IN 2017-2018

Karl Peltzer[1,2], MA Clin Psych, PhD, Dr Habil and Supa Pengpid[1,3,*], MPH, DrPH, MBA

[1]Department of Research Administration and Development, University of Limpopo, Turfloop, South Africa

[2]Department of Psychology, College of Medical and Health Science, Asia University, Taichung, Taiwan

[3]ASEAN Institute for Health Development, Mahidol University, Salaya, Phutthamonthon, Nakhon Pathom, Thailand

[*] *Correspondence*: Professor Supa Pengpid, ASEAN Institute for Health Development, Mahidol University, 25/25 Phutthamonthon Road 4, Salaya, Phutthamonton, Nakhon Pathom 73170, Thailand. Email: supaprom@yahoo.com.

Abstract

In this chapter we aimed to assess the associations between religiosity (affiliation, involvement, and intrinsic religiosity) and well-being indicators (self-rated health, happiness, and life satisfaction) among middle-aged and older adults in India. The cross-sectional sample consisted of 72,262 persons (45 years and older) from the 2017-2018 Longitudinal Ageing Study in India (LASI) Wave 1. The prevalence of Hindu religious affiliation was 81.9%, followed Muslim 11.7%, Christian 3.0%, Sikh 1.8% and other or none 1.7%. More than half of the participants (57.0%) do pooja or prayer every day, 14.0% attend religious services more than once a week or every day, 21.5% were involved in religious gatherings at least once a month, 34.9% had high spirituality or religiosity, and 79.2% considered religion as very important in their lives. The mean self-rated health status was 2.77 (range 1-5), mean happiness 2.48 (range 1-4), and mean life satisfaction 23.66 (range 5-35). In the adjusted ordered logistic regression analysis, daily pooja or prayer, higher spirituality/religiousness, and religious importance were significantly positively associated with self-rated health, happiness, and life satisfaction. Medium or high attendance of religious services was positively associated with self-rated health or with life satisfaction. Medium or high involvement in religious gatherings was positively associated with self-rated health or happiness. Compared to Hindus, Muslims and Sikhs had lower odds of self-rated health, Sikhs had higher odds of happiness, and Christians lower odds of life satisfaction. Daily pooja or prayer, higher spirituality/religiousness, and religious importance were significantly positively associated with self-rated health, happiness, and life satisfaction.

Introduction

In a study on well-being of older adults in India, "results suggest that normal activities of daily life, health, and social ties decline with advancing age, while life accomplishment remains stable over age. However, when all domains are integrated, well-being tends to fade out with advancing age" [1]. Several studies suggest that greater religiosity is associated with better well-being across the life course [2-4]. For example, stronger private devotion (devotional) and higher frequency of religious attendance (participatory) were both positively related to life satisfaction [5]. Most of the studies investigating the relationship between religiosity and well-being indicators, such as self-reported health, happiness and life satisfaction have been conducted in high-income countries [6-9].

There is a lack of research studying the association between religiosity variables (affiliation, involvement, and intrinsic religiosity) and well-being indicators, such as self-reported health, happiness and life satisfaction, in low- and middle-income countries, such as in India. In a pilot survey among older adults in India, attendance of religious function was associated with well-being [1], in a study among older adults in Columbia higher religiosity was associated with better self-rated [10], among older adults in Malaysia [11], intrinsic religiosity was positively associated with life satisfaction, and in a study among older adults from seven cities in Latin America or the Caribbean showed that those who considered "religion as very important were less likely to report fair or poor health compared to those who were less religious (somewhat important, not very important)" [12]. This study aimed to estimate the association between religiosity variables (affiliation, involvement, and intrinsic religiosity) and well-being indicators (self-reported health, happiness and life satisfaction) among middle-aged and older adults in India.

OUR STUDY

This secondary data analysis utilized data from the cross-sectional and nationally representative Longitudinal Ageing Study in India (LASI) Wave 1, 2017-2018; "the overall household response rate is 96%, and the overall individual response rate is 87%" [13]. In a household survey, "interview, physical measurement and biomarker data were collected from individuals aged 45 and above and their spouses, regardless of age" [13]. Specific details on the sampling approach are found elsewhere [13]. The study was approved by the "Indian Council of Medical Research (ICMR) Ethics Committee and written informed consent was obtained from the participants" [13].

Measures

Self-rated health status was sourced from the question, "In general, would you say your health is excellent, very good, good, fair, or poor?" Responses were coded as "1=poor, 2=fair, 3=good, 4=very good and 5=excellent" [13].

Happiness was assessed with the question, "How often did you feel happy?" Response options were: "1=Rarely or never (less than 1 day), 2=Sometimes (1 or 2 days), 3=Often (3 or 4 days), and 4=Most or all of the time (5–7 days)" [13].

Life satisfaction was measured with the 5-item Satisfaction With Life Scale (SWLS) [14]. Total scores ranged from 5-35, and were grouped into 5-9, 10-14, 15-19, 20-24, 25-29, and 30-35, with higher scores indicating higher life satisfaction [14]. Cronbach's alpha for the SWLS in this study was 0.86.

Exposure variables

Religious affiliation was sourced from the question, "What is your religion?" Response options were "None, Hindu, Muslim, Christian, Sikh, Buddhist/neo-Buddhist, Jain, Jewish, Parsi/Zoroastrian and Other, please specify…" [13].

Religious activities were assessed with three questions, "In the past year, how often have you …1) Done pooja or prayer? 2) Attended religious services (at temple/mosque/church, etc.)? and 3) Involved yourself in satsang/bhajan/kirtan/any religious gathering?" Response options ranged from 1=not at all to 6=every day [13].

Religiousness and spirituality was measured with four items from the Daily Spiritual Experience Scale (DSES) [15], e.g., "Do you think that you have a feeling of deep inner peace?" Responses ranged from 1=never to 5=every day in a week, and the summed scores were trichotomized to 4-7=low, 8-11=medium, and 12-20=high. Cronbach's alpha for the DSES in this study was 0.86.

Importance of religion was assessed with the item, "How important would you say religion is in your life?" Responses were dichotomized into 1=very important and 0=somewhat important or not too important [13].

Confounding variables

Level of education (none, some), age group (45-59 and 60 or more years), sex (male, female), marital status (currently married vs. widowed/divorced/separated/deserted/live-in relationship/never married), residence (rural, urban) [13]. *Current tobacco use* was sourced from two items, 1) "Do you currently smoke any tobacco products (cigarettes, bidis, cigars, hookah, cheroot, etc.)? and 2) Do you use smokeless tobacco (such as chewing tobacco, gutka, pan masala, etc.)?" [13]. *Heavy episodic alcohol use* was assessed with the question, "In the last 3 months, how frequently on average, have you had at least 5 or more drinks on one occasion?" [13]. and defined as "one to three days per month, one to four days per week, five or more days per week, or daily."

Data analysis

Descriptive statistics were applied to describe well-being and religiosity indicators. Univariate and multiple ordered logistic regression was utilized to assess the predictors of self-rated health status, happiness, and life satisfaction. Missing values were excluded, $p < 0.05$ showed significance, and no multi-collinearity was detected. Statistical analyses were conducted with STATA software version 15.0 (Stata Corporation, College Station, TX, USA), taking the complex study design into account.

FINDINGS

The sample consisted of 72,262 individuals (≥45 years) from India. The prevalence of Hindu religious affiliation was 81.9%, followed by Muslims

11.7%, Christians 3.0%, Sikhs 1.8% and other or none 1.7%. More than half of the participants (57.0%) do pooja or prayer every day, 14.0% attend religious services more than once a week or every day, 21.5% were involved in religious gatherings at least once a month, 34.9% had a high spirituality or religiosity, and 79.2% considered religion as very important in their lives. The mean self-rated health status was 2.77 (range 1-5), mean happiness 2.48 (range 1-4) and mean life satisfaction 23.66 (range 5-35) (see Table 1).

Table 1. Sample characteristics of middle and older adults in India, 2017-2018

Variable	Sample	Self-rated health	Happiness	Life satisfaction
		M (SD)	M (SD)	M (SD)
All	**72262**	**2.77 (1.0)**	**2.48 (1.0)**	**23.66 (7.5)**
Religious affiliation				
Hindu	52983 (81.9)	2.79 (1.0)	2.49 (1.0)	23.69 (7.5)
Muslim	8668 (11.7)	2.67 (1.0)	2.44 (1.0)	23.48 (7.2)
Christian	7216 (3.0)	2.76 (1.0)	2.39 (1.0)	22.40 (7.9)
Sikh	1999 (1.8)	2.66 (1.0)	2.72 (1.0)	25.04 (6.6)
Other or none	1392 (1.7)	2.82 (1.0)	2.53 (1.0)	24.21 (7.6)
Done pooja or prayer				
1-3 times/month or ≥1 times/year or not at all	14988 (23.8)	2.60 (1.0)	2.35 (1.0)	22.50 (7.6)
Once/week or ≥1/week	13919 (19.2)	2.77 (1.0)	2.41 (1.0)	22.80 (7.4)
Every day	43219 (57.0)	2.84 (1.0)	2.56 (1.0)	24.43 (7.3)
Attendance of religious services				
≥1 times/year or not at all	36760 (53.8)	2.67 (1.0)	2.43 (1.0)	23.12 (7.5)
1-3 times/month	25196 (32.2)	2.90 (1.0)	2.52 (1.0)	24.13 (7.3)
≥1/week or every day	10169 (14.0)	2.88 (1.0)	2.59 (1.0)	24.68 (7.5)
Involved in religious gathering				
Not at all	29650 (42.0)	2.71 (1.0)	2.43 (1.0)	23.36 (7.7)
≥1 times/year	26542 (36.5)	2.74 (1.0)	2.51 (1.0)	23.82 (7.1)
≥1-3 times/month-every day	15933 (21.5)	2.95 (1.0)	2.55 (1.0)	23.98 (7.5)
Spirituality/religiosity				
Low (4-7)	19844 (31.3)	2.62 (1.0)	2.22 (1.0)	21.44 (7.9)
Medium (8-11)	23427 (33.8)	2.79 (1.0)	2.42 (0.9)	23.74 (6.5)
High (12-20)	27069 (34.9)	2.90 (1.0)	2.78 (1.0)	25.58 (7.3)
Religion				
Not very important	13851 (20.8)	2.65 (0.9)	2.30 (1.0)	22.06 (7.6)
Very important	57675 (79.2)	2.81 (1.0)	2.53 (1.0)	24.09 (7.4)

Associations with well-being indicators

Table 2 describes the association between religious variables and well-being indicators in univariate ordered logistic regression (see Table 2).

Table 2. Unadjusted ordered logistic regression with well-being

Variable	Self-rated health	Happiness	Life satisfaction
	UOR (95% CI)	**UOR (95% CI)**	**UOR (95% CI)**
Religiosity variables			
Religious affiliation			
Hindu	1 (Reference)	1 (Reference)	1 (Reference)
Muslim	0.88 (0.83, 0.94)***	0.92 (0.82, 1.04)	0.94 (0.83, 1.06)
Christian	0.97 (0.81, 1.15)	0.85 (0.61, 1.17)	0.77 (0.59, 0.99)*
Sikh	0.87 (0.83, 0.93)***	1.54 (1.39, 1.72)***	1.30 (1.18, 1.44)***
Other or none	1.03 (0.93, 1.14)	1.09 (0.92, 1.29)	1.19 (1.00, 1.40)*
Done pooja or prayer			
1-3 times/month or ≥1	1 (Reference)	1 (Reference)	1 (Reference)
times/year or not at all	1.18 (1.13, 1.24)***	1.12 (1.01, 1.24)*	1.08 (0.99, 1.18)
Once/week or ≥1/week	1.27 (1.22, 1.32)***	1.48 (1.36 (1.61)***	1.56 (1.45, 1.67)***
Every day			
Attendance of religious services			
≥1 times/year or not at all	1 (Reference)	1 (Reference)	1 (Reference)
1-3 times/month	1.26 (1.21, 1.30)***	1.18 (1.09, 1.27)***	1.26 (1.17, 1.35)***
≥1/week or every day	1.23 (1.18, 1.29)***	1.32 (1.22, 1.44)***	1.46 (1.33, 1.60)***
Involved in religious gathering			
Not at all	1 (Reference)	1 (Reference)	1 (Reference)
≥1 times/year	1.04 (1.00, 1.07)*	1.15 (1.08, 1.23)***	1.06 (1.00, 1.13)
≥1-3 times/month-every day	1.28 (1.22, 1.33)***	1.26 (1.15, 1.38)***	1.11 (1.01, 1.23)*
Spirituality/religiosity			
Low (4-7)	1 (Reference)	1 (Reference)	1 (Reference)
Medium (8-11)	1.18 (1.13, 1.23)***	1.46 (1.35, 1.58)***	1.66 (1.53, 1.79)***
High (12-20)	1.32 (1.27, 1.37)***	2.87 (2.66, 3.10)***	2.74 (2.53, 2.97)***
Religion			
Not very important	1 (Reference)	1 (Reference)	1 (Reference)
Very important	1.17 (1.13, 1.22)***	1.52 (1.38, 1.67)***	1.52 (1.39, 1.67)***

UOR: Unadjusted Odds Ratio; CI: Confidence Interval; ***p<0.001, **p<0.01, *p<0.05.

Table 3. Adjusted ordered logistic regression with well-being

Variable	Self-rated health	Happiness	Life satisfaction
	AOR (95% CI)	AOR (95% CI)	AOR (95% CI)
Religiosity variables			
Religious affiliation			
Hindu	1 (Reference)	1 (Reference)	1 (Reference)
Muslim	0.85 (0.80, 0.91)***	0.95 (0.89, 1.00)	0.92 (0.82, 1.04)
Christian	0.90 (0.79, 1.03)	0.87 (0.72, 1.06)	0.69 (0.51, 0.92)*
Sikh	0.83 (0.78, 0.88)***	1.12 (1.05, 1.19)***	1.05 (0.95, 1.16)
Other or none	1.02 (0.92, 1.12)	0.99 (0.90, 1.08)	1.19 (1.00, 1.41)
Done pooja or prayer			
1-3 times/month or ≥1	1 (Reference)	1 (Reference)	1 (Reference)
times/year or not at all	1.05 (0.99, 1.10)	0.99 (0.92, 1.05)	0.90 (0.82, 1.00)
Once/week or ≥1/week	1.07 (1.03, 1.12)***	1.07 (1.01, 1.13)*	1.15 (1.05, 1.26)**
Every day			
Attendance of religious services			
≥1 times/year or not at all	1 (Reference)	1 (Reference)	1 (Reference)
1-3 times/month or once/week	1.10 (1.06, 1.14)***	0.96 (0.92, 1.00)	1.06 (0.97, 1.16)
≥1/week or every day	1.04 (0.99, 1.09)	0.98 (0.93, 1.03)	1.14 (1.02, 1.28)*
Involved in religious gatherings			
Not at all	1 (Reference)	1 (Reference)	1 (Reference)
≥1 times/year	0.98 (0.95, 1.02)	1.05 (1.02, 1.09)**	0.98 (0.92, 1.05)
≥1-3 times/month-every day	1.14 (1.08, 1.19)***	1.03 (0.97, 1.09)	0.89 (0.77, 1.01)
Spirituality/religiosity			
Low (4-7)	1 (Reference)	1 (Reference)	1 (Reference)
Medium (8-11)	1.11 (1.07, 1.16)***	1.19 (1.14, 1.24)***	1.59 (1.46, 1.72)***
High (12-20)	1.22 (1.18, 1.26)***	1.67 (1.61, 1.73)***	2.50 (2.31, 2.71)***
Religion			
Not very important	1 (Reference)	1 (Reference)	1 (Reference)
Very important	1.09 (1.05, 1.13)***	1.14 (1.08, 1.20)***	1.29 (1.17, 1.42)***
Confounding variables			
Sex			
Female	1 (Reference)	1 (Reference)	1 (Reference)
Male	1.09 (1.05, 1.13)***	0.99 (0.95, 1.03)	1.03 (0.95, 1.11)
Age in years			
45-59	1 (Reference)	1 (Reference)	1 (Reference)
60 or more	0.71 (0.69, 0.73)***	1.02 (0.98, 1.05)	1.22 (1.15, 1.30)***
Marital status			
Not married	1 (Reference)	1 (Reference)	1 (Reference)
Married	1.11 (1.07, 1.15)***	1.13 (1.08, 1.18)***	1.26 (1.15, 1.37)***
Education			
Some	1 (Reference)	1 (Reference)	1 (Reference)
None	0.97 (0.94, 1.01)	0.89 (0.86, 0.93)***	0.71 (0.66, 0.76)***

Variable	Self-rated health	Happiness	Life satisfaction
	AOR (95% CI)	**AOR (95% CI)**	**AOR (95% CI)**
Current tobacco use			
No	1 (Reference)	1 (Reference)	1 (Reference)
Yes	0.95 (0.93, 0.98)**	0.97 (0.94, 1.07)*	0.88 (0.83, 0.92)***
Heavy episodic drinking			
No	1 (Reference)	1 (Reference)	1 (Reference)
Yes	1.09 (0.98, 1.22)	1.01 (0.95, 1.07)	1.03 (0.90, 1.17)
Residence			
Rural	1 (Reference)	1 (Reference)	1 (Reference)
Urban	1.17 (1.13, 1.22)***	1.05 (1.01, 1.10)*	1.07 (0.98, 1.16)

AOR: Adjusted Odds Ratio; adjusted for all variables in the table; CI: Confidence Interval; ***p<0.001, **p<0.01, *p<0.05.

In the adjusted ordered logistic regression analysis, daily pooja or prayer, higher spirituality/religiousness, and religious importance were significantly positively associated with self-rated health, happiness, and life satisfaction. Medium attendance of religious services was positively associated with self-rated health and high attendance of religious services was positively associated with life satisfaction. High involvement in religious gathering was positively associated with self-rated health, and medium involvement in religious gathering was positively associated with happiness. Compared to Hindus, Muslims and Sikhs had lower odds of self-rated health, Sikhs had higher odds of happiness, and Christians lower odds of life satisfaction (see Table 3).

Discussion

In this national study of middle-aged and older adults in India, the study aimed to assess the associations between religiosity (affiliation, involvement, and intrinsic religiosity) and well-being indicators (self-rated health, happiness, and life satisfaction). Independent of confounding factors, religious activity (daily pooja or prayer, and/or attendance of religious services and/or involvement in religious gatherings), higher spirituality/religiousness, and religious importance were significantly positively associated with self-rated health, happiness, and life satisfaction.

These findings are in agreement with previous research among older adults in low- and middle-income countries that have found religiosity was associated with well-being in India [1], better self-rated health in Colombia [10] and seven cities in the Americas [12], and higher life satisfaction in Malaysia [11]. Some of the possible mechanisms of religious participation-well-being link may include "the promotion of healthy lifestyles by religious groups, facilitation of social support of religious organizations by and for members providing a schema of meaning" [16]. Furthermore, repetitive prayers may reinforce feelings of hope and optimism, increasing life satisfaction and happiness [17].

Compared to Hindus, Muslims and Sikhs scored lower on self-rated health, Sikhs scored higher on happiness and Christians scored lower on life satisfaction. Life expectancy at birth in India was the highest among Christians (68.1 years), followed by Muslims (66.0 years) and Hindus (65.0%) [18]. More research is needed to explore the differences in well-being indicators by religious affiliation in India. Compared to middle-aged adults (45-59 years), older adults (≥60 years) had lower self-rated health but higher life satisfaction. This result may be expected as health deteriorates with age, but life satisfaction may increase with age, as found in some previous studies [19]. Tobacco use was negatively associated with all three well-being indicators, as found previously in a study in India [1].

Study limitations

Although this was a national study of older adults in India, the study was limited by its cross-sectional design and the self-report of data collected. In additional limitation was that "happiness" was only assessed with one item. Future studies may include a happiness scale.

CONCLUSION

In this national study among middle-aged and older adults in India, religious activity (daily pooja or prayer, and/or attendance of religious services, and/or involvement in religious gatherings), higher spirituality/religiousness, and religious importance were significantly positively associated with self-rated health, happiness, and life satisfaction.

ACKNOWLEDGMENTS

The Longitudinal Aging Study in India Project is funded by the Ministry of Health and Family Welfare, Government of India, the National Institute on Aging (R01 AG042778, R01 AG030153), and United Nations Population Fund, India.

REFERENCES

[1] Ladusingh L, Ngangbam S. Domains and determinants of well-being of older adults in India. J Cross Cult Gerontol 2016;31(1):89-111. doi: 10.1007/s10823-016-9279-z. PMID: 26797966.

[2] Bodogai SI, Olah Ş, Roşeanu G. Religiosity and subjective well-being of the Central and Eastern European's elderly population. J Relig Health 2020;59(2):784-95. doi: 10.1007/s10943-018-0659-2.

[3] Koenig HG, King DE, Carson VB. Handbook of religion and health, 2nd ed. New York: Oxford University Press, 2012.

[4] Hoverd WJ, Sibley C. Religion, deprivation and subjective wellbeing: Testing a religious buffering hypothesis. IJW 2013;3(2):182–96.

[5] Ellison CG. Religious involvement and subjective well-being. J Health Soc Behav 1991;32(1):80-99.

[6] Kim HH, Jung JH. Ageism, religiosity, and wellbeing among older adults: Evidence from the European Social Survey (ESS4). Res Aging 2020:164027520953632 doi: 10.1177/0164027520953632.

[7] Zimmer Z, Jagger C, Chiu CT, Ofstedal MB, Rojo F, Saito Y. Spirituality, religiosity, aging and health in global perspective: A review. SSM Popul Health 2016;2:373-81. doi: 10.1016/j.ssmph.2016.04.009.

[8] Park J, Roh S, Yeo Y. Religiosity, social support, and life satisfaction among elderly Korean immigrants. Gerontologist 2012;52(5):641-9. doi: 10.1093/geront/gnr103.

[9] Wilmoth JD, Adams-Price CE, Turner JJ, Blaney AD, Downey L. Examining social connections as a link between religious participation and well-being among older adults. J Relig *Spiritual Aging* 2014;26(2-3):259-78, doi: 10.1080/15528030.2013.867423.

[10] Reyes-Ortiz CA, Payan C, Altamar G, Gomez F, Koenig HG. Religiosity and self-rated health among older adults in Colombia. Colomb Med 2019;50(2):67-76. doi: 10.25100/cm.v50i2.4012.

[11] Foong HF, Hamid TA, Ibrahim R, Haron SA. The association between religious orientation and life satisfaction in older adults living with morbidity and multimorbidity: a gender perspective in Malaysia. Psychogeriatrics 2020;20(6):891-9. doi: 10.1111/psyg.12614.

[12] Reyes-Ortiz CA, Pelaez M, Koenig HG, Mulligan T. Religiosity and self-rated health among Latin American and Caribbean elders. Int J Psychiatry Med 2007;37(4):425-43. doi: 10.2190/PM.37.4.f.

[13] International Institute for Population Sciences (IIPS), NPHCE, MoHFW, Harvard TH Chan School of Public Health (HSPH) and the University of Southern California (USC). Longitudinal Ageing Study in India (LASI) Wave 1, 2017-18, India Report. Mumbai: International Institute for Population Sciences, 2020.

[14] Diener E, Emmons RA, Larsen RJ, Griffin S. The Satisfaction With Life Scale. J Pers Assess 1985;49(1):71-5. doi: 10.1207/s15327752jpa4901_13.

[15] Underwood LG, Teresi JA. The Daily Spiritual Experience Scale: Development, theoretical description, reliability, exploratory factor analysis, and preliminary construct validity using health-related data. Ann Behav Med 2002;24:22-33.

[16] Idler EL. Religious observance and health: Theory and research. In: Schaie KW, Krause N, Booth A, eds. Religious influences on health and wellbeing in the elderly. New York: Springer, 2004:20-43.

[17] Lambert NM, Fincham FD, Braithwaite SR, Graham SM, Beach SRH. Can prayer increase gratitude? Psycholog Relig Spirituality 2009;1:139-49. doi: 10.1037/a0016731.

[18] Kumari M, Mohanty SK. Caste, religion and regional differentials in life expectancy at birth in India: cross-sectional estimates from recent National Family Health Survey. BMJ Open 2020;10(8):e035392. doi: 10.1136/bmjopen-2019-035392.

[19] Gana K, Bailly N, Saada Y, Joulain M, Alaphilippe D. Does life satisfaction change in old age: results from an 8-year longitudinal study. J Gerontol B Psychol Sci Soc Sci 2013;68(4):540-52. doi: 10.1093/geronb/gbs093.

In: Social and Health Issues …
Editors: S Pengpid, K Peltzer et al.
ISBN: 978-1-53619-937-6

Chapter 24

PERCEIVED AGE DISCRIMINATION AMONG OLDER ADULTS IN INDIA: RESULTS OF A NATIONAL SURVEY IN 2017-2018

Supa Pengpid*[1,2], *MPH, DrPH, MBA
and Karl Peltzer*[2,3,*], *MA Clin Psych, PhD, Dr Habil
[1]ASEAN Institute for Health Development, Mahidol University, Salaya, Phutthamonthon, Nakhon Pathom, Thailand
[2]Department of Research Administration and Development, University of Limpopo, Turfloop, South Africa
[3]Department of Psychology, College of Medical and Health Science, Asia University, Taichung, Taiwan

---

* *Correspondence*: Professor Karl Peltzer, Department of Research Administration and Development, University of Limpopo, Turfloop Campus, Private Bag X1106, Sovenga 0727, South Africa. Email: kfpeltzer@gmail.com.

Abstract

This study aimed to estimate the prevalence and correlates of perceived age discrimination among older adults in a national population survey in India. The sample included 52,933 older adults (≥50 years) from a cross-sectional national community-dwelling survey in India in 2017-2018. Results indicate that the prevalence of perceived age discrimination (PAD) was 9.5%, 9.7% among women, and 9.3% among men. In the adjusted logistic regression analysis, older age, no education and food insecurity were positively associated with PAD, while medium subjective socioeconomic status, Muslim, Christian and Sikh were negatively associated with PAD. In addition, in unadjusted analysis, belonging to Scheduled tribes and other backward classes were positively associated with PAD, while high subjective socioeconomic status, married, and urban residence were negatively associated with PAD. One in ten older adults in India experienced PAD, and several associated factors were identified that may be targeted to reduce age discrimination.

Introduction

Perceived discrimination can be defined as “a behavioural manifestation of a negative attitude, judgment, or unfair treatment toward members of a group”, such as age, gender, religion, caste, weight, physical disability, physical appearance, and financial status, and can be characterised as a form of stress [1]. Perceived age discrimination (PAD) is “defined as the individuals’ views and experiences reported about discrimination due to their age; thus, it refers to all older adults’ perceived differentiation based on age” [2]. PAD was found in a systematic review to significantly worse health outcomes [3]. Among older adults, PAD has been found to be fairly prevalent in the ‘western world’ or high-income countries [4]. For example, among older adults (≥52 years) in England, the prevalence of PAD was 34.8%, and USA 29.1% [5]. Among adults in 28 European countries, the mean prevalence of PAD was 34.5% [6]. In South Korea, among older adults (N = 812, 60-89 years), 48.1% had experienced one or more incidents of PAD [7]. However, little is known about PAD in rapidly ageing societies in low- and middle-income countries, such as India. Regarding the aged population (≥60 years), India is currently having the second largest older age population in the world [8], it was 7% of the total population in 2009 and is projected to increase to 20% in 2050 [9].

The proportion of age discrimination in different discriminatory situations was among older adults in England 17.7% less courtesy, 8.7% service setting, 11.1% less clever, 4.6% harassed and 8.7% medical setting [10]. In a German Ageing Survey (40-93 years), the prevalence of PAD in the work domain was 52.6%, in the medical care domain 37.0%, and in the social interactions domain (32.4%) [11].

Factors associated with age discrimination in older adults include older age [10, 12], men [5], higher education [10], lower education [12, 13], lower wealth status [10, 13], retired or not in employment [10], not married [12, 13)], belonging to a minority [13], residing in urban areas [7], functional disability and depressive symptoms [12]. Age discrimination legislation exists, for example in the USA and UK [5]. In India, "there is no codified law on age discrimination, and there is no designated statutory body that deals with matters pertaining to age discrimination. As a result, there is no statutory defense available, and only common law actions can be taken when cases of discrimination based on age are highly unjustified." [14]. To better understand and respond to PAD in India, it is necessary to identify these experiences at the national level. The objective of our study was to characterize PAD in a nationally representative sample of the Indian older adult population in terms of prevalence and correlates of PAD.

OUR STUDY

National cross-sectional data from the Longitudinal Aging Study in India (LASI) Wave 1, 2017-2018 were analyzed (individual response rate 87%) [15]. Face-to-face interviews were conducted by male and female trained research teams with individuals aged 45 and above and their female spouses, regardless of age, in a household survey from 35 states and union territories of India (excluding Sikkim). In this paper, we restricted our sample to 50 years and above. Field teams input responses directly into a laptop computer.

Details of the sampling strategy have been described elsewhere [15]. The "Indian Council of Medical Research (ICMR) Ethics Committee approved the study and written informed consent was attained from participants" [15].

Measures

Perceived age discrimination was assessed with the Everyday Discrimination Scale (short version) to assess discrimination in six different social situations, such as less courtesy, service setting, less clever, harassed, afraid, and medical setting [16]. Response options ranged from 1 = "never" to 6 = "almost every day", and were dichotomised to 'never' = 0 and 'ever' (collapsing those reporting 'less than once a year' or greater into one category) = 1. Participants that responded affirmative to any discrimination question were asked a follow-up question inquiring into the potential reasons for the discrimination. Response options were "age, gender, religion, caste, weight, physical disability, other aspects of physical appearance, financial status, and other" [16]. Participants who attributed any experience of discrimination to their age were defined as cases of perceived age discrimination [10].

Covariates consisted of education, age, sex, Caste/tribe, religious affiliation, urban and rural residence [15]. Scheduled tribes, Scheduled castes, and other backward classes have been historically disadvantaged due to various socio-economic factors like wealth or traditional occupation and are given reservation by the government of India [17]. Subjective socioeconomic status was assessed with the question, "Please imagine a ten-step ladder, where at the bottom are the people who are the worst off – who have the least money, least education, and the worst jobs or no jobs, and at the top of the ladder are the people who are the best off – those who have the most money, most education, and best jobs. Please indicate the number (1-10) on the rung on the ladder where you would place yourself" [15]. Steps 1 to 3 on the socioeconomic ladder were defined as low, 4-5 as medium, and 6-10 as high.

Food insecurity was assessed with four questions, 1) "In the last 12 months, did you ever reduce the size of your meals or skip meals because there was not enough food at your household? (Yes/No) 2) In the last 12 months, were you hungry but didn't eat because there was not enough food at your household? (Yes/No) 3) In the past 12 months, did you ever not eat for a whole day because there was not enough food at your household? 4) Do you think that you have lost weight in the last 12 months because there was not enough food in your household?" [15]. Any positive response to the four questions was scored as one.

Data analysis

Considering the clustered study design, data analyses were conducted with "STATA software version 15.0 (Stata Corporation, College Station, TX, USA)." Unadjusted and adjusted logistic regression analyses were used to calculate associations between independent variables and PAD. Variables with a significance level of 0.05 in univariate analyses were subsequently included in the multivariable model. In addition, adjusted logistic regression analyses were used to calculate associations between independent variables and PAD in six different discrimination situations. Covariates were selected based on previous literature review [5-7, 10, 12, 13]. *P*-values of below 0.05 were accepted as significant and missing values were excluded from the analysis.

FINDINGS

The sample included 52,933 older adults (50 years and older), 53.0% were female and 47.0% male. More than half of the participants (53.0%) had no formal education, and 69.0% were residing in rural areas. One in ten participants (9.9%) had food insecurity, 38.2% had low subjective socioeconomic status, and 70.1% were married. Majority were Hindu (82.4%) and 46.7% belonged to other backward classes. The prevalence of PAD was 9.5%, 9.7% among women, and 9.3% among men (see Table 1).

Associations with perceived age discrimination

In the adjusted logistic regression analysis, older age, no education, and food insecurity were positively associated with PAD, while medium subjective socioeconomic status, Muslim, Christian and Sikh were negatively associated with PAD. In addition, in unadjusted analysis, belonging to Scheduled tribes and other backward classes were positively associated with PAD, while high subjective socioeconomic status, married, and urban residence were negatively associated with PAD (see Table 2).

Table 1. Sample characteristics of older adults (≥50 years) in India, 2017-2018 (N = 52,933)

Variable	Variable specification	Sample	Perceived age discrimination
		%	%
All			**9.5**
Age in years	50-59	38.1	7.5
	60-69	36.2	10.1
	70-79	18.7	11.3
	80 or more	7.0	13.0
Sex	Female	53.3	9.7
	Male	46.7	9.3
Education	≥1 years	47.0	7.7
	No schooling	53.0	11.1
Subjective socioeconomic status	Low	38.2	11.4
	Medium	37.4	8.2
	High	24.4	8.5
Food insecurity	No	90.1	8.4
	Yes	9.9	18.8
Marital status	Not married	29.9	11.5
	Married	70.1	8.7
Caste/tribe	None of the below	25.1	8.2
	Scheduled tribe	19.4	10.3
	Scheduled caste	8.8	9.1
	Other backward class	46.7	10.2
Religious affiliation	Hindu	82.4	10.1
	Muslim	11.3	7.9
	Christian	2.8	5.5
	Sikh	1.8	3.5
	Other or none	1.7	6.9
Residence	Rural	69.0	10.1
	Urban	31.0	8.1

Table 2. Associations with perceived age discrimination

Variable	**Variable specification**	**COR (95% CI)**	***p*-value**	**AOR (95% CI)**	***p*-value**
Age in years	50-59	1 (Reference)		1 (Reference)	
	60-69	1.38 (1.12, 1.71)	0.003	1.32 (1.07, 1.6[illegible])	0.008
	70-79	1.57 (1.25, 1.96)	<0.001	1.45 (1.17, 1.80)	<0.001
	80 or more	1.83 (1.42, 2.37)	<0.001	1.60 (1.25, 2.04)	<0.001
Sex	Female	1 (Reference)		---	
	Male	0.95 (0.81, 1.11)	0.495		
Education	≥1 years	1 (Reference)		1 (Reference)	
	No schooling	1.50 (1.27, 1.78)	<0.001	1.29 (1.13, 1.47)	<0.001
Subjective socioeconomic status	Low	1 (Reference)		1 (Reference)	
	Medium	0.69 (0.62, 0.77)	<0.001	0.78 (0.69, 0.88)	<0.001
	High	0.72 (0.55, 0.95)	0.019	0.87 (0.68, 1.10)	0.232
Food insecurity	No	1 (Reference)		1 (Reference)	
	Yes	2.52 (2.15, 2.94)	<0.001	2.33 (2.00, 2.70)	<0.001
Marital status	Not married	1 (Reference)		1 (Reference)	
	Married	0.73 (0.64, 0.84)	<0.001	0.89 (0.78, 1.00)	0.057
Caste/tribe	None of the below	1 (Reference)		1 (Reference)	
	Scheduled tribe	1.28 (1.10, 1.48)	<0.001	1.02 (0.86, 1.21)	0.832
	Scheduled caste	1.11 (0.91, 1.36)	0.296	0.94 (0.74, 1.20)	0.605
	Other backward class	1.27 (1.08, 1.50)	0.005	1.16 (0.95, 1.41)	0.139
Religious affiliation	Hindu	1 (Reference)		1 (Reference)	
	Muslim	0.77 (0.62, 0.95)	0.015	0.77 (0.61, 0.98)	0.034
	Christian	0.52 (0.39, 0.70)	<0.001	0.52 (0.39, 0.70)	<0.001
	Sikh	0.33 (0.23, 0.46)	<0.001	0.34 (0.24, 0.48)	<0.001
	Other or none	0.67 (0.45, 0.99)	0.045	0.70 (0.47, 1.07)	0.098
Residence	Rural	1 (Reference)		1 (Reference)	
	Urban	0.78 (0.61, 0.99)	0.044	0.93 (0.74, 1.16)	0.507

COR = Crude Odds Ratio; AOR = Adjusted Odds ratio; CI = Confidence Interval.

Perceived age discrimination in different discriminatory situations

Among participants with less courtesy discrimination, 55.6% had PAD service setting discrimination, 59.6% had PAD, less clever discrimination, 55.4% had PAD afraid discrimination, 58.1% had PAD, harassed discrimination, 51.5% had PAD, and medical setting discrimination, 57.4% had PD (see Table 3).

Table 3. Age discrimination in different discrimination situations

Variable	<Courtesy	Service setting	<Clever	Afraid	Harassed	Medical setting
	N = 5250	N = 3174	N = 3668	N = 2593	N = 2848	N = 2858
	%	%	%	%	%	%
All	**55.6**	**59.6**	**55.4**	**58.1**	**51.5**	**57.4**
Age in years						
50-59	45.9	50.8	42.1	50.0	42.7	48.1
60-69	56.4	62.6	61.1	60.8	54.5	61.5
70-79	66.7	64.3	64.0	63.0	56.2	63.1
80 or more	78.8	81.2	79.2	75.8	73.1	71.3
Sex						
Female	58.3	62.9	59.4	61.3	55.5	59.6
Male	52.7	56.0	51.0	54.7	46.9	55.0
Education						
≥1 years	53.6	55.6	54.2	56.4	47.4	54.7
No schooling	57.0	61.9	56.1	59.2	54.2	59.0
Socioeconomic status						
Low	52.1	58.9	55.4	57.4	50.6	56.8
Medium	55.2	59.2	56.4	59.3	49.4	55.9
High	66.5	61.9	53.3	57.0	57.1	60.9
Food insecurity						
No	56.2	61.4	55.6	60.9	52.8	58.6
Yes	53.0	53.7	53.5	49.6	47.2	52.8
Marital status						
Not married	62.6	68.2	66.2	64.8	62.1	66.7
Married	52.3	55.9	50.7	55.3	47.1	53.4
Caste/tribe						
None of the below	59.9	62.9	55.2	60.3	52.7	58.4
Scheduled tribe	53.9	56.8	54.9	55.0	50.7	53.0
Scheduled caste	57.2	63.9	56.8	64.5	50.9	62.4
Other backward class	54.5	58.9	55.7	57.2	51.5	58.1
Religion						
Hindu	58.2	62.2	59.2	58.9	52.9	58.7
Muslim	43.0	45.0	35.8	51.9	45.9	50.3
Christian	35.6	43.6	46.3	48.3	32.0	38.2
Sikh	44.9	47.6	48.5	78.1	54.1	48.2
Other or none	49.1	45.2	29.3	62.9	39.0	53.5
Residence						
Rural	56.2	60.0	57.3	59.9	52.0	57.8
Urban	54.2	58.5	50.0	53.5	50.2	56.0

In adjusted logistic regression analyses, older age, no food insecurity, not married and Hindus were the most consistent in four to six discrimination situations. Men reported less age discrimination than women

Table 4. Associations with age discrimination in discrimination situations of less courtesy, service setting and less clever

Variable	<Courtesy		Service setting		<Clever	
	AOR (95% CI)	*p*-value	AOR (95% CI)	*p*-value	AOR (95% CI)	*p*-value
Age in years						
50-59	1 (Reference)		1 (Reference)		1 (Reference)	
60-69	1.50 (1.08, 2.08)	0.017	1.57 (1.22, 2.02)	<0.001	1.94 (1.49, 2.53)	<0.001
70-79	2.40 (1.76, 3.29)	<0.001	1.70 (1.08, 2.66)	0.021	2.28 (1.49, 3.50)	<0.001
80 or more	3.97 (2.66, 5.92)	<0.001	3.18 (1.93, 5.24)	<0.001	3.81 (2.36, 6.16)	<0.001
Sex						
Female	1 (Reference)		1 (Reference)		1 (Reference)	
Male	0.86 (0.62, 1.20)	0.382	0.87 (0.66, 1.14)	0.307	0.86 (0.65, 1.13)	0.284
Education						
≥1 years	1 (Reference)		1 (Reference)		1 (Reference)	
No schooling	1.31 (0.94, 1.83)	0.108	1.30 (0.96, 1.76)	0.096	1.01 (0.75, 1.36)	0.957
Socioeconomic status						
Low	1 (Reference)		1 (Reference)		1 (Reference)	
Medium	1.14 (0.86, 1.51)	0.373	1.06 (0.83, 1.36)	0.637	1.01 (0.78, 1.30)	0.965
High	1.97 (1.12, 3.47)	0.018	1.11 (0.78, 1.57)	0.561	0.88 (0.61, 1.25)	0.461
Food insecurity						
No	1 (Reference)		1 (Reference)		1 (Reference)	
Yes	0.86 (0.65, 1.12)	0.261	0.74 (0.56, 0.99)	0.042	0.85 (0.63, 1.14)	0.280
Marital status						
Not married	1 (Reference)		1 (Reference)		1 (Reference)	
Married	0.86 (0.59, 1.26)	0.433	0.73 (0.57, 0.95)	0.019	0.73 (0.57, 0.93)	0.010
Caste/tribe						
None of the below	1 (Reference)		1 (Reference)		1 (Reference)	
Scheduled tribe	0.76 (0.56, 1.02)	0.063	0.66 (0.47, 0.92)	0.014	0.84 (0.61, 1.18)	0.318
Scheduled caste	1.00 (0.67, 1.48)	0.985	1.06 (0.68, 1.65)	0.798	1.11 (0.73, 1.67)	0.628
Other backward class	0.84 (0.59, 1.20)	0.345	0.79 (0.58, 1.08)	0.134	1.08 (0.80, 1.47)	0.604

Table 4. (Continued)

Variable	<Courtesy		Service setting		<Clever	
	AOR (95% CI)	*p*-value	AOR (95% CI)	*p*-value	AOR (95% CI)	*p*-value
Religion						
Hindu	1 (Reference)		1 (Reference)		1 (Reference)	
Muslim	0.55 (0.32, 0.95)	0.033	0.43 (0.29, 0.64)	<0.001	0.39 (0.22, 0.71)	0.002
Christian	0.43 (0.27, 0.69)	<0.001	0.44 (0.25, 0.78)	0.005	0.62 (0.38, 1.02)	0.061
Sikh	0.55 (0.30, 1.01)	0.055	0.52 (0.19, 1.42)	0.202	0.63 (0.30, 1.33)	0.226
Other or none	0.67 (0.32, 1.40)	0.286	0.48 (0.17, 1.32)	0.153	0.31 (0.15, 0.65)	0.002
Residence		52393				
Rural	1 (Reference)		1 (Reference)		1 (Reference)	
Urban	1.03 (0.66, 1.60)	0.913	1.00 (0.69, 1.45)	0.999	0.94 (0.64, 1.39)	0.757

AOR = Adjusted Odds ratio; CI = Confidence Interval.

Table 5. Associations with age discrimination in discrimination situations of afraid, harassed and medical setting

Variable	Afraid		Harassed		Medical setting	
	AOR (95% CI)	*p*-value	AOR (95% CI)	*p*-value	AOR (95% CI)	*p*-value
Age in years						
50-59	1 (Reference)		1 (Reference)		1 (Reference)	
60-69	1.51 (1.16, 1.97)	0.002	1.48 (1.14, 1.93)	0.003	1.67 (1.28, 2.18)	<0.001
70-79	1.75 (1.10, 2.79)	0.018	1.69 (1.14, 2.49)	0.008	1.73 (1.08, 2.77)	0.022
80 or more	2.93 (1.71, 5.02)	<0.001	2.79 (1.72, 4.53)	<0.001	2.03 (1.24, 3.34)	0.005
Sex						
Female	1 (Reference)		1 (Reference)		1 (Reference)	
Male	0.75 (0.58, 0.96)	0.023	0.81 (0.64, 1.04)	0.102	0.96 (0.73, 1.27)	0.793
Education						
≥1 years	1 (Reference)		1 (Reference)		1 (Reference)	
No schooling	0.94 (0.71, 1.24)	0.649	1.19 (0.91, 1.57)	0.207	1.18 (0.86, 1.61)	0.311

Variable	Afraid		Harassed		Medical setting	
	AOR (95% CI)	*p*-value	AOR (95% CI)	*p*-value	AOR (95% CI)	*p*-value
Socioeconomic status						
Low	1 (Reference)		1 (Reference)		1 (Reference)	
Medium	1.01 (0.75, 1.34)	0.964	0.98 (0.76, 1.27)	0.883	0.94 (0.73, 1.22)	0.644
High	0.92 (0.63, 1.33)	0.654	1.35 (0.96, 1.89)	0.087	1.14 (0.78, 1.68)	0.503
Food insecurity						
No	1 (Reference)		1 (Reference)		1 (Reference)	
Yes	0.59 (0.45, 0.77)	<0.001	0.78 (0.61, 0.99)	0.039	0.80 (0.58, 1.10)	0.171
Marital status						
Not married	1 (Reference)		1 (Reference)		1 (Reference)	
Married	0.87 (0.65, 1.18)	0.374	0.66 (0.50, 0.89)	0.005	0.69 (0.53, 0.92)	0.010
Caste/tribe						
None of the below	1 (Reference)		1 (Reference)		1 (Reference)	
Scheduled tribe	0.80 (0.55, 1.15)	0.223	0.86 (0.61, 1.24)	0.426	0.76 (0.54, 1.08)	0.129
Scheduled caste	1.26 (0.80, 1.97)	0.322	0.96 (0.60, 1.53)	0.870	1.15 (0.73, 1.79)	0.555
Other backward class	0.88 (0.63, 1.22)	0.444	0.92 (0.65, 1.31)	0.659	0.97 (0.71, 1.32)	0.835
Religion						
Hindu	1 (Reference)		1 (Reference)		1 (Reference)	
Muslim	0.86 (0.56, 1.31)	0.470	0.71 (0.48, 1.06)	0.093	0.62 (0.42, 0.92)	0.016
Christian	0.53 (0.31, 0.91)	0.020	0.48 (0.27, 0.86)	0.014	0.46 (0.23, 0.92)	0.029
Sikh	2.34 (0.81, 6.73)	0.115	1.07 (0.48, 2.40)	0.865	0.70 (0.28, 1.72)	0.438
Other or none	1.16 (0.43, 3.13)	0.764	0.57 (0.23, 1.46)	0.246	0.93 (0.40, 2.14)	0.859
Residence						
Rural	1 (Reference)		1 (Reference)		1 (Reference)	
Urban	0.73 (0.51, 1.06	0.100	0.95 (0.68, 1.34)	0.783	0.98 (0.67, 1.44)	0.938

AOR = Adjusted Odds ratio; CI = Confidence Interval.

in the afraid discrimination situation. Older adults with high subjective socioeconomic status reported higher odds of age discrimination in the less courtesy situation, and Scheduled tribe high lower odds of age discrimination in the service setting (see Tables 4 and 5).

DISCUSSION

The study aimed to estimate the prevalence and correlates of perceived age discrimination in older adults in a national population survey in India in 2017-2018. Results show for the first time that the prevalence of PAD was 9.5% in India, which is lower than in previous studies among older adults in England (34.8%), USA (29.1%) [5] and South Korea (48.1%) [7]. A partial explanation for the differences in the prevalence of PAD may be related to the fact that the mean ages in the US study (71.1 years) [5], England (67.4 years) [5], South Korea (72.9 years) [7] were higher than in our study in India (63.4 years). However, comparing the prevalence of PAD among those 80 years and older, the prevalence of PAD (13.0%) in India was much lower than in the US study (31.3%) and in England (35.2%). In addition, in the South Korea study, PAD was assessed with multiple items, while in our study and the studies in USA and England, PAD was only assessed with one item. Assessing PAD with multiple items may increase the likelihood of any positive responses on PAD. Cross-cultural research on PAD seems to suggest that intergenerational living is more common in non-Anglo than in Anglo cultures, thereby decreasing the likelihood of PAD [18]. Similarly, Latina/o and Asian American participants reported engaging in more elder respect emphasising the cultural norm of intergenerational solidarity [19]. In India, the "intergenerational support domain received very high scores for most of the Indian states. This is due to the higher weight provided to the caring of grandchildren in the participation domain of active ageing. The joint family system is a popular practice in India that encourages intergenerational exchange in care and support" [20]. "The joint family model, defined as a group of people who generally live under one roof, share food cooked at one hearth, hold property in common, participate in common family worship, and are related to each other, is portrayed as a golden model that meets care requirements of older people in countries where formal support is limited" [20]. In another study in four Southeast Asian cultures (Singapore, Thailand, Taiwan and Philippines), respect for the elderly is changing, but respect towards the elderly remains a central value [21].

The proportion of age discrimination in different discriminatory situations was in this study higher than in the England study (55.6% less courtesy in this study vs. 17.7% in England), (59.6% vs. 8.7% service setting), (55.4% vs. 11.1% less clever), (51.5% vs. 4.6% harassed), and (57.4% vs. 8.7% medical setting) [10], and the German Ageing Survey (57.4% vs. 37.0% medical setting) and (55.6% vs. 32.4% less courtesy or social interactions [11]. These results show that our Indian sample experienced a high proportion of PAD in all discrimination situations.

Consistent with previous research [10, 12, 13], this study showed that older age and lower socioeconomic status (lower education, food insecurity, and lower subjective socioeconomic status) was associated with PAD. Compared to people with lower socioeconomic status, people with higher socioeconomic status (having some education, not having food insecurity, and higher subjective socioeconomic status) may be less likely to experience age discrimination due to lessor exposure to discriminatory situations or a greater sense of control [10].

While a previous study found a positive association between belonging to a minority in Europe and PAD [13], this study found an inverse association between religious minorities (Muslim, Christian and Sikh) and PAD. In a study in South Korea [7], urban residence was associated with PAD, while in this study in unadjusted analysis residing in rural areas was associated with PAD. Consistent with previous studies [12, 13], this survey showed that in unadjusted analysis married was protective against PAD. Unlike some previous research that found higher PAD in men than women [5], this study did not significant sex differences in the prevalence of PAD. In unadjusted analysis, compared to historically advantaged groups (none of the disadvantaged groups), historically disadvantaged groups (Schedule tribe and other backward classes) had higher odds of PAD. The Indian National policy for senior citizens [22] recognises that "the problems of elderly women are exacerbated by a lifetime of gender-based discrimination, compounded by other forms of discrimination based on class, caste, disability, illiteracy, unemployment and marital status. In recognizing the need for affirmative action in favour of the elderly, special attention will be necessary to older females so that they do not become victims of triple neglect and discrimination on account of gender, widowhood and age" [22]. According to a recent national action plan in India, "age-related discrimination in schemes/programmes for credit, marketing, medical insurance, etc. to senior citizens is reviewed, and discrimination against the senior citizen for availing opportunities or education will be removed. Elderly will be facilitated for reporting whenever they feel they have been discriminated against or abused" [23].

Strength and limitations of the study

Study strengths included the use of standardized measures adapted from the Health and Retirement Study and a large, nationally representative sample of middle-aged and older adults in India. The self-report of most data may have their limitations. It is possible that participants underreported age discrimination. PAD was only assessed with one item, and future studies should include several items. Due to the cross-sectional design of the study, we were unable to determine the direction of the assessed associations.

Conclusion

One in ten older adults in India experienced PAD, and several associated factors were identified. Factors associated with PAD were older age, no education, food insecurity, lower subjective socioeconomic status, and Hindus. These associated factors may be targeted in an effort to reduce PAD.

ACKNOWLEDGMENTS

The Longitudinal Aging Study in India Project is funded by the Ministry of Health and Family Welfare, Government of India, the National Institute on Aging (R01 AG042778, R01 AG030153), and United Nations Population Fund, India.

REFERENCES

[1] Pascoe EA, Smart Richman L. Perceived discrimination and health: a meta-analytic review. Psychol Bull 2009;135(4):531-54. doi: 10.1037/a0016059.

[2] Macnicol J. Age discrimination: An historical and contemporary analysis. Cambridge: Cambridge University Press, 2006.

[3] Chang ES, Kannoth S, Levy S, Wang SY, Lee JE, Levy BR. Global reach of ageism on older persons' health: A systematic review. PLoS One 2020;15(1):e0220857. doi: 10.1371/journal.pone.0220857.

[4] Van den Heuvel W. Discrimination against older people. Rev Clin Gerontol 2012;22(4):293-300. doi:10.1017/S095925981200010X

[5] Rippon I, Zaninotto P, Steptoe A. Greater Perceived Age Discrimi-nation in England than the United States: Results from HRS and ELSA. J Gerontol B Psychol Sci Soc Sci 2015;70(6):925-33. doi: 10.1093/geronb/gbv040.

[6] Ayalon L. Perceived age, gender, and racial/ethnic discrimination in Europe: Results from the European Social Survey. Educ Gerontol 2014; 40:7:499-517. doi: 10.1080/03601277.2013.845490.

[7] Kim IH, Noh S, Chun H. Mediating and moderating effects in ageism and depression among the Korean elderly: The roles of emotional reactions and coping reponses. Osong Public Health Res Perspect 2016;7(1):3-11. doi: 10.1016/j.phrp.2015.11.012. 8.

[8] Agarwal A, Lubet A, Mitgang E, Mohanty S, Bloom DE. Population aging in India: Facts, issues, and options, IZA Discussion Paper No. 10162, 2016. URL: http://ftp.iza.org/dp10162.pdf.

[9] Subaiya L, Bansod DW. Demographics of population ageing in India: Trends and differentials, BKPAI working paper No. 1. United Nations Population Fund (UNFPA), 2011. New Delhi, India. URL: https://www.researchgate.net/publication/316605954_Demographics_of_population_ageing_in_India.

[10] Rippon I, Kneale D, de Oliveira C, Demakakos P, Steptoe A. Perceived age discrimination in older adults. Age Ageing 2014;43(3):379-86. doi: 10.1093/ageing/aft146.

[11] Voss P, Wolff JK, Rothermund K. Relations between views on ageing and perceived age discrimination: a domain-specific perspective. Eur J Ageing 2016;14(1):5-15. doi: 10.1007/s10433-016-0381-4.

[12] Giasson HL, Queen TL, Larkina M, Smith J. Age group differences in perceived age discrimination: associations with self-perceptions of aging. Gerontologist 2017;57 (Suppl 2): S160-8. doi: 10.1093/geront/gnx070.

[13] van den Heuvel WJ, van Santvoort MM. Experienced discrimination amongst European old citizens. Eur J Ageing 2011;8(4):291-9. doi: 10.1007/s10433-011-0206-4.

[14] Pradhan A. Age Discrimination in the workplace: An Indian perspective, 2020. URL: https://vasitum.com/blog/featured/age-discrimination-in-the-workplace-an-indian-perspective/#:~:text=Since%20there%20is%20no%20codified,on%20age%20are%20highly%20unjustified.

[15] International Institute for Population Sciences (IIPS), NPHCE, MoHFW, Harvard TH Chan School of Public Health (HSPH) and the University of Southern California (USC). Longitudinal Ageing Study in India (LASI) Wave 1, 2017-18, India Report. Mumbai: International Institute for Population Sciences, 2020.

[16] Sternthal MJ, Slopen N, Williams DR. Racial disparities in health: How much does stress really matter? Du Bois Rev 2011;8(1):95-113. doi: 10.1017/S1742058X11000087.

[17] Legal Affairs. Issues of Social Justice: Scheduled Castes and Scheduled Tribes and Other Backward Classes – An unfinished national Agenda. URL: https://legalaffairs.gov.in/sites/default/files/IX.ISSUESOF%20SOCIAL%20JUSTICE%20%20SCHEDULED%20CASTES%20%20AND%20SCHEDULED%20TRIBES%20AND%20OTHER%20BACKWARD%20CLASSESAN%20UNFINISHED%20NATION.pdf.

[18] Campos ID, Stripling AM, Heesacker M. "Estoy viejo" [I'm old]: internalized ageism as self-referential, negative, ageist speech in the Republic of Panama. J Cross Cult Gerontol 2012;27(4):373-90. doi: 10.1007/s10823-012-9181-2.

[19] Sung K-T. Elder respect among American college students: exploration of behavioral forms. Int J Aging Hum Dev 2002; 55(4): 367–82. doi:10.2190/M1A4-FNBHAAVB-KCNY.

[20] Guntupalli AM, Chakraborty S. Active Ageing Index (AAI) in India: Is the approach used in European countries applicable to developing countries? In: Zaidi A, Harper S, Howse K, Lamura G, Perek-Białas J, eds. Building evidence for active ageing policies. Singapore: Palgrave Macmillan, 2018. https://doi.org/10.1007/978-981-10-6017-5_20.

[21] Ingersoll-Dayton B, Saengtienchai C. Respect for the elderly in Asia: Stability and change. Int J Aging Hum Dev 1999;48(2):113-30. doi: 10.2190/G1XR-QDCV-JRNM-585P.

[22] Ministry of Social Justice and Empowerment, Government of India. National Policy for Senior Citizens March 2011. URL: http://socialjustice.nic.in/writereaddata/UploadFile/dnpsc.pdf.

[23] Government of India Ministry of Social Justice and Empowerment. National Action Plan for Welfare of Senior Citizens (NAPSrC), 2020. URL: http://socialjustice.nic.in/writereaddata/UploadFile/NAPSrC.pdf.

SECTION II: ACKNOWLEDGMENTS

In: Social and Health Issues … ISBN: 978-1-53619-937-6
Editors: S Pengpid, K Peltzer et al.

Chapter 25

About the Editors

Supa Pengpid, MPH, DrPH, MBA is a Professor at the ASEAN Institute for Health Development, Mahidol University Thailand since June 2013. She holds a Masterof Sciences in Public Health (MSc), Doctor of Public Health (DrPH in 2001) both from Mahidol University and Master of Business Administration (MBA in 2010) from Regenesys Business School, South Africa. She is a public health expert especially in health behaviour and public health. Her main research interests are health behaviour interventions in areas of chronic diseases prevention, obesity management, alcohol, HIV, TB and sexuality education, gender based violence and health systems research. Email: supaprom@yahoo.com

Karl Peltzer, MA Clin Psych, PhD, Dr Habil is a Research Associate in the Department of Research Administration and Development, University of Limpopo in South Africa. His research focuses on health promotion, risk behaviour and disease prevention, and socio-behavioural interventions on public health subject areas of alcohol, tobacco, cancer, tuberculosis and HIV control, nutrition, physical activity, hypertension, mental health, injury and violence prevention in low- and middle-income countries. Email: kfpeltzer@gmail.com

Joav Merrick, MD, MMedSci, DMSc, born and educated in Denmark is professor of pediatrics, Division of Pediatrics, Hadassah Hebrew University Medical Center, Mt Scopus Campus, Jerusalem, Israel and Kentucky Children's Hospital, University of Kentucky, Lexington, Kentucky United States and professor of public health at the Center for Healthy Development, School of Public Health, Georgia State University, Atlanta, United States, the former medical director of the Health Services, Division for Intellectual and Developmental Disabilities, Ministry of Social Affairs and Social Services, Jerusalem, the founder and director of the National Institute of Child Health and Human Development in Israel. Numerous publications in the field of pediatrics, child health and human development, rehabilitation, intellectual disability, disability, health, welfare, abuse, advocacy, quality of life and prevention. Received the Peter Sabroe Child Award for outstanding work on behalf of Danish Children in 1985 and the International LEGO-Prize ("The Children's Nobel Prize") for an extraordinary contribution towards improvement in child welfare and well-being in 1987. In 2017 appointed a Kentucky Colonel by the Commonwealth of Kentucky, the highest honor the governor can bestow to a person. Email: jmerrick@zahav.net.il

In: Social and Health Issues … ISBN: 978-1-53619-937-6
Editors: S Pengpid, K Peltzer et al.

Chapter 26

About the ASEAN Institute for Health Development, Mahidol University, Salaya, Phutthamonthon, Nakhon Pathom, Thailand

The ASEAN Institute for Health Development (AIHD) was established in 1982 as the ASEAN Training Centre for Primary Health Care Development. It was a joint effort of Mahidol University, the Ministry of Public Health and the Department of Technical and Economic Cooperation (DTEC, now TICA) of the Royal Thai Government, with strong support from the Japan International Cooperation Agency (JICA).

AIHD is based on a forward-looking and conceptually challenging perspective on human resource development which aims to support the global strategy of "Health for all" through the primary health care approach advocated by the World Health Organization, an approach which is valid not only for Thailand but also other ASEAN countries.

AIHD has three key missions, namely education and training, technical services, and research and development, focusing on participatory community-based health and related program management, with a special emphasis on facilitating the paradigm shift from a "service-oriented" approach to a “development” approach in order to promote “Health for all” through human capacity building and community empowerment.

Vision

Center of excellence in research, education, professional services for innovative of sustainable health by 2020.

Mission

Provide transformative education for graduates to become leaders in health system management and sustainability. Enhance capacity related of public health workforce in relate to sustainable health development and develop innovative research for sustainable health.

Strategies

Excellence in research for health development models and sustainability. Transformative education. Innovative professional service for sustainable health and wxcellence in management for sustainable organization.

Website

www.aihd.mahidol.ac.th

In: Social and Health Issues … ISBN: 978-1-53619-937-6
Editors: S Pengpid, K Peltzer et al.

Chapter 27

About the Department of Research Administration and Development, University of Limpopo, Turfloop, South Africa

The Department of Research Administration and Development is a key Department at the University of Limpopo overseeing research performance across the university, developing and implementing policies aligned to the university's strategic plan (UL 2019 - 2023) goal 5, which is improving the university's research standing and status. The department further intends to accelerate professional, quality, efficient research output with the hope to generate funds for the university. Among its key research responsibilities, the department is responsible for managing and directing all aspects of planning, policy, performance, operational support for research and innovation activities and to implement technology transfer and intellectual property (IP) management strategy.

In: Social and Health Issues … ISBN: 978-1-53619-937-6
Editors: S Pengpid, K Peltzer et al.

Chapter 28

About the National Institute of Child Health and Human Development in Israel

The National Institute of Child Health and Human Development (NICHD) in Israel was established in 1998 as a virtual institute under the auspices of the Medical Director, Ministry of Social Affairs and Social Services in order to function as the research arm for the Office of the Medical Director. In 1998 the National Council for Child Health and Pediatrics, Ministry of Health and in 1999 the Director General and Deputy Director General of the Ministry of Health endorsed the establishment of the NICHD.

Mission

The mission of a National Institute for Child Health and Human Development in Israel is to provide an academic focal point for the scholarly interdisciplinary study of child life, health, public health, welfare, disability, rehabilitation, intellectual disability and related aspects of human development. This mission includes research, teaching, clinical work, information and public service activities in the field of child health and human development.

Service and academic activities

Over the years many activities became focused in the south of Israel due to collaboration with various professionals at the Faculty of Health Sciences (FOHS) at the Ben Gurion University of the Negev (BGU). Since 2000 an affiliation with the Zusman Child Development Center at the Pediatric Division of Soroka University Medical Center has resulted in collaboration around the establishment of the Down Syndrome Clinic at that center. In 2002 a full course on "Disability" was established at the Recanati School for Allied Professions in the Community, FOHS, BGU and in 2005 collaboration was started with the Primary Care Unit of the faculty and disability became part of the master of public health course on "Children and society". In the academic year 2005-2006 a one semester course on "Aging with disability" was started as part of the master of science program in gerontology in our collaboration with the Center for Multidisciplinary Research in Aging. In 2010 collaborations with the Division of Pediatrics, Hadassah Hebrew University Medical Center, Jerusalem, Israel around the National Down Syndrome Center and teaching students and residents about intellectual and developmental disabilities as part of their training at this campus.

Research activities

The affiliated staff have over the years published work from projects and research activities in this national and international collaboration. In the year 2000 the International Journal of Adolescent Medicine and Health and in 2005 the International Journal on Disability and Human Development of De Gruyter Publishing House (Berlin and New York) were affiliated with the National Institute of Child Health and Human Development. From 2008 also the International Journal of Child Health and Human Development (Nova Science, New York), the International Journal of Child and Adolescent Health (Nova Science) and the Journal of Pain Management (Nova Science) affiliated and from 2009 the International Public Health Journal (Nova Science) and Journal of Alternative Medicine Research (Nova Science). All peer-reviewed international journals.

National collaborations

Nationally the NICHD works in collaboration with the Faculty of Health Sciences, Ben Gurion University of the Negev; Department of Physical Therapy, Sackler School of Medicine, Tel Aviv University; Autism Center, Assaf HaRofeh Medical Center; National Rett and PKU Centers at Chaim Sheba Medical Center, Tel HaShomer; Department of Physiotherapy, Haifa University; Department of Education, Bar Ilan University, Ramat Gan, Faculty of Social Sciences and Health Sciences; College of Judea and Samaria in Ariel and in 2011 affiliation with Center for Pediatric Chronic Diseases and National Center for Down Syndrome, Department of Pediatrics, Hadassah Hebrew University Medical Center, Mount Scopus Campus, Jerusalem.

International collaborations

Internationally with the Department of Disability and Human Development, College of Applied Health Sciences, University of Illinois at Chicago; Strong Center for Developmental Disabilities, Golisano Children's Hospital at Strong, University of Rochester School of Medicine and Dentistry, New York; Centre on Intellectual Disabilities, University of Albany, New York; Centre for Chronic Disease Prevention and Control, Health Canada, Ottawa; Chandler Medical Center and Children's Hospital, Kentucky Children's Hospital, Section of Adolescent Medicine, University of Kentucky, Lexington; Chronic Disease Prevention and Control Research Center,

Baylor College of Medicine, Houston, Texas; Division of Neuroscience, Department of Psychiatry, Columbia University, New York; Institute for the Study of Disadvantage and Disability, Atlanta; Center for Autism and Related Disorders, Department Psychiatry, Children's Hospital Boston, Boston; Department of Pediatric and Adolescent Medicine, Western Michigan University Homer Stryker MD School of Medicine, Kalamazoo, Michigan, United States; Department of Paediatrics, Child Health and Adolescent Medicine, Children's Hospital at Westmead, Westmead, Australia; International Centre for the Study of Occupational and Mental Health, Düsseldorf, Germany; Centre for Advanced Studies in Nursing, Department of General Practice and Primary Care, University of Aberdeen, Aberdeen, United Kingdom; Quality of Life Research Center, Copenhagen, Denmark; Nordic School of Public Health, Gottenburg, Sweden, Scandinavian Institute of Quality of Working Life, Oslo, Norway; The Department of Applied Social Sciences (APSS) of The Hong Kong Polytechnic University Hong Kong.

Targets

Our focus is on research, international collaborations, clinical work, teaching and policy in health, disability and human development and to establish the NICHD as a permanent institute in Israel.

Contact

Professor Joav Merrick, MD, MMedSci, DMSc
National Institute of Child Health and Human Development,
Jerusalem, Israel.
Email: jmerrick@zahav.net.il

SECTION III: INDEX

INDEX

A

B

C

D

E

F

G

H

I

L

M

N

O

P

Q

R

S

T

U

V

W